Musculoskeletal Biomechanics

Paul Brinckmann, Ph. D.
Professor and Director
Institute for Experimental
Biomechanics
Universitätsklinikum Münster
Münster, Germany

Wolfgang Frobin, Ph. D.
Institute for Experimental
Biomechanics
Universitätsklinikum Münster
Münster, Germany

Gunnar Leivseth, M. D., Ph. D.
Professor
Department of Clinical Neurosciences
Faculty of Medicine
Norwegian University of
Science and Technology
Trondheim, Norway

Foreword by
Gunnar Andersson, M. D., Ph. D.

244 illustrations

Thieme
Stuttgart · New York

Library of Congress Cataloging-in-Publication Data

Brinckmann, Paul
[Orthopädische Biomechanik. English]
Musculoskeletal biomechanics / Paul Brinckmann,
Wolfgang Frobin, Gunnar Leivseth.
p. : cm.
Includes bibliographical references and index.
ISBN 3131300515 – ISBN 1-58890-080-0
1. Human mechanics. 2. Musculoskeletal system – Mechanical properties. 3. Orthopedics. I. Frobin, W. II. Leivseth, Gunnar. III. Title.
[DNLM: 1. Biomechanics. 2. Movement-physioloy. 3. Orthopedics. WE 103 B8580 2002]
QP303 B7513 2002
612.7'6-dc21   2001058204

Title of the German edition:
Orthopädische Biomechanik.
Published and copyrighted 2000
by Georg Thieme Verlag, Stuttgart,
Germany.

© 2002 Georg Thieme Verlag, Rüdigerstraße 14, D-70469 Stuttgart, Germany
Thieme New York, 333 Seventh Avenue, New York, NY 10001, USA.

Cover drawing by Martina Berge, Erbach

Typesetting by Satzpunkt Bayreuth GmbH, 95444 Bayreuth

Printed in Germany by Gulde Druck, Tübingen

ISBN 3-13-130051-5 (GTV)
ISBN 1-58890-080-0 (TNY)   1 2 3 4 5

WITHDRAWN

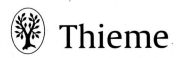

Thieme

Foreword

Orthopedic surgeons use biomechanical theory every day. It influences prevention, diagnosis, and treatment of most musculoskeletal injuries and diseases. Consider advising a patient with back pain about lifting, relating loss of range of motion of a joint to an internal joint derangement, or operating on a fracture using internal fixation: All should be based on sound knowledge of biomechanical principles. This book provides such basic knowledge and more. Written by well-known biomechanics experts with a long history of teaching and working with orthopedic surgeons and beautifully illustrated, it blends sound basic theory with applied biomechanical principles.

Most young orthopedic residents fear mathematical engineering theory. It can be made complex; it can also – as in this text – be made simple and relevant. Its application in daily practice should be intuitive. This requires that principles be learned, not memorized.

Dr. Brinckmann and his coauthors have written a superior treatise on the subject. In striking an appropriate balance, the book keeps you focused on the principles, while providing the background theory. Orthopedic surgeons and other health professionals with an interest in biomechanics are fortunate. Buy, read and enjoy.

Gunnar Andersson, M. D., Ph. D.
Chair, Department of Orthopedic Surgery
Rush-Presbyterian-St. Luke's Medical Center
Chicago, Illinois

Preface

Based on lectures, scientific papers, and publications, this book addresses readers from the disciplines of physiotherapy, rehabilitation, orthopedics, and biomechanical research. Its aim is accurately to present the lines of thought and procedures in orthopedic biomechanics, as well as the current state of knowledge of mechanical effects on the human locomotor system, though with only minimal reference to physics and mechanics and with the simplest possible mathematical calculations. The insight into the structure and function of the locomotor system gained from a mechanical aspect lays the foundation for understanding mechanisms of primary mechanical impairment and dysfunction and for treatment and rehabilitation concepts as well as for preventive measures.

The book is divided into four parts. Chapters 2–7 form an introduction into the fundamental aspects of physics and mechanics. These fundamentals are reiterated only to the extent necessary for an understanding of the chapters that follow. It would not hurt to have college textbooks on physics, geometry, and trigonometry to hand (if, indeed, anyone still has such books!). Proof is generally not provided for theorems in the field of mechanics or for mathematical formulae cited here. In such instances the reader will find the note "the proof is not detailed here." This indicates that the validity of the theorems or formulae is not obvious (sometimes far from obvious!), but has to be proven. (We trust such proof has been furnished correctly in the past by competent authors.)

Chapters 8–15 deal with the function and loading of joints and the mechanical properties of muscle, tendon, skin, and bone. Biomechanical discussions and model calculations are generally confined to two-dimensional problems and to systems without accelerated masses and inertial forces. For many problems, the static, two-dimensional case constitutes at least an acceptable approximation. The underlying mechanical facts usually come across vividly as well. For a number of problems of practical interest, for example, joint loads or pressure on articular surfaces, knowing the precise magnitude of the mechanical parameters is not of prime interest. Often it is more interesting to explore what changes can be induced by therapy, training, external aids, modified behavior, or ergonomic improvements at the workplace.

As stated above, simple calculations cannot be dispensed with when discussing mechanical aspects of the locomotor system. All calculations are explained step by step. It is quite conceivable that some readers may find this too simple (sorry!) and that others may find it takes some getting used to (sorry again!). Vector algebra is explained because the reader will come across it in scientific papers and textbooks. When dealing with forces and moments, vector notation is not used consistently throughout this book; preference is given to conveying the basic information as clearly as possible without forcing vector notation on to the reader. This will (hopefully) not result in confusion. Those who start performing calculations in the field of biomechanics will, in any case, soon get used to vector notation.

Appendix A illustrates the specifically biomechanical standpoint and the interaction of mechanical and non-mechanical factors with the examples of currently (and controversially) discussed problems of primary mechanical causes of disk prolapse, adaptation and remodeling of bones, and loading of the spine in standing compared to sitting. Appendix B deals with the mathematical description of translation and rotation in three-dimensional space. The description of orientation and location of objects is of interest in a number of biomechanical studies. New electromagnetic measurement devices, for example, deliver Euler angles to describe the orientation of a rigid body with respect to a reference coordinate system. This topic (and the associated problems) thus deserve a comprehensive description. The chapters comprising Appendix B are mathematically demanding. The aim is to provide the reader of the scientific literature with a guideline, at least, even if he has no intention of using the mathematical apparatus himself. Appendix B concludes with a chapter on errors. Consideration of error influences is an important, indispensable part of biomechanical research.

At the end of each chapter, a list of textbooks and review papers is recommended as further reading. References to scientific papers cited in the text or the figures are given without exception. The papers cited were selected because they were judged by the authors to be exceptionally interesting or especially instructive. Thus, the selection is certainly subjective, and no claim is made that the list of references is comprehensive. If complete coverage is needed, databases are easily accessible for this purpose nowadays. It must be kept in mind, however, that scientific work described in books or in new, specialized journals may only be incorporated into established databases with considerable delay, if at all. (Studying the original publications rather than just their abstracts and extracting new, up-to-date sources from their lists of references is thus neither outdated nor old-fashioned.)

The authors hope that this book will help the reader to understand past and current scientific work in the field of orthopedic biomechanics, to judge the scientific and practical relevance of such work, and to apply state-of-the-art knowledge in solving practical problems in the fields of physiotherapy, rehabilitation, and orthopedics. Perhaps it will also provide a stimulus for the reader's own, future commitment to biomechanical development and research.

The authors thank Mrs. Susan Griesbach, Münster, for her expert help in editing the English translation of the German version of this book and Mr. Charles Wolstenholme, Tromsø, for the careful design of the illustrations. The authors also wish to thank the Thieme publishing house and acknowledge the pleasant cooperation especially with the Executive Editor Mr. Clifford Bergman M. D. and the Production Director Mr. Gert A. Krüger in the preparation of this book.

Münster / Trondheim, January 2002

Paul Brinckmann
Wolfgang Frobin
Gunnar Leivseth

Contents

1 Musculoskeletal Biomechanics, an Important and Interesting Discipline at the Interface between Medical and Natural Sciences

A cursory view might convey the impression that the effects of mechanical factors on the human locomotor system are nowadays sufficiently well known, so that physiotherapy and orthopedics should focus their attention on other, more up-to-date issues. The basic patterns of posture and locomotion have remained essentially unchanged for many centuries, although exposure to physical exertion may have decreased at the workplace and increased in leisure- time activities in our generation compared with our parents or grandparents. What new findings are we to expect, with the basic laws of physics and mechanics having been discovered and formulated long ago? To preserve one's state of health, as it is sometimes called, it is enough to 'lead a healthy life', to 'keep one's body adequately trained' and to keep physical activity within the limits of 'not too much' and 'not too little'.

A closer look, however, tells us that our present understanding of the relation between mechanical influences and the health and functioning of our locomotor system is rather limited. What is especially fragmentary (if not missing completely) is knowledge of long-term effects that may have a crucial influence on quality of life. What effects, for example, on our state of health at age 55 to 70 years can be expected to result from exposure to physical exertion in athletics, or at the workplace, at an age of 15 to 30 years? Positive effects? Detrimental effects? No long-term effects at all? Can properties like muscle force, tendon strength, or bone density, acquired by physical training, be preserved over long periods of time? What precisely are the limits of 'excessively high' or 'excessively low' mechanical loading of joints, in particular for the spine, hip, or knee? Or, conversely, down to what limit is it sensible to relieve the load on one's body by refraining from certain tasks or by making use of ergonomic aids? In the search for answers to such questions, we come across many opinions, sometimes completely subjective, sometimes based on circumstantial evidence, but rarely supported by scientifically proven, hard evidence. It is quite possible that we are currently on the wrong track with respect to the mechanical loading of our locomotor system and that epidemiologists will be telling us one hundred years on what we have done wrong. A disconcerting thought!

Limitation of present knowledge is due to a number of factors:
- For a number of problems of interest, conducting direct experiments is out of the question for ethical reasons. Hypotheses on conditions leading to fatigue fractures of bones or prolapse of intervertebral disks cannot, for example, be tested on living subjects because of the risk of irreversible consequences. Invasive procedures for measuring force, pressure, or stress in the locomotor system are technically feasible and acceptable for test subjects only in exceptional cases.
- Mechanical effects on the locomotor system can only rarely be observed in isolation because of interference by other, non-mechanical influences in virtually all cases. Mechanically induced remodeling of bones, for example, is also subject to hormonal influences. The overlapping of mechanical and non-mechanical factors complicates the interpretation of empirical observations.
- Observations from cohorts of patients or cohorts recruited from certain workplaces are often difficult to evaluate because the living conditions and the working environment undergo continuous changes and the required observation periods of (usually) several years are difficult to achieve.
- The amount of relevant knowledge from animal experiments is limited because animals use their locomotor apparatus in a different fashion. For example, animals do not subject their lumbar spine, as well as their knee and hip joints, to the high loads resulting from erect stance and bipedal gait. In addition, animals do not function like humans and usually have a shorter life than humans. In the early days of anthropogenesis, humans rarely reached the age of 30 years. From the evolutionary point of view, tolerating everyday mechanical loading thus constitutes a new challenge for a subject over 30 years old.

In this situation we gain knowledge of the effects of mechanical influences from the following sources:

- The laws of mechanics permit forces and mechanical stress in the locomotor system to be calculated. However, assumptions and simplifications are indispensable to this aim because the spatial architecture of bones, muscles, tendons, and ligaments, as well as the material properties of the tissues, are often unknown in detail. Furthermore, the strategy of our neuromuscular system regulating the action and co-activation of muscles is largely unknown. Calculations dealing with simplified models of the body are designated biomechanical 'model calculations'. Due to the assumptions made and the simplifications introduced, the range of validity of the results has always to be examined critically.

- Experiments can be performed in the laboratory (*in vitro*) on bone, cartilage, muscles, and other tissues. Unfortunately, some tissues or organs cannot be preserved long enough in the laboratory for long-term effects of mechanical factors to be explored. For example, one can try to simulate loading modes of lumbar spine specimens resulting in disk prolapse being induced by one single load cycle. Performing repeated loadings in order to simulate *in vivo* loads on intervertebral disks occurring over periods of months or years is not practical, as the material properties of the disks will change during the course of the experiment. When evaluating results from experiments *in vitro*, it has always to be considered whether, and to what extent, the experimental set up and protocol actually correctly reflected conditions *in vivo* (or at least to an acceptable approximation).

- Experimentation with living cells, for example studying the influences of stress or strain on bone-depositing or bone-resorbing cells, is a comparatively new field. Due to the interaction of mechanical and non-mechanical factors, observations from cell cultures are, however, not necessarily equally valid throughout the human body. Exercise programs aimed at increasing bone density in the elderly cannot be based solely on observations of mechanical conditions leading to calcium excretion in cell cultures. Nevertheless, important new knowledge is expected to emerge from the field of cell biology.

- Experiments with volunteers are a stroke of luck for biomechanical research. Athletes, for example, volunteer to submit to high loading, and upper tolerance limits of the tissues, or influences on bone architecture and density, can be investigated in such cohorts. To clarify potential effects of high loading, however, it is not sufficient to investigate only elite athletes, as was almost exclusively the case in the past. A complete picture of the effects of high mechanical loading in athletics is provided only if elite athletes are supplemented by all those subjects who quit high-performance training prematurely for any reason.

- Investigations on cohorts of patients or subjects from selected workplaces are indispensable. Anecdotal evidence of the effect of mechanical factors is, however, insufficient. Such studies merely give some indication. Sound, convincing epidemiological studies must compare selected cohorts with control cohorts (case-control studies) or, even better, be designed as prospective studies. Changes in the environmental as well as in the working conditions, long observation periods and problems in assembling (and keeping together) sufficiently large cohorts pose considerable problems for epidemiological studies.

To understand the effect of mechanical influences on maintenance of the state of health and to enable prophylactic measures to be planned, both the mechanical loads and the mechanical properties of the organs have to be explored. If the intention is, for example, to improve the compressive strength of vertebral bodies, a) the type of loading *in vivo* and b) the parameters determining vertebral strength in the loading mode of interest must be known. Only then can specific measures to improve strength be designed. This is, however, only the first step. Mere speculation is insufficient; it remains to be seen whether or not the proposed protocol really is successful.

For these reasons, a large amount of space in this book is given to the determination of the load on muscles, tendons, bones, and joints. The intention is not to discuss the loading of all joints in the body. The fact is rather that the presentation is limited to the highly loaded joints: shoulder, lumbar spine, hip, and knee. The reflections and model calculations discussed in the context of these joints may also serve as models for the mechanical aspects of cervical and thoracic spine, jaw, arm, hand, ankle, and foot. The chapters on mechanical properties of muscle and bone are closely related to those on joint loading. The forces that load the joints are essentially generated by muscles and transmitted by tendons. Bones must withstand these forces.

Research in orthopedic biomechanics is demanding and exciting due to the intricate interrelation of mechanical and non-mechanical influences on the locomotor system. It is inevitable that specific problems sometimes demand specialized and advanced knowledge from other fields such as physics, theoretical mechanics, metrology, informatics, statistics, cell biology, and theoretical and clinical medicine. Such problems can be dealt with only in an interdisciplinary fashion (which makes things more interesting and stimulating).

Complaints caused by (or, to be more cautious, potentially caused by) mechanical factors are widespread. The causes, sequence of events, treatment protocols and long-term prognosis are, however, often not fully understood. In such cases, advice on prevention is not well-founded. Because clinical problems affect many people, orthopedic biomechanics is not only an interesting but also an important discipline. Many examples from the history of medicine demonstrate that fundamental progress was triggered by (sometimes long-term) observations of individual cases. This requires a 'trained eye', and this book is aimed at assisting this training. The long-term follow-up of subjects or patients, based on observations of their environment, their work, and the success of physiotherapeutic, or orthopedic, treatment offers great potential for progress. It is a rewarding activity!

Further reading

Textbooks on musculoskeletal and orthopedic biomechanics

Burstein AH, Wright TM. *Fundamentals of orthopaedic biomechanics. Baltimore:* Williams & Wilkins; 1994

Dvir Z (ed). *Clinical Biomechanics.* New York: Churchill Livingstone; 2000

Frost HM. *Orthopaedic biomechanics.* Springfield: Thomas; 1973

Kassat G. *Biomechanik für Nicht-Biomechaniker. Alltägliche bewegungstechnisch-sportpraktische Aspekte.* Bünde: Fitness Contur; 1993

Mow VC, Hayes WC (eds). *Basic orthopaedic biomechanics.* 2nd ed. Philadelphia: Lippincott-Raven; 1997

Nigg BM, Herzog W (eds). *Biomechanics of the musculo-skeletal system.* 2nd ed. Chichester: Wiley; 1999

Nordin M, Frankel VH (eds). *Basic biomechanics of the musculoskeletal system.* 3rd ed. Philadelphia: Lippincott Williams & Wilkins 2001

Panjabi MM, White AA. *Biomechanics in the musculoskeletal system.* New York: Churchill Livingstone; 2001

Radin EL, Simon SR, Rose RM, Paul IL. *Practical biomechanics for the orthopedic surgeon.* New York: Wiley; 1979

Special topics

Adams M, Bogduk N, Burton K, Dolan P. *The biomechanics of back pain.* New York: Churchill Livingstone; 2002

Brand PW, Hollister AM. *Clinical mechanics of the hand.* St.Louis: Mosby; 1999

Cavanagh PR, Ulbrecht JS. Biomechanics of the diabetic foot: a quantitative approach to the assessment of neuropathy, deformity and plantar pressure. In: Jahss MH (ed). *Disorders of the foot and ankle.* Vol 2. 2nd ed. Philadelphia: Saunders 1991

Chaffin DB, Andersson GBJ, Martin BJ. *Occupational biomechanics.* 3rd ed. New York: Wiley; 1999

Chao EYS, An KN, Cooney III WP, Linscheid RL. *Biomechanics of the hand. A basic research study.* River Edge: World Scientific; 1989

Debrunner HU, Jacob HAC. *Biomechanik des Fusses.* 2nd ed. Stuttgart: Enke; 1998

Hecker R. *Physikalische Arbeitswissenschaft.* Berlin: Köster; 1998

Johnson AT. *Biomechanics and exercise physiology.* New York: Wiley; 1991

Kumar S (ed.). *Perspectives in rehabilitation ergonomics.* London: Taylor & Francis; 1997

Kumar S (ed.). *Biomechanics in Ergonomics.* London: Taylor & Francis; 1999

Mann RA. Overview of foot and ankle biomechanics. In: Jahss MH (ed). *Disorders of the foot and ankle.* Vol 1. 2nd ed. Philadelphia: Saunders; 1991

Martin RB, Burr DB, Sharkey NA. *Skeletal tissue mechanics.* New York: Springer; 1998

van Eijden TMGJ. Biomechanics of the mandible. *Crit Rev Oral Biol Med* 2000; **11**: 123–36

Winter DA. *Biomechanics and motor control of human movement.* 2nd ed. New York: Wiley; 1990

Reference books

Abé H, Hayashi K, Sato M (eds.). *Data Book on Mechanical Properties of Living Cells, Tissues, and Organs.* Tokyo: Springer; 1996

Bronzino JD (ed.). *The biomedical engineering handbook.* Boca Raton: CRC Press; 1995

Nelson EW, Best CL, McLean WG. *Engineering mechanics. Statics and dynamics.* 5th ed. McGraw-Hill, New York 1998

Spiegel MR, Liu J. *Mathematical handbook of formulas and tables.* 2nd ed. McGraw-Hill, New York 1999

Wirhed R. *Sport-Anatomie und Bewegungslehre.* 2nd ed. Stuttgart: Schattauer; 1994

Yamada H. *Strength of Biological Materials.* Baltimore: Williams & Wilkins; 1970

2 Basic Concepts from Physics and Mechanics

Basic concepts like force, moment, mechanical stress, energy, or work are unambiguously defined in physics and mechanics; there is no difference in meaning of these concepts in the field of biomechanics. A detailed treatise of the laws of mechanics and material properties can be found in any textbook on physics or mechanics. This chapter reiterates only those items that are important for an understanding of later chapters in this book; they are illustrated by examples from the human body.

When discussing biomechanical problems in orthopedics or physiotherapy, the term 'mechanical load' (or, briefly, 'load') is frequently used. In its strict sense (as used in this book), the term 'load' designates a force or a moment. For example, it may designate the force transmitted by a joint or the bending moment exerted on a bone. When used in this way, loading by a force is measured in newtons [N], and loading by a moment in newton meters [Nm]. The term 'mechanical load' is, however, occasionally used in the literature to designate some mechanical effect on the biological tissues. It is up to the reader to find out what is actually meant. When used in this fashion, 'mechanical loading' of cartilage or skin might, for example, designate pressure, friction, or deformation. Obviously these are quite different effects that require their own specific description and evaluation. To avoid confusion, it is preferable to adhere strictly to the well-defined mechanical terms when discussing biomechanical problems; only in rare instances are new technical terms required.

Force

Forces can be neither measured nor observed directly; forces are merely a theoretical concept of physics. However, effects of forces are measurable and observable. As an effect of a force the acceleration or deformation of a body can be observed. Newton's second law

$$F = m \cdot a$$

describes the relation between a mass m, its acceleration a and the force which effected the acceleration (Fig. 2.1). Mass is measured in units of kilograms [kg]. The acceleration is the temporal change in velocity. Velocity is measured in units of meters per second [m/s], and the temporal change in velocity in units of meters per second squared [m/s²]. Since the units ('dimensions') on both sides of an equation must be identical, force is thus measured in units of 'kilogram · meter/second squared' [kg · m/s²]. This unit has been given its own name and is termed newton [N].

One example: A body of 5 kg mass may have zero velocity at the beginning of the observation period and a velocity of 20 m/s one second later. In the observation period, the object has thus been accelerated by 20 m/s per second = 20 m/s². On the assumption that the velocity increased linearly in the observation period, the force that effected the acceleration is calculated as $F = 5 \cdot 20$ kg · m/s² = 100 N.

In anticipation of the following chapter (vector algebra) it has to be pointed out that Newton's second law is really an equation between the vector of the force **F** and the vector of the acceleration **a**.

$$\mathbf{F} = m \cdot \mathbf{a}$$

In this form, the law states that the magnitude of the acceleration is proportional to the magnitude of the force. The mass m is the factor of proportionality. As an equation between two vectors, Newton's law states in addition that the acceleration is effected in the direction of the force.

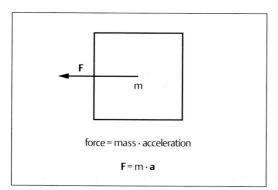

force = mass · acceleration

$$F = m \cdot a$$

Fig 2.1 Effect of a force: acceleration of a mass. Newton's second law relates the force **F**, the mass m and the acceleration **a**.

The deformation of a body by a force is illustrated in Fig. 2.**2** by the example of a coil spring. When loaded by a force, the spring shortens. For an elastic spring the relation between the force and the deformation is given by Hooke's law

$$F = c \cdot dL/L$$

In this equation L designates the initial length of the spring and dL its change in length. L and dL are stated in units of meters [m]. The value of the constant c depends on the material properties and the form of the spring. c designates how much the spring deforms under a given force, i.e. whether the spring is 'hard' or 'soft'. Note: elastic deformation is only one of several types of deformation. The plastic deformation of a piece of chewing gum is likewise effected by a force; the relation between force and deformation is described by an equation differing from Hooke's law.

Experience shows that when a body 1 exerts a force F_{12} on a body 2, the body 2 exerts a force F_{21} of equal magnitude but opposite direction on body 1 (Newton's third law)

$$F_{12} = -F_{21}$$

In the static case, i.e., when no accelerated movements occur, force and counteracting force add up to zero. In the example shown in Fig. 2.**3** the downward directed gravitational force of the mass is of equal magnitude and opposite in direction to the upward directed force of the spring.

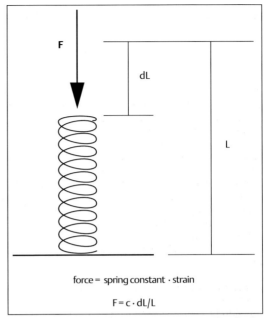

force = spring constant · strain

$$F = c \cdot dL/L$$

Fig. 2.2 Effect of a force: deformation of a body. Hooke's law relates the force F, the initial length L and the change in length dL of the spring.

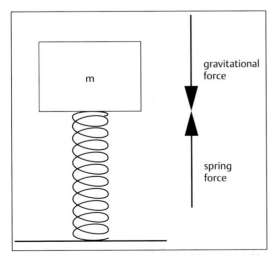

Fig. 2.3 Illustration of Newton's third law. In equilibrium, the gravitational force and the elastic force of the spring are opposingly directed and equal in magnitude.

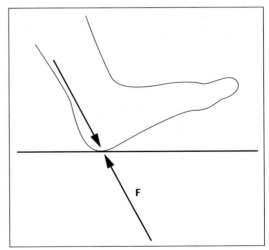

Fig. 2.4 When the foot hits the floor, a force **F** decelerates and also deforms the foot. An equal but opposite force is directed from the foot on to the floor. This force deforms the floor.

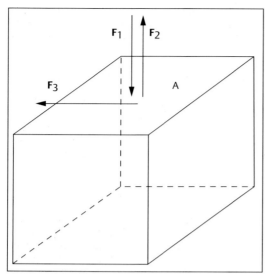

Fig. 2.**5** A force directed perpendicular to a surface (**F**$_1$ or **F**$_2$) is described as a compressive or tensile force, depending on its direction. A force acting parallel to a surface (**F**$_3$) is called a shear force.

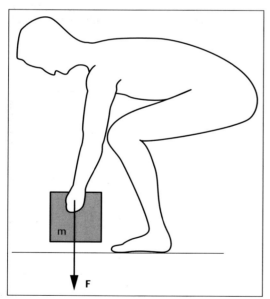

Fig. 2.**6** Illustration of the effect of inertia. When holding the mass, the gravitational force F = m · g acts. In this formula, m denotes the mass and g the gravitational acceleration. When the mass is lifted with an upward directed acceleration a, the inertial force m · (–a) acts in addition. In this moment, the hand feels a downward directed force of F = m · (g + a). While lifting, the object appears to be 'heavier' compared with mere holding.

Both effects of a force, acceleration and deformation, can be observed in the course of the gait cycle when the heel strikes the floor (Fig. 2.**4**). After a heel strike, the velocity of the body decreases; in addition, the heel deforms. Deceleration (negative acceleration) of the body and deformation of the heel are caused by a force exerted from the floor on to the foot. There is an equal, opposite force from the foot on the floor. This force deforms the floor. The deformation of a concrete floor is small, but still measurable. The deformation of an elastic floor in a gymnasium can be seen with the naked eye.

Forces in specified directions with respect to a given surface bear additional designations (Fig. 2.**5**). A force directed perpendicularly on to a surface is designated as compressive force. A force directed perpendicularly away from the surface is designated as tensile force. A force acting in or parallel to the plane of the surface is designated as shear force.

In the dynamic case, i.e. when accelerated movements are encountered, inertial forces come into play. If the acceleration of a mass m equals a, the inertial force amounts to

$$\mathbf{F} = m \cdot (-\mathbf{a})$$

The inertial force has the magnitude m · a and its direction is opposite to the direction of the acceleration. Fig. 2.**6** illustrates the effect of the inertial force (or inertia) when lifting a mass from the floor. During lifting, the acceleration is directed upwards. The inertial force is directed downwards and is of magnitude m · a. In the initial phase of lifting, the object thus appears to be 'heavier' when compared to simply holding it.

Inertial forces become apparent when the human body is decelerated (i.e. negatively accelerated), for example, when hitting the floor after jumping from a wall or gymnastic apparatus. The magnitude of the force between the body and the floor depends on the acceleration a. The acceleration can be calculated approximately by dividing the change in velocity Δv by the time interval Δt required to decelerate the body

$$a \approx \Delta v / \Delta t$$

This approximation rests on the assumption that the magnitude of the acceleration is constant during the time interval Δt. With a given change in velocity, a short time interval for deceleration will result in a larger inertial force; a longer time interval will result in a smaller inertial force. When hitting the floor with a straight leg, the time interval required to decelerate the body will be short and the force between floor and foot will be accordingly high. If the time interval for decelerating the body is prolonged, either by bending the knees or by a deformable (compliant) gym floor, the magnitude of the inertial force will be smaller. Decreasing an inertial force by prolongation of the time interval available for acceleration (or deceleration) is known as 'damping'.

In many biomechanical problems gravitational forces play an important role. The gravitational force is always directed perpendicularly downwards; its magnitude is given by

$$F = m \cdot g$$

In this equation, m designates the mass, given in kilograms [kg]. g is a constant, determined from free fall or pendulum experiments, called 'gravitational acceleration'. g has the numerical value of 9.81 [m/s²]. It follows that a mass of 1 kg exerts a gravitational force of $1 \cdot 9.81$ kg $\cdot$ m/s² = 9.81 N. If errors of the order of 2 % are deemed negligible (as is usually the case in orthopedic biomechanics), the numerical value of g can be rounded off to 10.0 [m/s²]. Thus the gravitational force (or 'weight') of a mass of 1 kg amounts (when rounded) to 10.0 N. Colloquially, the terms 'mass' and 'weight' are used synonymously. Strictly speaking, this usage is not correct. The mass of a body is given in kilograms [kg], and its weight in newtons [N]. In everyday life, the imprecise use of these technical terms does not give rise to any misunderstanding. In biomechanical calculations, however, the weight of a mass must always be expressed in newtons, as the product m·g. Otherwise the dimension as well as the numerical value of the result will be faulty.

A three-dimensional, solid body of mass m can be thought to be composed of n small volume elements with masses m_i (i = 1, 2, 3, ... n). Gravity exerts a force on each of these masses. To arrive at a simple description of the effect of gravity on the whole body, a special point, the 'center of gravity', is defined where the mass of the whole body is imagined to be concentrated. Gravity then acts at this point of mass m. The method used to determine the location of the center of gravity is illustrated in Fig. 2.**7,** using the example of a flat disk. For the purpose of calculation, the disk is imagined to be composed of i small, quadratic elements of mass m_i. The x- and y-coordinates of the center of gravity X_{cg} and Y_{cg} are then calculated from

$$X_{cg} = \Sigma \, m_i \cdot X_i/m$$
$$Y_{cg} = \Sigma \, m_i \cdot Y_i/m$$

In these formulae X_i and Y_i designate the coordinates of the elements with masses m_i; m is the total

mass of the body. Σ is the mathematical summation sign. The sum has to be extended over all n elements m_i from i = 1 to i = n. Explicitly, the first equation reads

$$X_{cg} = (m_1 \cdot X_1 + m_2 \cdot X_2 + m_3 \cdot X_3 + ... + m_n \cdot X_n)/m$$

If the location of the center of gravity of a three-dimensional object is to be calculated, the object is imagined to be composed of small volume elements (cubes). X_{cg} and Y_{cg} are calculated as stated above. The z-coordinate of the center of gravity is given by

$$Z_{cg} = \Sigma \, m_i \cdot Z_i/m$$

Alternatively, the location of the center of gravity of a solid body can be found experimentally. Fig. 2.**8** illustrates a practicable procedure (one of several possible choices) using the example of the flat disk. If the disk is suspended from a thin thread, the center of gravity at rest is known to be located perpendicularly below the point of fixation. (If this were not the case, the disk would oscillate without reaching a resting position.) By suspending the disk from two different points of fixation, the location of the center of gravity can be determined unequivocally. To the same end, a three-dimensional object has to be suspended from three different points of

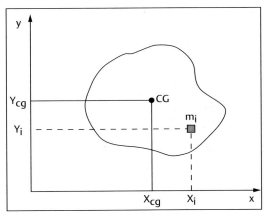

Fig. 2.7   Calculation of the location of the center of gravity CG of a flat disk. For the purpose of calculation, the disk is imagined to be composed of small, quadratic elements of mass m_i. The coordinates of the center of gravity are obtained by summation (or integration) over all elements multiplied by their respective distances from the axes and divided by the total mass m of the disk.

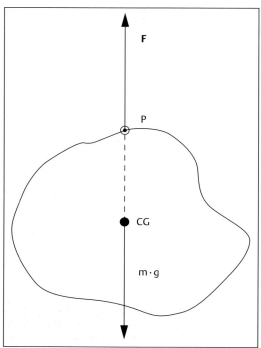

Fig. 2.8 Experimental determination of the position of the center of gravity of a disk. In static equilibrium the tensile force in the suspending thread and the gravitational force of the mass of the disk are equal and opposite. The center of gravity is located somewhere along the dotted line below the point of suspension. When the disk is suspended from a second point, the center of gravity is determined by the intersection of the two lines.

fixation, which must not lie in the same plane. It has to be stressed that the center of gravity is merely a calculated point that allows for the effects of gravitational force on the body in question to be described simply. The center of gravity need not coincide with a material point of the body. For example, the center of gravity of a torus (circular ring) lies in the center of the torus, i.e. at a location where there is no mass.

▨ Moment

The moment effected by a force can be defined in different ways, as a number or as a vector. (See the following chapter on vector algebra.) If calculations are limited to two-dimensional problems where the axis of rotation is perpendicular to the plane of interest, the moment can be defined simply as a (positive or negative) number

$$M = \pm L \cdot F$$

In this equation L is the magnitude of the perpendicular distance of the line of action of the force from the fulcrum (the point where the axis of rotation intersects the plane). The line of action is an imaginary line in the direction of the force, running through the point of force exertion. F is the magnitude of the force. In the context of orthopedic biomechanics, the distance L is also called the 'moment arm' of the force **F**. In precise mathematical notation, where the bars indicate the magnitude (positive value) of distance and force, we can write

$$M = \pm |L| \cdot |\mathbf{F}|$$

Alternatively, the moment can be given as a product of the distance L_1 of the point of force exertion from the fulcrum, the sine of the angle φ between the direction of the force and the line connecting the point of force exertion and the fulcrum and the magnitude of the force

$$M = \pm |L_1| \cdot \sin\varphi \cdot |\mathbf{F}|$$

In this equation, φ is the smaller of the two angles between the direction of the force and the distance line. φ is $\leq 90°$ and the numerical value of $\sin\varphi$ lies between 0 and +1. In the case of a distance line perpendicular to the direction of the force, φ equals 90° and $\sin\varphi$ equals +1; the two definitions of M above are thus identical.

Fig. 2.**9** illustrates the definition of moment. The gravitational force F = m · g of the mass m held in the hand exerts a moment M with respect to the axis of rotation in the center of the condylus humeri

$$M = L \cdot F = L_1 \cdot \sin\varphi \cdot F = L \cdot m \cdot g$$

L and L_1 form the side and the base of a right-angled triangle; thus L equals $L_1 \cdot \sin\varphi$.

If the moment is defined as a product of the magnitudes of distance and force (and not as a product of vectors; see the following chapter on vector algebra), a further rule for obtaining the positive or negative sign of the moment has to be followed. If the force effects a rotation in a clockwise direction, the moment is counted as positive; if the force effects a counterclockwise rotation, the moment is given a negative sign. In the example given in Fig. 2.**9** the force effects a rotation in clockwise direction. This moment is positive. In graphic illustrations the moments defined as numbers (and not as vectors) are depicted by curved arrows with the arrowhead pointing in the direction of the rotation. It has to be pointed out that, for historical reasons, the direction of rotation of positive moments (i.e. clockwise) does not match the definition of positive angles. Angles are counted as positive when rotation is in a counterclockwise direction.

As with forces, moments cannot be observed or measured directly; only their effects can be observed. These effects are the acceleration of a rotational motion or the deformation of a body in torsion or bending. The relationship between a moment and accelerated rotation of a body is given by

$$M = I \cdot \alpha$$

In this equation I denotes the moment of inertia of the body in relation to the axis of rotation. I depends on the distribution of the mass of the body with respect to the axis of rotation. A mass m concentrated at a point located at a distance L from the axis has a moment of inertia equal to $m \cdot L^2$. A three-dimensional object can be imagined to be composed of small volume elements with masses m_i; the moment of inertia is the sum of the contributions of all masses m_i multiplied by their squared distance from the axis of rotation. In other words, if the shape and the distribution of the mass of the object are known, the moment of inertia can be calculated. The moment of inertia has the dimension $[kg \cdot m^2]$. The moment of inertia is valid only for the specified axis; if the location or the direction of the axis relative to the object is changed, the moment changes as well. Formulae used to calculate the moment of inertia of regularly shaped objects with respect to their axes of symmetry are listed in reference books on mechanical engineering.

α designates the angular acceleration. Angular acceleration is the temporal change in angular velocity ω, which in turn is the temporal change in the angle of rotation. Angles are measured in degrees or radians; angles are dimensionless quantities. A full rotation of 360° corresponds to an angle of 2π radian (π = 3.14159...); accordingly 1 radian corresponds to an angle of 57.2958°. If angles are measured in radians, angular velocity is measured in 'radian per second' [1/s]. The unit of angular acceleration is then 'radian per second squared' [1/s^2]. Analogous to the resistance of a mass to linear acceleration, the inertial force, the quantity $I \cdot (-\alpha)$, describes the resistance of a body to accelerated rotation. This quantity has the magnitude $I \cdot \alpha$ and opposes the moment that causes the angular acceleration.

In the scientific literature, moments of inertia of segments of the human body (head, arms, trunk, etc.) are usually not tabulated in units of $kg \cdot m^2$. Instead, the so-called radius of gyration, i, is used.

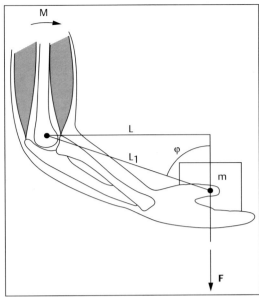

Fig. 2.**9**   Moment M of the gravitational force of the mass held in the hand in relation to the axis of the elbow joint located in the center of the condylus humeri. For calculation of the moment, either the perpendicular distance L of the axis from the line of action of the force, or the distance L_1 from the axis to the point of force exertion (the center of gravity of the mass) can be used. In the second case, the product of distance and force has to be multiplied by the sine of the angle φ between L_1 and the direction of the force.

From the radius of gyration i and the mass m of the segment the moment of inertia I can be calculated as

$$I = i^2 \cdot m$$

The advantage of this formula is that it is very easy to allow for different body masses in biomechanical calculations. It has to be kept in mind, however, that i represents the geometrical shape and the mass distribution of the body segment. To employ the mass simply as a scale factor assumes that body segments of different subjects are geometrically similar. This is only a (sometimes crude) approximation; consider for example the shape of the thighs of different subjects.

Fig. 2.**10** illustrates the effects of a moment: angular acceleration and torsional deformation. If a mass m is attached to the rope around the wheel, the wheel is loaded by a moment of the magnitude

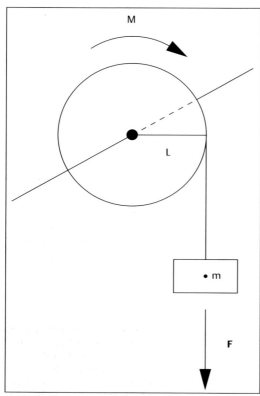

Fig. 2.**10** Illustration of the effects of a moment: accelerated rotation and/or torsional deformation. Under the influence of the force on the rope slung around the wheel, the wheel will undergo an accelerated rotation. If the wheel was fixed to the axis, the axis would be twisted.

$L \cdot F = L \cdot m \cdot g$. The wheel performs an accelerated rotation. If the wheel was fixed (non revolving) to the axis, application of the moment would result in a torsional deformation of the axis. For a thin axis of elastic material the relation between the moment M and the angle of torsion φ is given by

$$M = c \cdot \varphi$$

c is a constant that depends on the properties of the material, the cross section, and the length of the axis. (The equation is analogous to that describing the deformation of a spring under a force.)

Fig. 2.**11** illustrates a situation where a torsional deformation of the lower extremity occurs. When the ski hits an obstacle, a sideways directed force F applied at a distance L from the long axis of the leg exerts a moment $L \cdot F$ on the leg. First the leg is rotated; but since the range of rotational movement in the ankle, knee and hip joints is small, a torsional deformation of the leg results. If the ski is long and the force is high, the resulting moment may be large enough to effect a torsional fracture of the tibia or to rupture the ligaments of the knee.

The forces in Figs 2.**9**–2.**11** not only exert moments but at the same time effect a linear acceleration of the human body or the wheel and axis structure. If, by contrast, two forces of equal magnitude but opposing direction load a body, the forces effect a moment (provided the forces are not applied at the identical point), but the sum of the forces equals zero. In this case, the two forces exert a 'pure' moment. Fig. 2.**12** illustrates this with the example of a beam loaded by a pair of forces (force couple). The moment is the sum of the moments exerted by the two forces and amounts to

$$M = 2 \cdot L \cdot F$$

According to the sign convention quoted above, this moment has a positive sign.

A single force F that loads a body at a distance L from the fulcrum (Fig. 2.**13**) can be replaced by a pure moment $2 \cdot (L \cdot 1/2\,F) = L \cdot F$ and a force F exerted at the fulcrum. This decomposition is advantageous if the linear acceleration of the whole set-up and the angular acceleration are to be investigated separately.

When dealing with objects whose length is large compared with the dimensions of their cross sections (for example, beams or long bones), moments that load the objects in certain directions bear specific designations. A moment which twists a beam about its long axis is called 'torsional moment' or 'torque'. A moment that bends the beam is called 'bending moment'. In Fig. 2.**14** the force F on the free end of the angulated beam exerts a bending

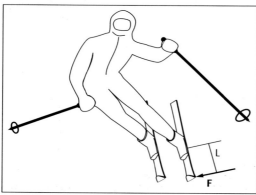

Fig. 2.**11** A laterally directed force F applied at the distance L from the leg exerts a moment $L \cdot F$ on the leg. The leg will rotate and eventually deform in torsion.

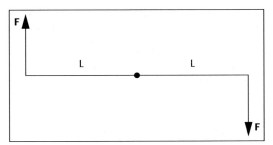

Fig 2.**12** If two forces of equal magnitude but opposing direction act on a body, the sum of the forces equals zero. If the two forces are neither applied at the same point nor act along the same line, the pair of forces effects a moment on the body. In the example shown, the moment in relation to the fulcrum of the beam amounts to 2 · L · F.

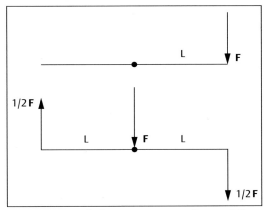

Fig. 2.**13** A single force **F** acting at a distance L from the fulcrum can be replaced by a pure moment L · F and a force **F** acting at the fulcrum. In both cases a force **F** and a moment L · F act on the body; the two loading modes are identical.

moment on part a and a bending as well as a torsional moment on part b of the beam. According to the definition of the moment, the bending moment increases in part a with increasing distance from the point where the force is exerted. The same is true for part b; the highest bending moment occurs at the location where the beam is fixed at the wall. By contrast, the torsional moment is constant over the length of part b. (The reason is that the distance between the point where the force is applied and the long axis of part b does not change along the length of part b.)

Depending on the point of application, forces may effect linear and torsional deformation as well as linear and rotational acceleration at the same time. In the example given in Fig. 2.**14**, the force **F** acts as a shear force on all cross sections of the beam (including the cross section where the beam is fixed at the wall). According to Newton's second law the whole set-up of beam and wall is accelerated by the force **F**. (The fact that the wall does not move downwards is due to the opposingly directed force from the earth on to the wall.)

In simple cases the pressure on an interface can be calculated directly from the definition. If a rigid body lies with a plane side on a plane surface (Fig. 2.**15**) the pressure may be assumed to be uniform over the whole area A of the interface. When loaded by a force F directed perpendicular to the surface, the pressure is calculated as p = F/A. If the force remains constant and the area A is increased, the pressure decreases in proportion to the increase in area.

Pressure

Pressure describes in detail how force is transmitted from one object to another via an interface. Pressure is defined as 'force perpendicular to an interface divided by the area of the interface'

$$p = F/A$$

In this equation force F is inserted in newtons [N] and the area A in square meters [m^2]. The unit of pressure [N/m^2] bears the name pascal [Pa].

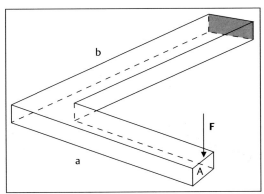

Fig. 2.**14** A force **F** on an angulated beam exerts different moments on the different parts of the beam. The force exerts a bending moment on section a, and a bending as well as a torsional moment (torque) on section b.

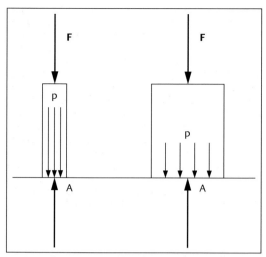

Fig 2.**15** Illustration of the definition of pressure. Pressure p is defined as force **F** perpendicular to an interface divided by the area A of the interface. In simple cases, the pressure can be directly determined from its definition. In the case of a plane surface between rigid bodies, p = F/A. If the area is increased (with the force kept constant), the pressure decreases.

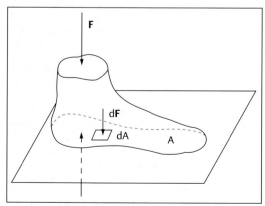

Fig. 2.**16**   Even in the case of a plane interface between the bare foot and the floor, the pressure dF/dA is not uniform over the contact area. A pressure distribution exists. The pattern of the pressure distribution and the location of the maximum and minimum pressure depend on the architecture of the hard and soft tissues of the foot. The mean pressure over the area of contact is F/A.

Plane areas of contact are rarely encountered between the human body and its environment or between articulating bones. And even if the interface is planar, as between the bare foot and the floor (Fig. 2.**16**), experience tells us that the pressure does not assume identical values at different points of the contact area. In the case of the foot it is obvious why the pressure has different values at different locations. The fraction of the force d**F** which is transmitted by each small element dA of the contact area (i.e., the local pressure dF/dA) depends on the architecture of the bones and ligaments and on the thickness and mechanical properties of the tissues of the sole of the foot. If the pressure is not uniform over the interface area, the term 'pressure distribution' is used.

Calculation of the pressure distribution under the sole of the foot is a complicated problem and can be expected to produce approximate values only. There is, however, a simple, exact formula that can be employed (in this, as well as in similar cases) to calculate the order of magnitude of the pressure. The term 'mean pressure' denotes the mean value of the pressure, averaged over the pressure distribution on the interface. The mean pressure p_{mean} can be calculated by dividing the force F by the projected area A_{proj}

$$p_{mean} = F/A_{proj}$$

The projected area is the area that is seen when looking along the direction of the force on to the interface area. In the example given in Fig. 2.**16**, the projected area is the contact area between foot and floor (the gravitational force pointing perpendicularly downwards). When standing on one leg the magnitude of the force **F** equals the weight (gravitational force) of the body.

The formula for calculating the mean pressure is of practical importance in biomechanics. In complicated arrangements where the true pressure distribution could hardly be calculated, the mean pressure gives, at least, an impression of the magnitude of the pressure to be expected at the interface. Knowing the mean of a pressure distribution implies that the pressure in some locations will be higher and in other locations lower than the mean pressure. Furthermore, the formula implies that the mean pressure increases or decreases in proportion to the force. If, for example, the force on a joint can be diminished by a change of posture or external loading, the mean pressure on the joint surface is expected to decrease in proportion. (Strictly speaking, this is only true if the shape of the pressure-transmitting joint surface remains unchanged under the change of force; in good approximation this is often the case.) Conversely, an increase in the

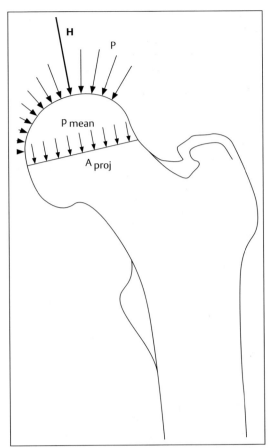

Fig 2.**17** The pressure is not uniform over the contact area of acetabulum and femoral head. Given a force **H** between acetabulum and head, the mean pressure on the joint surface can be calculated as a quotient of the force H and the 'projected' area of the joint surface A_{proj}. The projected area is the area that is seen from the direction of the force. In the case of the hip joint, the projected area is a circle with the radius of the femoral head.

force-transmitting interface area can be expected to decrease the pressure. Employing compliant supports in hospital beds to protect sensitive skin regions makes use of this effect; the exact shape of the pressure distribution between body and mattress need not be known in such a case.

Fig. 2.**17** illustrates how the formula for the mean pressure can be employed to estimate the pressure on the articular surface of the hip joint. The pressure on the surfaces of the femoral head and the acetab-

ulum is suspected (correctly) not to be uniform; the theoretical approach to this complicated problem is dealt with below in the chapter on mechanical aspects of the hip joint. To estimate the magnitude of the pressure, the force between acetabulum and head is divided by the projected area of the joint surface. Viewed from the direction of the force, the projected area of the joint is a circle with a radius r of the femoral head. (A closer look shows that this is not strictly true, due to the femoral head not being completely covered laterally by the acetabulum.) With a femoral head radius of 2.5 cm, the projected area A_{proj} amounts to $\pi \cdot r^2 = 3.14 \cdot 0.000625$ m^2. Assuming a joint load of 1500 N, the mean pressure on the articular surface is calculated as $1500/(3.14 \cdot 0.000625)$ N/m$^2 = 7.6 \cdot 10^5$ Pa = 0.76 MPa.

Mechanical stress

When a force acts on a body, a deformation in the direction of the force is observed (Fig. 2.**18**). Compressive or tensile forces shorten or stretch the body; shear forces effect an angular deformation. The deformation changes the relative locations of atoms or molecules within the material. This gives rise to internal forces (rejection and attraction) of electrical origin, which balance the external forces.

The mechanical stress on the surface of a small cube-shaped volume element of a loaded body (Fig. 2.**19**) is defined as the fraction of the force dF transmitted via the surface dA divided by this surface area. If the force dF is directed perpendicular to the surface dA, there is a compressive or tensile stress σ. If the force dF runs parallel to the surface dF, there is a shear stress τ. (The definition of compressive stress on an imaginary inner surface is identical with the definition of pressure on an external surface. The terms 'pressure' and 'compressive stress' have identical meanings. They are measured in the same unit [Pa].)

In static mechanical equilibrium, stresses on opposite sides of a cube-shaped volume element are equal in magnitude but opposite. Different values of compressive, tensile, and shear stress may exist on the three pairs of opposing surfaces of the cube. The state of mechanical stress of a cube-shaped volume element is thus uniquely described by six numbers (three compressive or tensile stresses, three shear stresses). It has to be pointed out that the stress on the surface of a volume element imagined to be cut from a body depends on the spatial orientation of the element with respect to the body. If (with the loading mode left unchanged) a different orientation of the volume element in Fig. 2.**19** were chosen, different values of the stress on

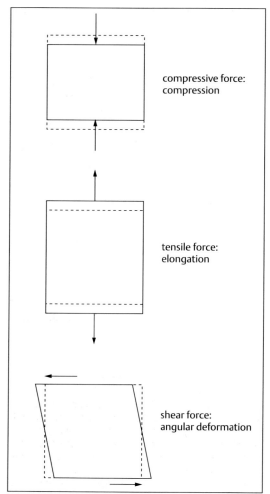

compressive force:
compression

tensile force:
elongation

shear force:
angular deformation

Fig 2.**18** A force effects a deformation of a body; in static equilibrium internal forces balance the external force. The deformation occurs in the direction of the force, but simultaneous, additional deformations in other directions are possible. A tensile force effects elongation, a compressive force results in compression, and a shear force causes an angular deformation.

the surfaces of the cube would be found. The stress values at different orientations are interrelated; conversion formulae (not quoted here, see textbooks on properties of materials) allow the change in stresses to be calculated depending on the orientation.

In simple cases it is possible to employ the definition of stress for a straightforward calculation of

the stress. In the example given in Fig. 2.**19** with the body loaded by a compressive force $\mathbf{F}_1$ and a shear force $\mathbf{F}_2$, the stress may be assumed to be uniform over any internal surface parallel to the outer surface A. Under this assumption, the compressive stress σ and the shear stress τ on the surface dA of a cube-shaped volume element oriented parallel to the outer surface A, amount to

$$\sigma = F_1/A$$
$$\tau = F_2/A$$

Mechanical effects on the tissues of the human body depend, ultimately, not on the forces but on the pressure on the surfaces of joints or skin and on the internal stresses in bones, tendons, muscles, or other organs. The pressure on surfaces and the stresses within a material depend a) on the magnitude of the load, b) on the loading mode (i.e., the way forces and moments are applied), c) on the geometrical shape of the organs, and d) on the material properties of the tissues. It follows that pressure or mechanical stress is altered by changing the external loading, by changing the shape and architecture of organs, or by changing the material properties of the tissues. In the human body, however, the last two of these procedures are only rarely applicable. The easiest way is to try to influence the external loading and the mode of load transmission to the human body. Obviously, it makes a big difference whether a needle is pressed (with equal force) with its pointed or blunt end against a fingertip. Influencing the load and the loading mode is of practical importance when the aim is a temporary or permanent reduction of the pressure on joint surfaces.

▉ Mechanical work, energy and power

Mechanical work E is defined as 'force times distance'; the distance L is to be measured in the direction of the force $\mathbf{F}$

$$E = F \cdot L$$

Mechanical work has the dimension 'newton times meter' [Nm]. This unit bears the name joule [J].

If a person lifts a mass m by a distance L, the human body performs mechanical work $F \cdot L = m \cdot g \cdot L$ [Nm] on the mass. The energy to produce this work stems from chemical processes in the muscles. The muscles, however, also consume chemical energy in situations involving no mechanical work, for ex-

Fig. **2.19** Loading a body results in mechanical stress within the volume of the body. The mechanical stress on the surface of a cube imagined to be cut from the volume of the body is defined as the fraction of the force dF transmitted through the surface dA of the cube. If the force dF is directed perpendicular to the surface dA, the stress is termed compressive or tensile stress; if the force is directed parallel to the surface, the stress is termed shear stress. For reasons of mechanical equilibrium the stresses on opposite sides of a cube are equal and opposite. Stresses on adjacent sides of the cube can be different. In a given loading situation the stresses depend on the spatial orientation of the cube; the stresses in different orientations can be obtained by mathematical conversion. In the case of a simple geometry of the body and a simple loading configuration, the stresses can be calculated directly from their definitions.

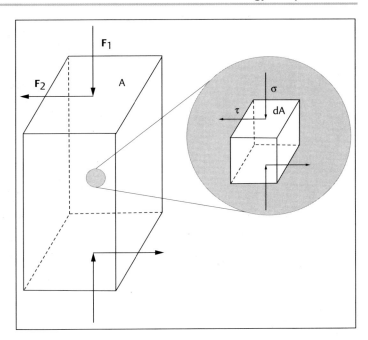

ample, in isometric contraction when holding a weight. For this reason, the energy consumption of muscles is usually not equal to the mechanical work performed by the muscles.

The kinetic energy of a body moving in linear direction amounts to

$$E = 1/2 \, m \cdot v^2$$

In this formula m denotes the mass and v the velocity of the body. In the case of a rotational movement the kinetic energy amounts to

$$E = 1/2 \, I \cdot \omega^2$$

In this equation I denotes the moment of inertia and ω the angular velocity. In both cases kinetic energy is measured in units of $[kg \cdot m^2/s^2]$. By inserting the dimension of the force $[N = kg \cdot m/s^2]$ we see that the dimension of the kinetic energy equals the dimension of mechanical work [Nm]. Energy and work are mechanically the same entity; the kinetic energy of a body can be regarded as the sum of the mechanical work performed in order to reach its velocity.

Potential mechanical energy is stored energy that can be converted into other forms of energy. For example, a mass lifted to a height h above ground level has a potential energy of

$$E = m \cdot g \cdot h \, [Nm]$$

By letting the mass fall, this energy can be converted into kinetic energy (and, on hitting the ground, ultimately into thermal energy i.e., heat). In the same way, the deformation energy stored in a deformed spring can be converted into other forms of energy when the spring is released.

Mechanical power P is defined as mechanical work per unit time. Thus, power is measured in units of [Nm/s]. This unit bears the name watt [W]. For a translational motion, this definition is equivalent to the definition of power as product of the force and the velocity $F \cdot v$ [Nm/s]. For a rotational motion, power can be defined as product of the moment and the angular velocity $M \cdot \omega$ [Nm/s]. The three definitions are equivalent; the dimension of power [Nm/s] is of course identical irrespective of the definition. The product of moment and angular velocity characterizes, for example, the power generated or absorbed by the muscles moving a joint. The product of power and time, or in case of a temporal variation of the power the integral $\int P dt$ extended over the time interval of interest, equals the energy. For a joint this quantifies the energy generated or absorbed by the muscles within the observation time.

Stability and instability

A mechanical system is designated as 'stable' if a small external perturbation leaves the system essentially unchanged. In contrast, the system is called 'unstable' if a small perturbation suffices to change it completely. A sphere at the deepest point of a bowl is in a stable state, because a small kick will let the sphere roll back and forth but the sphere will remain within the bowl. A sphere on the top of a mountain will be in an unstable state because upon a small kick the sphere will roll down and not return to its initial location. In physical terms, stability or instability of a state are characterized by the potential energy. A stable state is characterized by a (relative) minimum of its potential energy. In the example discussed, energy is required to displace the sphere from the deepest point of the bowl. An unstable state is characterized by a (relative) maximum of its potential energy. If the state is changed (if the sphere rolls downhill), energy is released and converted, for example, into kinetic energy or heat.

The stability (insensitiveness to small perturbations) of the position of a joint or the posture of the body is usually provided by activating muscles. In erect stance, for example, muscles are activated to limit postural sway and to guarantee that the center of gravity is located above the area of support, thus preventing falls (unstable postures). Activation of muscles, as well as co-contraction of agonists and antagonists, invariably leads to an increase in joint loading and joint stiffness (resistance to movement). The increased loading and stiffness is the price paid for the increase in stability.

In the context of medical problems, the term 'instability' is sometimes employed in an imprecise fashion. For example, a joint with a range of motion larger than normal may be designated 'unstable'. The correct designation in this case should be 'hypermobile'. By contrast, a shoulder joint whose humeral head has a tendency to dislocate from the glenoid cavity is a truly unstable joint.

Further Reading

Alonso M, Finn E. *Physics.* Addison Wesley, Harlow 1996
Nelson EW, Best CL, McLean WG. *Engineering mechanics. Statics and dynamics.* 5th ed. McGraw-Hill, New York 1998

3 Vector Algebra

Some physical quantities are comprehensively described by a single number, in some cases in combination with a positive or negative sign. Such quantities are termed scalars. Examples are: mass [kg], length or distance [m], volume [m^3] or temperature [degree]. There are other physical quantities that are not completely described by quoting their magnitude; a full description requires specification of a direction in a plane or in space. To describe a force unambiguously, for example, it is not sufficient to give the magnitude of the force. The direction of the force must be given as well. Other physical quantities that have to be described by their magnitude as well as by their direction are the location of a point with respect to another point, a velocity, an acceleration, or a moment. Physical quantities that are described by a magnitude and a direction are termed vectors.

The forces acting on a body or the motion of a body are often illustrated graphically. In such illustrations, the vectors (forces, changes of location, velocities, or accelerations) are depicted by arrows of different lengths and orientations in planes of interest or in three-dimensional space. In the two-dimensional case, where all vectors lie in the same plane, the graphical representation also allows simple operations like addition or subtraction of vectors to be performed by means of ruler and pencil. For many problems in biomechanics, the limited accuracy of such 'graphical illustrations' and 'graphical calculations' is adequate.

Alternatively, vectors are represented by their components. The components are vectors in the direction of the x-, y- and z-coordinate axes. The magnitude and direction of the components are described by positive or negative numbers, depending on whether the component vectors point in the positive or negative direction of the coordinate axes. The representation of vectors by their components must be used if products of vectors are to be calculated; unlike for addition or subtraction, there is no simple graphical procedure for multiplication of vectors. For precise or extensive vector calculations, especially when employing computers, the component representation of vectors is always used. This does not preclude the possibility of results being presented subsequently in graphical format.

To designate vectors, the following convention is adhered to in this book: vectors are designated by bold type. **F**, for example, designates a force vector. If more than one force is being dealt with, an index 1, 2, etc. may be added, e.g. **F**$_1$ or **F**$_2$. A character as index, for example **F**$_i$, is used if all forces in a given set-up are meant or if the sum of all forces **F**$_1$, **F**$_2$, ... **F**$_n$ from i = 1 to i = n is to be calculated. The magnitude of a vector is designated by a character in ordinary type; F, for example, designates the magnitude of the force vector **F**. Alternatively, the magnitude of a vector **F** may be designated as |**F**|; F and |**F**| have identical meaning. The components of a vector in relation to a right-handed rectangular xyz-coordinate system are designated by the indices x, y and z; for example **F**$_x$, **F**$_y$, and **F**$_z$.

The trigonometric functions sine, cosine, and tangent

When breaking down vectors into components or multiplying vectors by vectors, trigonometric functions come into play. This chapter serves to remind the reader of the definition of these functions. Those who remember the meaning of these sufficiently well from their schooldays can go straight to the next section.

Sides a and b of a right-angled triangle enclose the 90° angle (Fig. 3.**1**); side c opposite this angle is termed the hypotenuse. In relation to the angle α between b and c, side a is termed 'opposite' and side b 'adjacent'. The trigonometric functions sine, cosine, and tangent describe the quotients of the lengths of the sides of right-angled triangles dependent on the angle α. Using quotients of side lengths makes sense because all right-angled triangles with an angle α between the hypotenuse and the adjacent side are geometrically similar (see Fig. 3.**1**, upper illustration). In other words, for all right-angled triangles with an angle α between the hypotenuse and the adjacent side, the value of the quotient a/b is identical, irrespective of the actual size of the triangles.

The sine of an angle α is defined as

$$\text{sine of } \alpha = \text{opposite/hypotenuse}$$
$$\sin \alpha = a/c$$

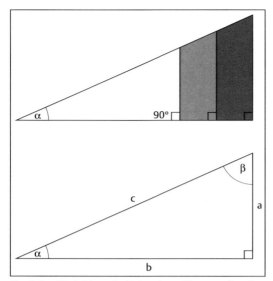

Fig. 3.1 All right-angled triangles with an angle α between the hypotenuse c and the adjacent side b are geometrically similar. The quotients of the adjacent and opposite sides a and b with the hypotenuse c define the trigonometric functions sine and cosine of angle α; the quotient of a and b defines the tangent of angle α.

The cosine of an angle α is defined as

$$\text{cosine of } \alpha = \text{adjacent/hypotenuse}$$
$$\cos \alpha = b/c$$

The tangent of an angle α is defined as

$$\text{tangent of } \alpha = \text{opposite/adjacent}$$
$$\tan \alpha = a/b$$

Of course the definitions hold for the angle β as well. The sine of the angle β in Fig. 3.**1** is defined as

$$\text{sine of } \beta = \text{opposite/hypotenuse}$$
$$\sin \beta = b/c$$

Analogous definitions hold for the cosine and the tangent of angle β.

Trigonometric functions are frequently employed because many geometrical problems can be reduced to problems with right-angled triangles. If some elements (side lengths, angles) of a right-angled triangle are known, the remaining elements can be calculated trigonometrically.

Example 1: The length of the hypotenuse c and the angle α between the hypotenuse and one side are known. Trigonometric functions allow the lengths of sides a and b to be calculated. The definitions given above yield

$$b = c \cdot \cos\alpha$$
$$a = c \cdot \sin\alpha$$

Example 2: Angle α and the length of side b are known. The lengths of sides a and c are calculated by

$$a = b \cdot \tan\alpha$$
$$c = b/\cos\alpha$$

Numerical values of sine, cosine, and tangent can be found in mathematical tables or by means of a pocket calculator. In addition to sine, cosine, and tangent, the inverse functions are stored in calculators. In mathematical formulae the inverse functions of sine, cosine, and tangent are termed asin, acos, and atan. The inverse functions are the angles that correspond to quotients of side lengths of right-angled triangles: asin is the angle α that belongs to a given quotient of the lengths of sides a and c; by analogy, the same applies to acos and atan. Given the length of two sides of a right-angled triangle, the angle between the two sides can be determined using inverse trigonometric functions.

Example 3: The lengths of sides a and b are known. The angle α between sides c and b is calculated by

$$\alpha = \text{atan } (a/b)$$

On the buttons of pocket calculators, the inverse functions asin, acos, and atan are often designated as $\sin^{-1}$, $\cos^{-1}$, and $\tan^{-1}$. (This is an awkward designation, because the symbol '$^{-1}$' is normally used to indicate '1.0 divided by …'. $\sin^{-1}\alpha$, however, does not designate $1.0/\sin\alpha$ but the inverse function of the sine, i.e. the angle α belonging to a given value of the sine.)

As quotients of lengths of the sides of right-angled triangles, trigonometric functions are defined only for angles up to 90°. In this domain sine, cosine and tangent have (as quotients of lengths) positive values. It has been advantageous, however, to extend the definition of trigonometric functions up to an angle of 360°. The generalized definition relates to quotients of lengths at the 'unit circle' (Fig. 3.**2**). The unit circle is a circle whose radius (distance OC) is equal to 1. The magnitude of the sine of an angle is equal to distance BC, the magnitude of the cosine is equal to distance OB, and the magnitude of the tangent is equal to distance AD. The functions, however, bear different positive or negative signs depending on the quadrant in which OC

Table 3.**1**   Signs for sine, cosine, and tangent for angles between 0° and 360°

Quadrant	Angles	Sine	Cosine	Tangent
I	0° to 90°	+	+	+
II	90° to 180°	+	–	–
III	180° to 270°	–	–	+
IV	270° to 360°	–	+	–

is located. Quadrants I to IV are parts of the plane as partitioned by a rectangular coordinate system.

The signs for trigonometric functions are listed in Table 3.**1**. In the example shown in Fig. 3.**2** (α = 125°), the sine of the angle α is positive; the cosine and the tangent are negative. The reader might like to confirm that, for angles up to 90°, defining trigonometric functions based on quotients of sides of right-angled triangles is identical to basing them on lengths at the unit circle.

Angles are quoted in different units, in degrees or radians. Expressed in degrees, a full rotation corresponds to 360°; expressed in radians, a full rotation corresponds to $2 \cdot \pi$ = 6.2831 radians (correct to four decimal places). It follows that 1 radian corresponds to 57.2958°. The degree is preferred in practice; computerized calculation programs usually use the radian.

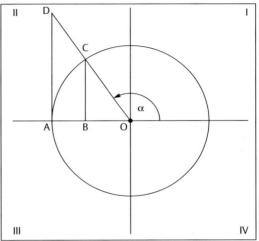

Fig. 3.**2**   Definition of trigonometric functions by distances at the unit circle (circle with radius OC = 1). For a given angle α (measured in an counterclockwise direction) the length of BC equals the magnitude of the sine, the length of OB equals the magnitude of the cosine, and the length of AD equals the magnitude of the tangent. Sine, cosine, and tangent bear positive or negative signs, depending on in which of quadrants I to IV the radius OC is located.

▨ Representation of vectors

In graphical illustrations, a vector is represented by an arrow (Fig. 3.**3**). The length of the arrow indicates the magnitude of the vector. The magnitude of a vector is a positive quantity (there are no arrows with a negative length). In order to infer the magnitude of a vector from a graphical representation, the scale factor of the representation must be known. If, for example, the arrow represents a force, it must be known how many centimeters of its length correspond to 1 N. The direction of the vector and its sense of direction are given by the direction of the arrow and the arrowhead respectively. In a plane, the direction of the arrow can be given by the angle α between the arrow and the x-axis of a rectangular xy-coordinate system. In a plane, a vector is fully described by its magnitude and its direction. In three-dimensional space, an additional angle has to be given; this is usually the angle between the vector and the z-axis of a rectangular xyz-coordinate system.

Alternatively, a vector can be represented by its components in relation to a xyz-coordinate system.

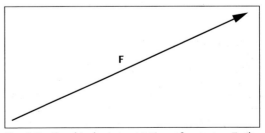

Fig. 3.**3**   Graphical representation of a vector **F**: the length of the arrow designates the magnitude of the vector. The direction of the arrow and the arrowhead denote the direction of vector **F**.

A vector **F** is then given by the vector sum of its components

$$\mathbf{F} = F_x \cdot \mathbf{e}_x + F_y \cdot \mathbf{e}_y + F_z \cdot \mathbf{e}_z$$

In this formula $\mathbf{e}_x$, $\mathbf{e}_y$ and $\mathbf{e}_z$ designate unit vectors. Unit vectors are vectors of length one in the direction of the coordinate axes. F_x, F_y and F_z are numbers which may be positive or negative. The x-component $F_x \cdot \mathbf{e}_x$ of the vector **F** is a vector in the direction of the x-axis (Fig. 3.**4**). The length of the vector component equals the magnitude (the positive value) of F_x; the sense of direction of the vector component (the direction in which the arrow points) is given by the sign of F_x. For example, $5.0 \cdot \mathbf{e}_x$ designates a vector component of length 5.0 pointing in the positive x-direction; $-2.0 \cdot \mathbf{e}_x$ designates a vector component of length 2.0 pointing in the negative x-direction. The same applies analogously to the other components of **F**.

In commonly used symbolic notation the component representation of a vector **F** is given by

$$\mathbf{F} = \begin{bmatrix} Fx \\ Fy \\ Fz \end{bmatrix}$$

In this notation, the unit vectors do not appear explicitly. The brackets indicate that the components of the vector **F** are calculated by multiplying the numbers F_x, F_y and F_z by the unit vectors. If only vectors in the xy-plane are being dealt with, the z-component is always equal to zero. In this case, the third component can be omitted and the vector may be represented just by the two numbers F_x and F_y.

The numbers F_x, F_y and F_z are known as the 'coordinates' of the vector **F**. It has become usual to refer to F_x, F_y and F_z as 'components' of the vector **F** as well. Strictly speaking, this is not correct, because components of a vector are vectors and not numbers. On the other hand, the somewhat casual use of the term 'component' prevents confusion with the 'coordinates' of a point relative to a coordinate system. In the following, the term 'component' is used in this casual fashion with the aim of avoiding any confusion.

Fig. 3.5 shows the symbolic representation of vectors using the example of two vectors $\mathbf{F}_1$ and $\mathbf{F}_2$ in the xy-plane. The axes of the rectangular coordinate system are scaled. The components of the vectors are the projections of the vectors on the axes; the signs of the coordinates give the direction of the components (the z-components in this example are equal zero)

$$\mathbf{F}_1 = \begin{bmatrix} +5.0 \\ +3.0 \\ 0.0 \end{bmatrix}$$

$$\mathbf{F}_2 = \begin{bmatrix} +3.0 \\ -4.0 \\ 0.0 \end{bmatrix}$$

Of course, this representation is valid for all vectors, not only for forces. A distance vector $\mathbf{L}_1$ in the

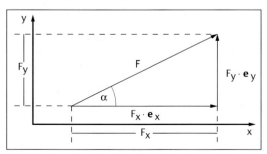

Fig. 3.4 In a plane the direction of a vector can be specified by the angle α with respect to the x-axis of an xy-coordinate system. Alternatively, the vector may be specified by its component vectors $F_x \cdot \mathbf{e}_x$ and $F_y \cdot \mathbf{e}_y$. $\mathbf{e}_x$ and $\mathbf{e}_y$ are unit vectors (vectors of length 1) pointing in the direction of the coordinate axes; F_x and F_y are numbers which may be positive or negative.

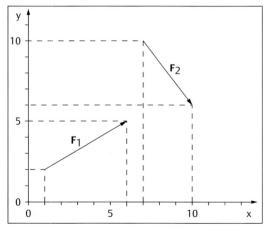

Fig. 3.5 Representation of vectors by specification of their components. The components of vectors $\mathbf{F}_1$ and $\mathbf{F}_2$ are given by the projections on the x- and y-axis. In the example shown $F_{1x} = +5$, $F_{1y} = +3$, $F_{2x} = +3$, $F_{2y} = -4$.

xy-plane, pointing from the point $(x = 1, y = 2)$ to the point $(x = 6, y = 5)$ is represented by

$$\mathbf{L}_1 = \begin{vmatrix} +5.0 \\ +3.0 \\ 0.0 \end{vmatrix}$$

The components of a vector (or rather, to be precise, we should say, 'the coordinates of a vector') can be calculated from its magnitude and its direction. In the two-dimensional case (Fig. 3.**4**)

$$F_x = |\mathbf{F}| \cdot \cos \alpha$$

$$F_y = |\mathbf{F}| \cdot \sin \alpha$$

Conversely, the angle α can be determined when the components F_x and F_y are known

$$\alpha = \operatorname{atan}(F_y / F_x)$$

The relation between the components and the magnitude of a vector is given by

$$|\mathbf{F}| = \sqrt{F_x^{\,2} + F_y^{\,2}}$$

This formula derives from Pythagoras' theorem. The components F_x and F_y, together with the vector, form a right-angled triangle. In a right-angled triangle

$$\text{hypotenuse}^2 = \text{adjacent side}^2 + \text{opposite side}^2$$

$$c^2 = a^2 + b^2$$

$$c = \sqrt{a^2 + b^2}$$

It must be pointed out that the location of the origin of a vector (the starting point of the arrow) is not specified by its magnitude and direction. The three vectors depicted in Fig. 3.**6** have the same magnitude (length) and the same direction; they represent an identical vector. It follows that, when drawn, a vector may be shifted parallel to, or along, its direction. Since magnitude and direction remain unchanged by this procedure, it remains the same vector. On the other hand, a mechanical state may well be altered when a vector is shifted. We expect different effects when an identical force vector is applied at different points of a body. The force might induce a linear translation and/or a rotation. To describe the effect of a force on a body it is not sufficient merely to communicate the force vector (magnitude and direction); the point of force application must be given as well.

▦ Addition of vectors: graphical procedure in the two-dimensional case

A specific rule, differing from the usual one for adding up pure numbers, is required for adding physical quantities that are characterized by magnitude and direction (i.e. vectors). Fig. 3.**7** illustrates the graphic procedure for adding up vectors, the parallelogram law of vector addition. Two coplanar forces of different magnitude and direction act on an object. The resultant force (i.e. the sum of the two forces) is to be determined. In its upper diagram Fig. 3.**7** shows an 'anatomical' set-up. A simplified 'model' (middle diagram) has to be derived before the problem can be solved. The directions of the forces are inferred from the outlines of the human bodies. The contact areas of the hands, by which the forces are actually transmitted, are replaced by the points of application of the forces. If no further details of force transmission are known, the points of force application are located centrally between the contact areas of the hands. In later chapters of this book the directions of muscle forc-

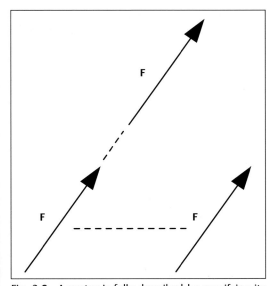

Fig. 3.6 A vector is fully described by specifying its magnitude, direction, and sense of direction. The origin of the vector (in the case of a force vector: the point of force application) is not covered by this description. Thus, the three arrows shown, all of identical length and identical direction, represent the same vector.

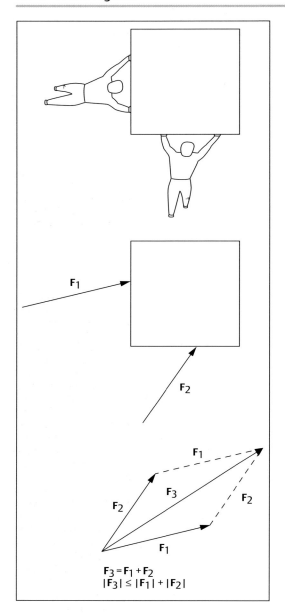

Fig 3.7 Illustration of the addition of two vectors in a two-dimensional situation, employing the parallelogram law of vector addition. Two forces are exerted at the object shown in the upper diagram. To arrive at the total force, a simplified 'model' of the set-up has to be established (middle diagram). To apply the parallelogram law (lower diagram), vector F_2 is shifted parallel to itself and along its direction until its origin is located at the tip of the arrowhead of F_1. The base of the triangle formed by F_1 and (the shifted) F_2 is the sum vector F_3. If F_1 is shifted to the tip if F_2, the identical sum vector F_3 is reached. Both triangles together form a parallelogram. The direction of the sum vector F_3 coincides neither with the direction of F_1 nor with the direction of F_2; the magnitude of F_3 is in general not equal to the sum of the magnitudes of F_1 and F_3.

es in biomechanical models are inferred in an identical fashion, from the anatomical direction of the muscles. Areas of insertion of muscles and tendons are represented by single points, usually by the center of the area of insertion.

To obtain the vector sum (Fig. 3.**7**, lower diagram), F_2 is shifted parallel to itself and along its own direction until the origin of F_2 coincides with the tip of F_1. The base in the triangle formed by F_1 and (the shifted) F_2 is the vector sum (also termed the 'resultant') F_3. The identical result is obtained if F_1 is shifted until its origin coincides with the tip of F_2. Again, the vector sum is given by the base of the triangle formed by F_2 and (the shifted) F_1. The two triangles form the so-called parallelogram of forces. It is obvious that the direction of the resultant F_3 (the diagonal of the parallelogram) coincides neither with the direction of F_1 nor with the direction of F_2. The magnitude of the resultant (length of the arrow) F_3 is always smaller than or, at most,

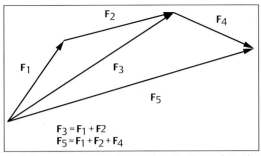

$$F_3 = F_1 + F_2$$
$$F_5 = F_1 + F_2 + F_4$$

Fig 3.9   In order to add up vectors $\mathbf{F}_1$, $\mathbf{F}_2$, and $\mathbf{F}_4$, the parallelogram law is applied twice. First $\mathbf{F}_1$ and $\mathbf{F}_2$ are added; in a second step $\mathbf{F}_4$ is added. The vector sum $\mathbf{F}_3$ of $\mathbf{F}_1$ and $\mathbf{F}_2$ does not need to be constructed explicitly. The sum vector $\mathbf{F}_5$ can be determined by joining $\mathbf{F}_1$, $\mathbf{F}_2$ and $\mathbf{F}_4$ to form a polygon.

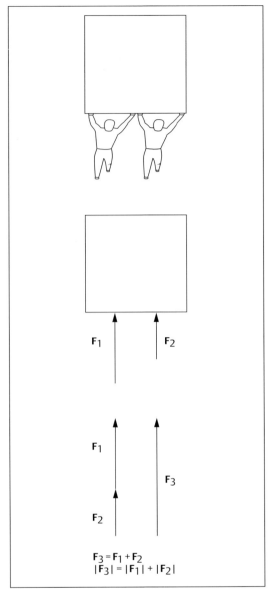

$$F_3 = F_1 + F_2$$
$$|\mathbf{F}_3| = |\mathbf{F}_1| + |\mathbf{F}_2|$$

Fig. 3.8   In the special case of two parallel vectors $\mathbf{F}_1$ and $\mathbf{F}_2$ the magnitude of the sum vector $\mathbf{F}_3$ is equal to the sum of the magnitudes of $\mathbf{F}_1$ and $\mathbf{F}_2$. The direction of $\mathbf{F}_3$ equals the direction of $\mathbf{F}_1$ and $\mathbf{F}_2$.

equal to the sum of the magnitudes of the vectors $\mathbf{F}_1$ and $\mathbf{F}_2$.

In the case of two parallel vectors, the construction of the vector sum is very simple. Fig. 3.**8** shows

in its upper drawing the 'anatomical' set-up and in its middle one the simplified model representing the forces exerted by vectors $\mathbf{F}_1$ and $\mathbf{F}_2$. The lower drawing shows the addition of these vectors according to the rule given above. In the case of two parallel vectors, the parallelogram of forces shrinks to a straight line. The diagonal in this 'parallelogram' is obtained simply by joining vectors $\mathbf{F}_1$ and $\mathbf{F}_2$. In this special case the direction of the vector sum $\mathbf{F}_3$ is seen to equal the direction of the two vectors; the magnitude of the vector sum $\mathbf{F}_3$ is given by the sum of the magnitudes of the two vectors $\mathbf{F}_1$ and $\mathbf{F}_2$. In the special case of parallel vectors (but only in this situation), the magnitudes of vectors may be added together arithmetically to provide the magnitude of the vector sum.

If more than two vectors are to be added, the parallelogram law of vector addition is applied repeatedly (Fig. 3.**9**). In order to add $\mathbf{F}_1$, $\mathbf{F}_2$, and $\mathbf{F}_4$, $\mathbf{F}_1$ and $\mathbf{F}_2$ are added first; in a second step $\mathbf{F}_4$ is added to the sum vector $\mathbf{F}_3$. $\mathbf{F}_5$ designates the resultant vector. It should be noted that it is ultimately not necessary to draw $\mathbf{F}_3$ explicitly. In order to add up vectors $\mathbf{F}_1$, $\mathbf{F}_2$, and $\mathbf{F}_4$ it is sufficient to join the three vectors to form a polygon. The sum vector $\mathbf{F}_5$ then points from the origin of $\mathbf{F}_1$ to the tip of $\mathbf{F}_4$.

If vectors to be added up form a closed polygon, this is the same as saying that the vector sum equals zero. Fig. 3.**10** illustrates this for vectors $\mathbf{F}_6$, $\mathbf{F}_7$, and $\mathbf{F}_8$. Between the arrowhead of $\mathbf{F}_8$ and the origin of $\mathbf{F}_6$ there is no space: the resultant is a vector of zero length. A situation where the sum of all forces equals zero is met in static equilibrium. On a drawing this is shown by the fact that the vectors of all forces applied form a closed polygon.

Subtracting one vector from another requires no new rule. Let us assume that the difference

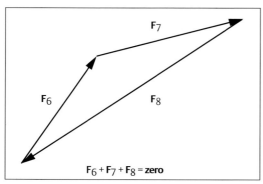

$$F_6 + F_7 + F_8 = \textbf{zero}$$

Fig 3.**10** If vectors to be added up form a closed polygon, it shows that the vector sum equals zero.

$$\mathbf{F}_{11} = \mathbf{F}_{10} - \mathbf{F}_{9}$$

is to be calculated. This difference can also be written as the sum

$$\mathbf{F}_{11} = \mathbf{F}_{10} + (-\mathbf{F}_{9})$$

$-\mathbf{F}_{9}$ designates a vector having an identical orientation but the opposite direction to $\mathbf{F}_{9}$. To show this graphically, we have to draw the arrowhead on the opposite end of the vector. (In numerical representation, this means that the vector coordinates change their sign, see the following section.) Vectors $\mathbf{F}_{10}$ and $-\mathbf{F}_{9}$ may now be added according to the scheme shown in Fig. 3.**7**.

Addition of vectors: numerical procedure

The numerical rule for adding vectors is based on the addition of the components (or, more precisely, on the addition of the coordinates). The x-, y- and (in the three-dimensional case) z-components of the sum vector are obtained by adding the respective x-, y- and z-components of the vectors to be added up. In the case of vectors $\mathbf{F}_1$ and $\mathbf{F}_2$ being added up, the components of the sum vector $\mathbf{F}_3$ are obtained from

$$F_{3x} = F_{1x} + F_{2x}$$
$$F_{3y} = F_{1y} + F_{2y}$$
$$F_{3z} = F_{1z} + F_{2z}$$

Fig. 3.**11** illustrates this rule for the two-dimensional situation (and also shows the graphical procedure for addition). In the example given, the components of vectors $\mathbf{F}_1$ and $\mathbf{F}_2$ are

$$F_{1x} = 4$$
$$F_{1y} = 1$$
$$F_{2x} = 2$$
$$F_{2y} = 3$$
$$F_{1z} = 0$$
$$F_{2z} = 0$$

For the vector sum $\mathbf{F}_3$ it holds that

$$F_{3x} = F_{1x} + F_{2x} = 4 + 2 = 6$$
$$F_{3y} = F_{1y} + F_{2y} = 1 + 3 = 4$$
$$F_{3z} = F_{1z} + F_{2z} = 0 + 0 = 0$$

in symbolic notation

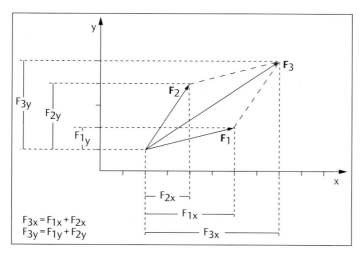

$$F_{3x} = F_{1x} + F_{2x}$$
$$F_{3y} = F_{1y} + F_{2y}$$

Fig 3.**11** In order to add vectors $\mathbf{F}_1$ and $\mathbf{F}_2$ numerically, the x- and y-components are added separately to give the x- and y-components of the sum vector $\mathbf{F}_3$. The same rule applies to the z-components in the thee-dimensional situation.

$$\mathbf{F}_3 = \begin{bmatrix} 4.0 \\ 1.0 \\ 0.0 \end{bmatrix} + \begin{bmatrix} 2.0 \\ 3.0 \\ 0.0 \end{bmatrix} = \begin{bmatrix} 6.0 \\ 4.0 \\ 0.0 \end{bmatrix}$$

As described above, the magnitude and direction of $\mathbf{F}_3$ can be calculated from its components.

Decomposition of a vector into vector addends

In the same way that a number can be broken down into addends, for example the number 10 into the addends 4 and 6, a vector can be decomposed, into two or more vector addends. The prerequisite is that the vector sum of the addends equals the original vector. The representation of a vector by components, by vectors in the direction of the coordinate axes, is one example of decomposition. In general, vectors pointing in arbitrary directions can be broken down. In Fig. 3.**9**, vector $\mathbf{F}_5$ can be imagined to be decomposed into vectors $\mathbf{F}_1$, $\mathbf{F}_2$, and $\mathbf{F}_4$.

It should be pointed out that the decomposition of a vector is, in principle, totally arbitrary. Like breaking down a number arbitrarily into addends, for example the number 10 into 1 + 9, or 3 + 5 + 2, and so on, a vector may also be decomposed into arbitrary addends. Decomposition makes sense only if specific problems have to be dealt with. Fig. 3.**12** gives an example in which the force $\mathbf{F}$ exerted by the foot on to the floor is decomposed into the addends $\mathbf{V}$ and $\mathbf{H}$ (the vector sum of $\mathbf{V}$ and $\mathbf{H}$ being equal to $\mathbf{F}$). The problem here is to evaluate risk of an accident. The downward bend of the floor depends on the vertically directed force $\mathbf{V}$. The risk of slipping on the floor depends on the relation between the horizontally directed force $\mathbf{H}$ and the friction between foot and floor. (The frictional force is given by $|\mathbf{V}|$ multiplied by the coefficient of friction.)

Multiplication of vectors: scalar product and vector product

The rules for multiplying vectors always employ the components of the vectors. Unlike addition, no graphic procedures exist for multiplication. While there is only one type of multiplication between numbers, vectors $\mathbf{A}$ and $\mathbf{B}$ can be multiplied in two different ways, by the 'scalar' product (i.e. 'A times B')

$$\mathbf{C} = \mathbf{A} \cdot \mathbf{B}$$

or by the 'vector' or 'cross' product (i.e. 'A cross B')

$$\mathbf{C} = \mathbf{A} \times \mathbf{B}$$

The result of the scalar product of two vectors $\mathbf{A}$ and $\mathbf{B}$ is a number C. C is calculated from the components of the two vectors as

$$C = A_x \cdot B_x + A_y \cdot B_y + A_z \cdot B_z$$

It can be shown (the proof is not presented here) that C amounts to

$$C = |\mathbf{A}| \cdot |\mathbf{B}| \cdot \cos\varphi$$

φ being the angle between vectors $\mathbf{A}$ and $\mathbf{B}$. Depending on the relative directions of $\mathbf{A}$ and $\mathbf{B}$, $\cos\varphi$ may assume positive or negative values; thus the scalar product may be positive or negative. If the two vectors are oriented perpendicular to each other, the scalar product equals zero.

The result of the vector product (cross product) of two vectors $\mathbf{A}$ and $\mathbf{B}$ is a vector $\mathbf{C}$. The components of $\mathbf{C}$ are calculated from the components of $\mathbf{A}$ and $\mathbf{B}$ as

$$C_x = A_y \cdot B_z - A_z \cdot B_y$$
$$C_y = A_z \cdot B_x - A_x \cdot B_z$$
$$C_z = A_x \cdot B_y - A_y \cdot B_x$$

It can be shown (the proof is not presented here) that vector $\mathbf{C}$ is perpendicular to the plane spanned by vectors $\mathbf{A}$ and $\mathbf{B}$. The magnitude of $\mathbf{C}$ is given by

$$|\mathbf{C}| = |\mathbf{A}| \cdot |\mathbf{B}| \cdot |\sin\varphi|$$

φ is the angle through which vector $\mathbf{A}$ is to be rotated in the direction of vector $\mathbf{B}$. The sense of direction of $\mathbf{C}$ is given by the sign of $\sin\varphi$. Fig. 3.**13**

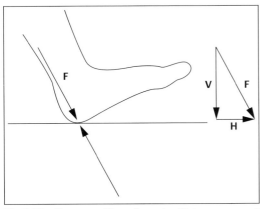

Fig. 3.**12**   Decomposition of a vector **F** into component vectors **H** and **V**. Addition of **H** and **V** reproduces **F**.

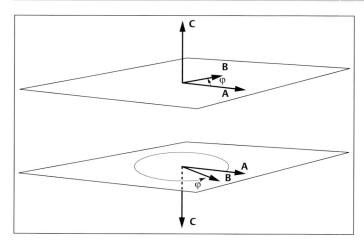

Fig 3.**13**   Representation of the vector product (cross product) **C** of vectors **A** and **B**. **C** is perpendicular to the plane spanned by **A** and **B**. The sense of direction of **C** is given by the sign of sinφ. The angle φ is counted counterclockwise from **A** to **B**. For angles above 180° sinφ is negative. For this reason the product vectors **C** in the upper and lower diagrams point in opposite directions.

illustrates this for the case where the angle φ between **A** and **B** is smaller, and also for the case where the angle φ is larger, than 180°. For angles larger than 180° sinφ is negative; for this reason the sense of direction of vector **C** in the lower diagram of Fig. 3.**13** points downward.

The direction of **C** can be visualized by the 'right hand' rule (Fig. 3.**14**). If thumb and forefinger point in the directions of vectors **A** and **B** (not necessarily running perpendicular to each other), the middle finger of the right hand running perpendicular to the thumb and the forefinger points in the direction of **C**. This right hand rule also serves to define a right-handed xyz-coordinate system. If **A** points in x-direction and **B** in y-direction, **C** points in the direction of the z-axis of the right-handed xyz-system.

Alternatively, the direction of **C** can be visualized by the rule illustrated in Fig. 3.**15**. Vector **C** runs perpendicular to the plane spanned by vectors **A** and **B**. The direction of **C** is given by the direction of the thumb if the fingers are bent in the sense of rotation of the angle φ from **A** to **B** around **C**. The reader may (at the risk of a slight contortion of the right hand) convince himself that both rules give the identical result.

The moment which had been defined in Chapter 2 in simplified form as 'force times perpendicular distance of the line of force action from the fulcrum' is really a vector, the vector product of the distance vector L_1 and the force vector **F**

$$M = L_1 \times F$$

The distance vector L_1 designates the distance (comprising the sense of direction) from the fulcrum to the point of application of the force. The vector **M** is perpendicular to the plane spanned by L_1 and **F**. Its magnitude amounts to

$$|M| = |L_1| \cdot |F| \cdot |\sin\varphi|$$

In the illustration shown in Fig. 3.**16** the distance vector L_1 points from the axis to the center of gravity of the mass hung on the rope slung around the wheel. Alternatively, the moment can be defined by employing the perpendicular distance vector **L** from the fulcrum to the line of action of the force

$$M = L \times F$$

Fig. 3.**14**   Right hand rule. If thumb and forefinger of the right hand point in the direction of **A** and **B**, the middle finger held at an angle of 90° with respect to the plane of **A** and **B** points in the direction of **C**.

Both definitions yield the same result. For φ equal to 90° and sinφ equal to 1, the first formula merges into the second formula. The magnitude of the mo-

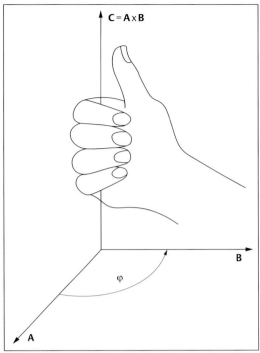

Fig. 3.**15** Right hand rule, alternative version. **C** points in the direction of the thumb if the fingers of the right hand are bent around **C** in the direction of the angle φ between **A** and **B**.

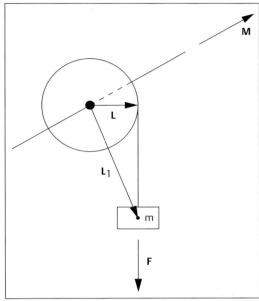

Fig. 3.**16** Illustration of the moment vector **M**. Gravity exerts a force on the mass hung on the rope slung around the wheel. The gravitational force **F** is applied at the center of gravity of the mass. The distance vector **L₁** points from the axis to the point of force application. The moment **M** is a vector, given by the vector product (cross product) of the distance vector and the force vector: **M** = **L₁** × **F**. **M** is oriented perpendicular to the plane spanned by **L₁** and **F**. The sense of direction of **M** can be determined by the right hand rule. In the diagram **M** is depicted by an arrow in the direction of the axis. Alternatively, **M** can be expressed by the vector **L** pointing from the axis to the line of force action and the force: **M** = **L** × **F**.

ment vector is identical to the value of the moment in its simplified version as defined in Chapter 2

$$M = L \cdot F$$

where L and F have to be inserted as positive numbers.

In order to compare the two definitions, vector **M** is shown in Figure 3.**16**. As determined by the right hand rule, **M** points in the direction of the axis of rotation. If the rope were suspended from the other side of the wheel, the moment vector would point in the opposite direction. By contrast, in the simplified definition (see Fig. 2.**10**) the moment is visualized by a bent arrow pointing in the direction of rotation. The reader is reminded again that, when calculating vector products, counterclockwise angles are positive. However, in the simplified definition a moment is counted positive if the rotation caused by the moment occurs in clockwise direction.

Those readers who are familiar with the rules of vector multiplication will always prefer to define a moment as the vector product of a distance vector and a force vector. If the rules for vector multipli-

cation are adhered to, no separate sign conventions have to be kept in mind (as with the simplified definition). The correct positive or negative signs result 'automatically'. As the distance vector, vector **L₁** from the fulcrum to the point of force application is used. It is not necessary to determine vector **L** pointing from the fulcrum perpendicular to the line of action of the force, because by definition the angle φ between **L₁** and **F** is taken into account by the vector product.

▨ Further reading

Rich B, Schmidt PA. *Geometry*. 3rd ed. McGraw-Hill, New York 1999.

Spiegel MR. *Vector analysis and an introduction to tensor analysis*. McGraw-Hill, New York 1959

Spiegel MR, Liu J. *Mathematical handbook of formulas and tables*. 2nd ed. McGraw-Hill, New York 1999

4   Translation and Rotation in a Plane

Describing body movements is a frequently occurring problem in orthopedic biomechanics. An example of such a movement is the forward bending of the trunk in order to grasp an object from the floor. At the beginning, the trunk is erect (initial state); at the end it is bent forward (final state). Other examples of movements are the relative motion of adjacent vertebrae while bending forward or the motion of the lower leg in relation to the upper leg when walking. A 'movement description' can be achieved by stating a set of numbers that communicates the magnitude of the motion and allows the final state to be unequivocally constructed if the initial state is known (and *vice versa*).

In the field of mechanics, the analysis of motions has physical and geometrical aspects. The physical aspects deal with the forces and moments required to generate a specified motion. The description of spatial location and orientation is a geometrical problem. Textbooks on analytic geometry deal at length with the geometric description of motion. These textbooks require knowledge of coordinate systems as well as of vector and matrix analysis. The algebraic tools are not only of theoretical interest; they are indispensable to all investigations where motions are measured. If, for example, the motion of the lower extremity in the course of walking is to be described from series of photographs or video images, a geometrical relationship between the measurement apparatus (camera) and the object (leg) needs to be established. This is accomplished by coordinate systems (camera and laboratory systems). In addition, geometrical relations between the image of the object in consecutive frames must be established. This is accomplished using vector and matrix analysis.

Initially, however, algebra can be dispensed with by analyzing the motion occurring in a plane graphically, using a pair of compasses and a ruler. This is the content of this chapter. (For measurements and calculations, especially in three dimensions, algebraic methods have to be used, see Chapters B1 and B2.) Objects moving in a plane are assumed to be rigid (i.e., not deformable). It follows that the shape of the objects (internal distances and angles, size) remains unchanged under the influence of the forces or moments that caused the movement. The assumptions of bodies being rigid and movement being confined to a plane are model assumptions frequently used in orthopedic biome-

chanics. For example, the motion of lower leg and thigh when walking can be described in the sagittal plane with these two assumptions in mind. In reality, lower leg and thigh are not rigid bodies, like the limbs of a puppet, as they change their shape noticeably when moving. In addition, the motion in question, in reality, is not confined to the sagittal plane.

To describe the motion of a rigid body in a plane it is not necessary to describe the motion of all points of the body; it is sufficient to describe the motion of two specific points on the body. In what follows, these points will be termed 'landmarks'. This term is used because, in many practical applications, markers are affixed to the bodies to be observed. The markers are constructed so as to be clearly visible in film, video, or radiographic images. If two markers are fixed on a rigid body, a reference system is created. The location of all points of the body can be unequivocally specified in relation to this reference system. It follows that, if the location (or the changed location over time) of the landmarks is known, the location (or changed location over time) of all other points of the body is known as well. For this reason, the description of plane motion of a rigid body may be confined to describing the motion of two landmarks.

Translation

A motion that moves all points of a body on straight lines over identical distances is termed 'linear movement' or 'translation'. In Fig. 4.1 two markers P and Q are fixed to a body. The body is moved along a straight line. At the end of the motion their location is designated by P' and Q'. Since, by definition, all points of the body have been moved along straight lines and over identical distances, the lines PP' and QQ' are parallel and of equal length. Since the body was assumed to be rigid (i.e. not deformable), the lines PQ and P'Q' are of equal length as well. It follows that the points P,P',Q',Q form the corners of a parallelogram. In other words, if the initial and the final state of the motion are known and if the points P, P', Q', Q (in that order) form the corners of a parallelogram, the movement can be interpreted as a translation. Fig. 4.1 shows the identical vectors PP' = **t** and QQ' = **t**. The magnitude and direction of **t** characterize the translation.

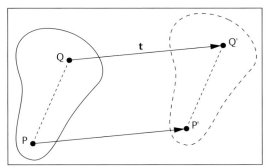

Fig. 4.1 Translation in a plane. To determine location and orientation of a body in a plane, knowledge of the location of at least two landmarks on the body is required. In this figure as well as in the following figures, the solid outline designates the initial state of the body, and the dashed outline the final state. A translation shifts all points of the body by the same distance in the same direction. The shift is characterized by the translation vector **t**.

Rotation

A rotation is characterized by the fact that all points of a body move on concentric circles with the identical angle of rotation around a center of rotation. In Figs 4.**2a** and 4.**2b** the landmarks P and Q move along arcs of circles to P′ and Q′. In Fig. 4.**2a** the center of rotation C is located within the boundary and in Fig. 4.**2b** outside the boundary of the rotating body. In both cases the angle between the lines PQ and P′Q′ equals φ. The rotation has a sense of direction; accordingly the angle of rotation may be positive or negative. A positive angle characterizes

a rotation in a counterclockwise direction, a negative angle characterizes a rotation in a clockwise direction. A plane rotation is unequivocally specified by the location of the center of rotation and the angle of rotation.

If the initial and final states of the body are known, the position of the center of rotation and the angle of rotation may be reconstructed (Figs 4.**3a** and 4.**3b**). Points P and P′ as well as Q and Q′ lie on arcs of circles around the (as yet unknown) center of rotation C. If lines PP′ and QQ′ are bisected perpendicularly, the center of rotation C is located at the intersection of these perpendicular bisectors (Fig. 4.**3a**). The assumption underlying this construction is that the perpendicular bisectors are differently orientated. In the special case of identical orientation (Fig. 4.**3b**) points P, Q and the center of rotation C lie on a straight line. In this case the center of rotation C is given by the intersection of the lines PQ and P′Q′. In both cases the angle of rotation is given by the angle between the lines PQ and P′Q′.

Combined translation and rotation

In general, a motion may be combined from translation and rotation. In the example given in Fig. 4.**4** the body is rotated in a first step around C by an angle φ in a counterclockwise direction. Through this rotation, points P and Q are moved on arcs of circles to P′ and Q′. In a second step the body is moved along a straight line. The final locations of the landmarks are P″ and Q″. The translation is characterized by the translation vector **t** = Q′Q″. If the initial and final state of the motion are known, the angle of rotation φ can be obtained by rotating the body in the final state around an arbitrarily chosen center of rotation C until the lines connect-

Fig. 4.2a Rotation in a plane. All points are rotated about the center of rotation C by the identical angle of rotation φ; the points move on arcs of concentric circles around the center of rotation. In the diagram, the direction of rotation is indicated by an arrow. In the example shown, the center of rotation is located within the boundary of the body.

Fig. 4.2b Rotation in a plane. In this example the center of rotation is located outside the boundary of the body.

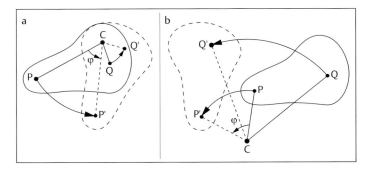

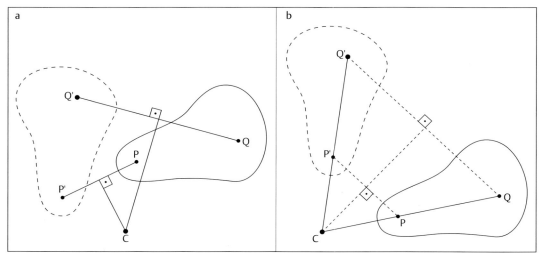

Fig. 4.**3a** Construction of the location of the center of rotation of a plane rotation (standard case). Perpendicular bisectors are constructed on the lines connecting the landmarks in the initial and final states. In the standard case these lines are not parallel. The center of rotation is located at the intersection of the perpendicular bisectors.

Fig. 4.**3b** Construction of the location of the center of rotation of a plane rotation (special case). In the special case, when the landmarks and the center of rotation lie on a straight line, the perpendicular bisectors coincide. In this case the center of rotation is located at the intersection of the lines through P and Q and P′ and Q′ respectively.

ing the landmarks are parallel. In a second step a translation may be performed until the landmarks coincide. The translation vector thus obtained depends on the preceding choice of the location of the center of rotation C; in general it is not identical with **t**. In other words: when describing a motion combined from rotation and translation, only the angle of rotation is unequivocally determined; the

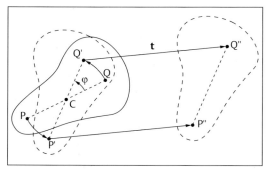

Fig. 4.**4** Plane motion, combined from rotation and translation. In the first step the body (landmarks P and Q) is rotated through an angle φ around the center of rotation C (landmarks P′ and Q′); in the second step the body is translated as indicated by the translation vector **t** (landmarks P″ and Q″).

contribution of translational motion depends on the choice of the center of rotation C.

For plane motions the following noteworthy theorem holds. Any motion resulting from a combination of translation and rotation can be described by a single rotation. This 'substitute' rotation occurs around a center of rotation differing from the original center of rotation but with the identical angle of rotation φ. Fig. 4.**5** shows the body in the same initial and final state as in Fig. 4.**4**. The construction of the substitute center of rotation C_s is performed using the same rule as illustrated in Fig. 4.**3**: the intersection of the perpendicular bisectors erected over the chords of concentric circles is the center of rotation of the substitute rotation.

The fact that an identical change of location of a body may be described either by a pure rotation or by a combination of translation and rotation emphasizes that the description of a motion provides no information on the actual course of the motion between the initial and the final state. In other words, if only the initial and the final location of a body are known, the actual motion between these locations may have varied considerably. Which description to choose in a given situation – a pure translation or a combination of translation and rotation – depends on the biomechanical model adopted. If, for example, a body is known to move around an axis (for example, the lower leg around the axis of the knee joint), the motion is likely to be described by a pure rotation. If translational or rotational movements are suspected to occur simultaneously or in sequence over time (for example, dorsoventral shift and rotation of a lumbar vertebra when bending forward) the observed motion is likely to be decomposed into a translational and a rotational part.

Instantaneous center of rotation

More detailed information about the course of a motion can be obtained if it is divided into many small (differential) consecutive steps rather than just considering a (possibly distant) final state in relation to the initial state. This is illustrated by describing the motion of the knee joint in the sagittal plane by a pure rotation. The sequence of very small (differential) motion steps of the tibia in relation to the femur is characterized by the instantaneous center of rotation and the associated small (differential) angles of rotation. During the course of the motion, the center of rotation is seen to change its location. The motion, in its total range from maximal extension to maximal flexion, is then described by the path of the instantaneous center of rotation. To avoid any misunderstanding it is pointed out that the term 'instantaneous center of rotation' is sometimes employed to describe not only differential rotations but also (inaccurately) rotations with finite angles. If, for example, two radiographs of the knee joint taken in very different states of bending are compared, the change in location of the tibia with respect to the femur can certainly be described by constructing a center of rotation according to the rule illustrated in Fig. 4.**5**. In the case of a large angle between the initial and the final state it would not be correct, however, to refer to this center as an 'instantaneous center'.

The motion of the tibia with respect to the femur occurs in good approximation in a plane. The motion is guided by the cruciate ligaments (Menschik, 1987). Figure 4.**6** shows two states of the knee joint characterized by index 1 (extension, solid outline) and index 2 (flexion, tibia shown in broken outline). The anterior cruciate ligament originates in the dorsal part of the condylus femori at B and inserts ventrally into the tibia at B_1 or B_2. The posterior cruciate ligament originates in the anterior part of the condylus femori and inserts dorsally into the tibia at A_1 or A_2. Defined by these points of insertion, the lengths of the ligaments are ac = BB_1 = BB_2, pc = AA_1= AA_2. The distances between the insertion points are d = AB and e = A_1B_1 (Fig. 4.**7**). The point where the ligaments cross in exten-

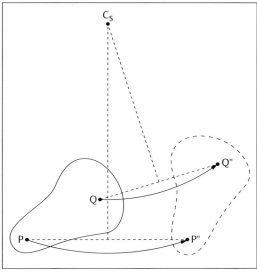

Fig 4.5 Location of the substitute center of rotation C_s for the combined motion illustrated in Fig. 4.4. The location of the substitute center of rotation was constructed according to the rule illustrated in Fig. 4.**3**.

sion is designated C_1, and in flexion, C_2. Menschik's model assumes that the lengths of the cruciate ligaments and the distances between their insertion points remain unchanged during the course of the motion. Under this assumption, the points of intersection C_1 and C_2 are, as shown below, the instantaneous centers of rotation. Since points C_1 and C_2 do not coincide in the extended and flexed posture, it is obvious that no single center of rotation exists in the knee joint: the location of the instantaneous center of rotation depends on the flexion angle of the joint.

To substantiate the claim that the point of intersection of the cruciate ligaments represents the instantaneous center of rotation, let us imagine the femur (points A, B) to be fixed and the tibia to be rotated by a small angle into flexion (Fig. 4.**7**, labels as in Fig. 4.**6**). In the course of this motion points B_1 and A_1 of the tibia are moved to B_1' and A_1'. In accordance with the rule for constructing the center of rotation, perpendicular bisectors are erected over the lines B_1B_1' and A_1A_1'. Since the insertion points of the anterior cruciate ligament (B_1 or B_1') as well as the insertion points of the posterior cruciate ligament (A_1 or A_1') move on arcs of circles around B and A, the perpendicular bisectors run through A and B. The point of intersection of the perpendicular bisectors lies within a polygon de-

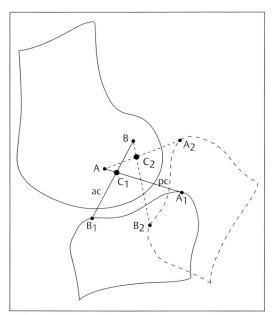

Fig. 4.**6** Motion of the knee joint as guided by the cruciate ligaments (Menschik, 1987). The knee joint is shown in extension (solid outline, points A, B, A_1, B_1, C_1) as well as in maximal flexion (position of the tibia shown in broken outline, points A, B, A_2, B_2, C_2). The anterior cruciate ligament ac runs from B to B_1 or to B_2. The posterior cruciate ligament pc runs from A to A_1 or A_2. The ligaments intersect at C_1 or C_2. The points of intersection of the ligaments are the instantaneous centers of rotation in extension and flexion. When moving from extension to flexion, the instantaneous center of rotation moves from C_1 to C_2.

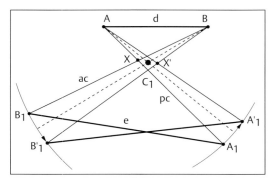

Fig. 4.**7** Determination of the instantaneous center of rotation of the knee joint. If the knee joint is imagined to perform a minute flexion movement, the center of rotation is located at C_1, according to the rule illustrated in Fig 4.**3**. ac and pc designate the lengths of the cruciate ligaments; d and e are the distances between their insertion points on the femur and tibia. Within the limits of a very small (differential) rotational movement, the constructed point C_1 coincides with the points of intersection X and X_1 of the ligaments. It follows that the intersection of the cruciate ligaments coincides with the instantaneous center of rotation.

fined by the intersections of the lines BB_1, BB'_1, AA_1 and AA'_1. If the angle of rotation is reduced to a very small (differential) amount, B'_1 moves towards B_1 and A'_1 towards A_1. At the same time, the point of intersection X' (intersection of AA'_1 with BB'_1) as well as the constructed point C_1 move towards point X (intersection of AA_1 with BB_1). This shows that the point of intersection of the cruciate ligaments gives the location of the instantaneous center of rotation. Using the same arguments it can be demonstrated that C_2 designates the instantaneous center of rotation for the flexed knee. From maximal extension to maximal flexion the instantaneous center of rotation moves along a curve that is determined by the points of intersection of the cruciate ligaments.

The rolling/gliding kinematics of two articulating bones can be qualitatively inferred from the location of the center of rotation relative to the contact area of the joint. When the center of rotation is located at the contact area, pure joint surface rolling occurs. Rolling is characterized by the fact that the point of contact moves during the course of rolling (e.g., the rolling of a wheel on a rail: the center of rotation is the point of contact between wheel and rail; this point moves as the wheel rolls). If the center of rotation is located far away from the point of contact, a lesser amount of surface rolling relative to gliding will occur. We thus infer from the location of the center of rotation of the knee joint that the relative motion of femur and tibia is a combination of rolling and gliding.

Error influences when describing a motion

If the center of rotation is located at a distance from a body, it becomes increasingly difficult to discriminate a rotation by a small angle from a pure translation. In Fig. 4.**8** the translational motion is depicted by the vector **t** pointing from P to P'_t and the rotational motion by the arc b of the circle from P to P'_r. If the vector **t** is kept constant and the center of rotation moves away from P, the radius r of the circle increases and the angle φ decreases. At the same time the arc b of the circle adapts more and more to the translation vector **t** and the distance d

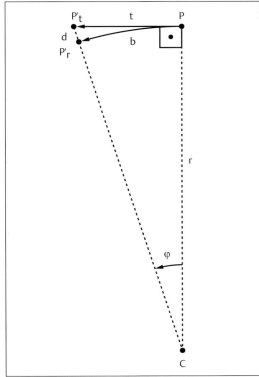

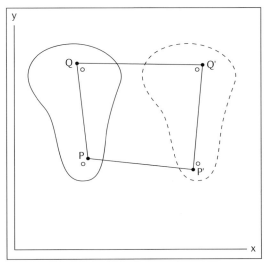

Fig. **4.9** Example of the influence of measurement errors on the description of a motion. In the example shown, only a translation took place in reality. The x- and y-coordinates of the landmarks P, Q, P', and Q' can be measured on an xy-digitizing table only with errors of magnitude σ. For this reason, the measured locations of the landmarks (solid circles) deviate slightly from their true locations (open circles). Unlike the error-free case, the measured landmarks no longer lie on the corners of a parallelogram (cf. Fig. 4.1). To an uncritical observer the measured angle between lines PP' and QQ' simulates a rotation. In such cases, comparison of the calculated measurement error with the measured angle allows the degree of probability that a rotation took place to be determined.

Fig. **4.8** Translation as limiting case of a rotation with the center of rotation shifted to infinity. Point P is shifted by the translation vector **t** to P'_t. Alternatively, P is shifted along the arc b of a circle around a remote center of rotation C to P'_r. If the center of rotation moves farther away from P, the radius r will increase and the angle φ will decrease. At the same time the arc b of the circle adapts more and more to the translation vector **t** and the distance d between the points P'_t and P'_r becomes smaller and smaller. In the end, there is no difference between a pure translation and a rotation about a center located in infinity.

between points P'_t and P'_r becomes smaller and smaller. If the center of rotation moves away to infinity, there will be no difference between rotational motion along the arc of a circle and translational motion. In other words: a translation can theoretically be described by a rotation about a center of rotation located in infinity.

The very minor difference between translation and rotation in the case of a large radius and a small angle of rotation demands caution when interpreting measured data. As measurement errors can never be avoided, a translation may be erroneously

interpreted as a rotation. In Fig. 4.**9** the body is assumed in reality to have performed only a translation. The location of the two landmarks can, however, be measured only with certain errors. Due to the measurement error the lines P'P and QQ' in Fig. 4.**9** are not parallel. An uncritical observer might conclude that the body had been rotated.

The magnitude of the simulated angle of rotation for the set-up shown in Fig. 4.**9** can be estimated in a model calculation. For this purpose the measurement error for the coordinates of the landmarks on an xy-digitizing table is assumed to amount to σ (equal in x and y direction). The measurement error Δγ (measured in radians) of the angle between PP' and QQ' then amounts to

$$\Delta\gamma = \pm\, 2\sigma/L$$

To reach this estimate (see Chapter B3) the distances PP' = L_1 and QQ' = L_2 are assumed to be approximately equal; L is the mean of L_1 and L_2. If the measured angle is not larger than the value calculated by the above formula, the apparent rotation is probably an artifact rather than real. (If the error of measurement of an angle between lines PQ and P′Q′ is to be determined, the same formula is valid; in this case L is the mean of PQ and P′Q′.)

As a practical application of the above formula, we can estimate the measurement error for the change of orientation of a vertebra from two radiographs taken in flexion and extension. Two small metallic markers may be located in the mid plane of the vertebra, 35 mm apart. The measurement error for the coordinates of the markers is assumed to amount to 0.5 mm. It follows that the uncertainty of the angle of rotation amounts to $\pm (2 \cdot 0.5/35) \cdot 57.2958$ or approximately $\pm 1.6°$. (The factor $360/2\pi = 57.2958$ converts the error given in radians into degrees.) If the uncertainty is to be reduced, either the locations of the markers must be measured with greater precision (smaller σ) or the distance between the markers must be increased (larger L). Another approach is to increase the number of markers; for more information on this topic see Chapter B3. In a similar way the uncertainty when determining the location of a center of rotation can be estimated. In general it holds true that the measurement of a rotation can be accepted as reliable only when the center is located not too far from the body.

Inevitable measurement errors for the coordinates of landmarks, and the difficulty of discriminating between translation and rotation in the case of small angles of rotation, result in complications if it is tried to trace a motion very precisely by dividing the path into many small segments. Let us imagine a body that in reality moves along a smooth curve. Repeated measurements of the body's location at short intervals splits the path into segments. On average the direction of the segments follows the true curve but due to measurement errors the direction of individual segments may deviate irregularly from the true (unknown) value. If an attempt were made to describe the motion in each segment of the path by a center and an angle of rotation, a large scatter would probably be found for the location of these centers. Since a zigzag curve of an instantaneous center of rotation cannot be interpreted meaningfully, it is necessary in such cases to smooth the curve mathematically before describing the motion. However, one is now confronted with the problem of selecting a smoothing algorithm (i.e., an appropriate mathematical procedure) that leaves the underlying, original curve unchanged.

To summarize: the motion of a body in a plane may be a translation, a rotation, or a combination of the two. Translation is described by the translation vector **t**; rotation is described by the location of the center of rotation and the angle of rotation. A motion composed of translation and rotation can always be described by a single rotation around a substitute center of rotation. For a given motion, the angle of rotation φ remains the same, no matter whether the motion is described by a single rotation, or by a combination of rotation and translation. It must be emphasized that the description of motion merely establishes a geometrical relationship between the final and the initial states of a body, in terms of its location and orientation. The description does not tell us in detail by which path the body moved from the initial to the final state.

Literature

Scientific papers quoted in the text or the figures

Menschik A. *Biometrie. Das Konstruktionsprinzip des Kniegelenks, des Hüftgelenks, der Beinlänge und der Körpergröße.* Berlin: Springer; 1987

5 Mechanical Equilibrium

The forces developed by muscles and those transmitted by joints can be measured directly only in exceptional cases. Biomechanical model calculations have to be relied upon to a large extent to gain an impression of the magnitude of these forces and to learn in which situations they assume maximal or minimal values. If the body is at rest (or if no accelerated movement occurs) the conditions of mechanical equilibrium allow an unknown moment and an unknown force to be determined. This is usually the moment effected by muscles equilibrating an external moment and the joint force transmitted between the bones of a joint.

Conditions of static mechanical equilibrium

The conditions of mechanical equilibrium read: 'a body is in static equilibrium if it experiences no accelerated translation (linear motion) and no accelerated rotation. In static equilibrium the sum of all external forces and the sum of all external moments acting on the body are equal to zero'

$$\sum_{i=1}^{i=n} \mathbf{F_i} = \mathbf{0}$$

$$\sum_{i=1}^{i=n} \mathbf{M_i} = \mathbf{0}$$

In these equations, $\mathbf{F_i}$ and $\mathbf{M_i}$ designate the vectors of the forces and moments acting on the body (from outside). The symbol Σ is the mathematical sum sign. The vector sums extend over all forces $\mathbf{F_i}$ and moments $\mathbf{M_i}$ from $\mathbf{F_1}$ to $\mathbf{F_n}$ and $\mathbf{M_1}$ to $\mathbf{M_n}$.

The validity of these equations can be seen immediately. If the sum of all forces were not equal to zero, a resultant force (unequal to zero) would act on the body. The body would then be linearly accelerated and, in contrast to the assumption, not be in static equilibrium. The analogous argument holds for the sum of the moments. If the sum of all moments were not equal to zero, a resultant moment (unequal to zero) would act on the body. The body would then undergo an accelerated rotation and would thus not be in static equilibrium. It follows that if a body is seen to perform no accelerated translation or rotation (in the simplest case: if

the body is at rest), the sum of all forces and the sum of all moments must be zero. Additionally, in the two-dimensional dynamic case, when accelerated translations and/or rotations occur, the conditions of mechanical equilibrium remain valid if the sum of the forces is extended over the inertial force $m \cdot (-\mathbf{a})$ and the sum of the moments over the term $I \cdot (-\alpha)$. In these expressions $\mathbf{a}$ and α designate the linear and angular acceleration; m designates the mass and I the moment of inertia of the body with respect to a given axis passing through the center of gravity.

If in static equilibrium the vector sums of all forces and all moments are equal to zero, the sums of the components of these vectors with respect to an xyz-coordinate system must be zero as well. For the x-, y- and z-components of the forces it holds in static equilibrium that

$$\Sigma \mathbf{F_{ix}} = \mathbf{0}$$
$$\Sigma \mathbf{F_{iy}} = \mathbf{0}$$
$$\Sigma \mathbf{F_{iz}} = \mathbf{0}$$

The sums are to be extended over all components of the forces acting on the body. In the two-dimensional case (i.e. in the majority of problems discussed in this book) all z-components of the forces equal zero.

Similar equations hold for the components of the moments

$$\Sigma \mathbf{M_{ix}} = \mathbf{0}$$
$$\Sigma \mathbf{M_{iy}} = \mathbf{0}$$
$$\Sigma \mathbf{M_{iz}} = \mathbf{0}$$

If the discussion is limited to the two-dimensional case, where the vectors of the forces and the distances lie in the xy-plane, the x- and y-components of the moments are always equal to zero. The z-components are not equal to zero because moments are defined as vector products of forces and distances.

If in the two-dimensional case a moment is defined as 'product of the magnitude of the force times the magnitude of the distance from the center of rotation,' the equilibrium condition for the moments reads

$$\Sigma \, M_i = \pm \, L_1 \cdot F_1 \pm L_2 \cdot F_2 \pm L_3 \cdot F_3 \ldots = 0$$

In this equation, F_i designates the magnitudes of the forces, and L_i the magnitudes of the perpendicular distances of the points of force application from the center of rotation. The ± signs remind the reader that, in this formulation, the moments are numbers and not vectors; according to the sign convention for moments, these numbers may be positive or negative.

In order to check whether or not the equilibrium condition for moments is fulfilled in a given loading situation, it is not compulsory for the distances L_i in the above equation to be the distances from the points of force application from a specified center of rotation. The point to which the distances L_i are related can rather be chosen arbitrarily. The following theorem is valid (the proof is not presented here): 'If the sum of the moments related to a reference point equals zero, the sum also equals zero if the moments are related to another, arbitrarily chosen point'. Relating the moment arms to a specific point, e.g. to the center of rotation, serves only to simplify the calculation. In the latter case, the moment of the force transmitted via the center of rotation (i. e., the joint force) can be omitted from the sum. The moment of this force equals zero because the distance to the reference point equals zero; hence this moment does not contribute to the sum of the moments.

Synonymous with this equation is the equation

$$|L_1| \cdot |F_1| - |L_2| \cdot |F_2| = 0$$

For the purpose of illustration, the magnitudes of all vectors are explicitly written in this equation. It follows that

$$L_2 \cdot F_2 = L_1 \cdot F_1$$

Thus, the unknown moment $L_2 \cdot F_2$ is obtained. If the distances L_1 and L_2 are known, the magnitude of the force F_2 can be obtained as well

$$F_2 = \frac{L_1 \cdot F_1}{L_2}$$

Example: calculation of an unknown force in the state of static equilibrium

Fig. 5.**2** illustrates the calculation of an unknown force employing the equilibrium condition of forces. Forces exerted by three persons act on a body; these forces are represented by vectors $\mathbf{F}_1$, $\mathbf{F}_2$ and $\mathbf{F}_3$. Initially $\mathbf{F}_1$ and $\mathbf{F}_2$ are known, $\mathbf{F}_3$ is unknown. In

Example: calculation of an unknown moment in the state of static equilibrium

Fig. 5.**1** illustrates the determination of an unknown moment employing the equilibrium condition of moments. The beam may rotate about a center of rotation. Vectors $\mathbf{F}_1$ and $\mathbf{F}_2$ represent the forces applied by the two subjects; F_1 and F_2 are their magnitudes. The xy-coordinate system is oriented so that both forces point in y-direction. L_1 and L_2 are the perpendicular distances of the points of force application from the center of rotation (the moment arms). Initially F_1 is known; F_2 and thus the moment $L_2 \cdot F_2$ are unknown.

In static equilibrium, i.e., if no accelerated rotation is observed, the sum of all moments must be equal to zero. If we describe moments by numbers (i. e., by simple products of distance and force and not by vectors) and keep the sign convention for moments in mind (a negative sign for the moment of $\mathbf{F}_2$ because this moment effects a counterclockwise rotation), we obtain

$$L_1 \cdot F_1 - L_2 \cdot F_2 = 0$$

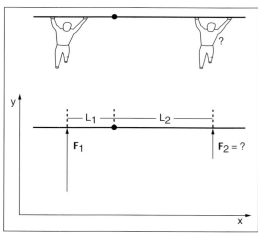

Fig. 5.**1** Example of the determination of an unknown moment in the state of static equilibrium. The beam may rotate about a center of rotation. Vectors $\mathbf{F}_1$ and $\mathbf{F}_2$ represent the forces applied by the two subjects; F_1 and F_2 are their magnitudes. L_1 and L_2 are the perpendicular distances of the points of force application from the center of rotation (the moment arms). In equilibrium it holds that $L_1 \cdot F_1 - L_2 \cdot F_2 = 0$. The signs of the moments are chosen according to the sign convention for moments. From this equation the unknown moment $L_2 \cdot F_2$ can be obtained.

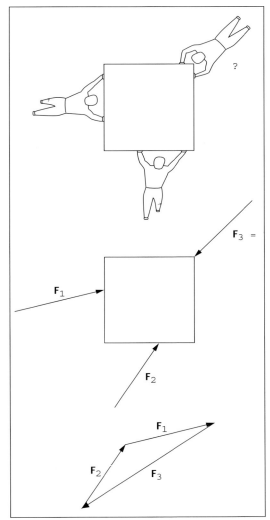

sentation vectors $\mathbf{F}_1$ and $\mathbf{F}_2$ have been added. The magnitude and direction of $\mathbf{F}_3$ is equal to the that of the sum of $\mathbf{F}_1$ and $\mathbf{F}_2$, but its sense of direction is opposed to the sense of direction of that sum. Vectors $\mathbf{F}_1$, $\mathbf{F}_2$, and $\mathbf{F}_3$ form a closed triangle. This is equivalent to the result that the vector sum of the forces equals zero. Note: the equilibrium condition of forces allows an unknown force to be determined but not the point of application of that force.

Alternatively, the problem can be solved numerically. For this purpose, the x- and y-components of vector $\mathbf{F}_3$ are calculated from the respective components of vectors $\mathbf{F}_1$ and $\mathbf{F}_2$. In static equilibrium

$$F_{1x} + F_{2x} + F_{3x} = 0$$
$$F_{1y} + F_{2y} + F_{3y} = 0$$

The resolution for the required components (coordinates) F_{3x} and F_{3y} is then

$$F_{3x} = -F_{1x} - F_{2x}$$
$$F_{3y} = -F_{1y} - F_{2y}$$

Example: calculation of the joint force of a beam balance in static equilibrium

To illustrate the principle of calculating joint forces in the human body by means of the equilibrium conditions, the joint force of a simple mechanical instrument, a beam balance, can be calculated (Fig. 5.**3a**). For reasons of clarity, the pointer of the beam balance (though essential to the mechanical functioning of the balance) is not shown in the illustration. In the state of static equilibrium the unknown force $\mathbf{F}$, which equilibrates an external gravitational force of 10 N, and the joint force $\mathbf{O}$, which supports the beam at the center of rotation, are to be calculated. The xy-coordinate system is oriented so that the forces to both sides of the axis of rotation of the beam point into the negative y-direction; the x-components of these forces equal zero. Related to applications in the human body treated in later chapters, force $\mathbf{F}$ represents the muscle force which equilibrates an external moment, and force $\mathbf{O}$ the joint force, i.e. the force transmitted from bone to bone in a joint.

In a first step (Fig. 5.**3b**) the magnitude of force $\mathbf{F}$ is calculated using the condition of the equilibrium of moments (the moment 1·F bears a negative sign according to the sign convention for moments: this moment effects a counterclockwise rotation)

$$2 \cdot 10 - 1 \cdot F = 0 \text{ Ncm}$$
$$1 \cdot F = 20 \text{ Ncm}$$
$$F = 20 \text{ N}$$

Fig. 5.2 Example of the determination of an unknown force in mechanical equilibrium. The unknown force $\mathbf{F}_3$ must be opposingly equal to the sum of the forces $\mathbf{F}_1$ and $\mathbf{F}_2$ in order that the sum of all forces be equal to zero. In the graphical representation this means that vectors $\mathbf{F}_1$, $\mathbf{F}_2$ and $\mathbf{F}_3$ form a closed triangle.

static equilibrium the sum of all forces must be equal to zero

$$\mathbf{F}_1 + \mathbf{F}_2 + \mathbf{F}_3 = \mathbf{0}$$

For the sum of all forces to equal zero, the unknown force $\mathbf{F}_3$ must be equal and opposite to the sum of $\mathbf{F}_1$ and $\mathbf{F}_2$. Thus magnitude and direction of $\mathbf{F}_3$ are unequivocally determined. In the graphic repre-

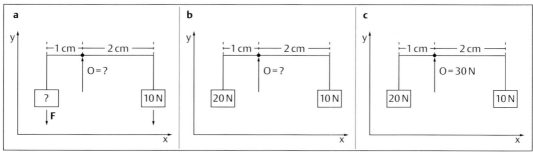

Fig. 5.3a Determination of the joint force **O** of a beam balance loaded on one side by a known weight and on the other side by an initially unknown weight **F**.

Fig 5.3b Step 1: determination of the moment of the force **F** employing the condition of the equilibrium of moments. If the moment arms are known, the compo-

nents of **F** can be determined. This results in $F_x = 0$ N, $F_y = -20$ N.

Fig. 5.3c Step 2: determination of the joint force **O** from the equilibrium condition of forces. This results in $O_y = +30$ N; the x-component of **O** equals zero.

Since force **F** points into the negative y-direction, the result can also be expressed by the components (coordinates) of this force

$$F_x = 0 \text{ N}$$
$$F_y = -20 \text{ N}$$

In the second step (Fig. 5.**3c**) the y-component of the joint force **O** is calculated from the equilibrium of forces

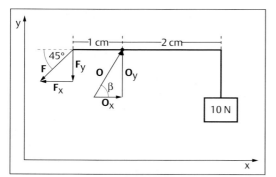

Fig. 5.4 Determination of the joint force **O** of a beam balance loaded on one side by a known weight and on the other by an initially unknown force **F**, directed at 45° with respect to the horizontal. One way to solve the problem is to calculate the x- and y-components of **F** and **O** separately. With moment arms equal to those in Fig. 5.3 we obtain (as we have done already there) $F_y = -20$ N and $O_y = +30$ N. Given the angle of 45° it follows that $F_x = -20$ N. In equilibrium O_x must be op-posingly equal to F_x: $O_x = +20$ N. From O_x and O_y the magnitude and direction of **O** can be obtained.

$$O_y + F_y - 10 = 0 \text{ N}$$
$$O_y - 20 - 10 = 0 \text{ N}$$
$$O_y = 10 + 20 \text{ N}$$
$$O_y = 30 \text{ N}$$

The y-component of force **O** equals +30 N. The pos-itive sign indicates that the vector of joint force **O** points into the positive y-direction. In this exam-ple, the x-component of force **O** equals zero.

If force **F**, which equilibrates the moment exert-ed by the gravitational force, is not directed in y-direction (Fig. 5.**4**) the easiest way to solve the problem is to first calculate the x- and y-compo-nents of forces **F** and **O**; from the components O_x and O_y, the magnitude and direction of vector **O** can then be obtained. With respect to applications in the human body discussed in later chapters, this example represents the case where the muscle force required for the equilibrium of moments is not directed parallel to the external force. In the set-up shown in Fig. 5.**4** the force **F** is assumed to act at an angle of 45° with respect to the long axis of the beam. With moment arms equal to those in Fig. 5.**3** the equilibrium of moments is (as was the case there)

$$F_y = -20 \text{ N}$$
$$O_y = +30 \text{ N}$$

Note: One might wonder why force F_x does not contribute to the sum of moments. The moment of the x-component of force **F** equals zero because this force component points along the direction of the beam and thus though the center of rotation.

Given the angle of force **F** to the x-axis and with knowledge of vector $F_y \cdot \mathbf{e}_y$, vector $F_x \cdot \mathbf{e}_x$ is specified as well. Solving for F_x means constructing the missing side of the triangle formed by $\mathbf{F}$, $F_x \cdot \mathbf{e}_x$ and $F_y \cdot \mathbf{e}_y$ while the direction of $\mathbf{F}$ and the magnitude of $F_y \cdot \mathbf{e}_y$ are known. If, as assumed here, the angle equals 45°, both sides of the triangle are of equal length.

$$F_x = F_y/\tan 45°$$
$$F_x = -20 \text{ N}$$

The magnitude of the force $\mathbf{F}$ is calculated from

$$|\mathbf{F}| = \sqrt{F_x^2 + F_y^2} = \sqrt{20^2 + 20^2} = 28.3 \text{ N}$$

In the state of static equilibrium the sum of the x-components of all forces must be equal to zero. The gravitational force on the right-hand side of the beam does not contribute to this sum because this force points into y-direction. With $F_x = -20$ N it follows that

$$F_x + O_x = 0 \text{ N}$$
$$O_x = 20 \text{ N}$$

The magnitude O of the joint force $\mathbf{O}$ is calculated from its components

$$|\mathbf{O}| = \sqrt{30^2 + 20^2} = 36.1 \text{ N}$$

The angle β between the joint force and the x-axis is calculated from

$$\beta = \text{atan} (O_y/O_x)$$

In the case discussed here, the angle amounts to β = 56.3°

We should add that the same problem could have been solved in another way. As a first step the moment arm of $\mathbf{F}$, i.e. the perpendicular distance of the line of action of $\mathbf{F}$ from the center of rotation, could have been calculated. From the equilibrium condition of moments the magnitude F of this force is then obtained. In the second step, the joint force $\mathbf{O}$ is determined graphically or numerically applying the condition of equilibrium of forces.

When attempting to determine joint forces in the human body, the situation occasionally arises that the direction of a muscle force equilibrating an external force is almost (but not exactly) equal to the direction of the external force. To illustrate such a case, it is assumed in Fig. 5.**5** that the force $\mathbf{F}$ deviates by 10° from the direction of the y-axis. With distances equal to those in Fig. 5.**4** and a gravitational force (pointing in y-direction) of 10 N on the right-hand side of the beam, the identical formulae as for the case shown in Fig. 5.**4** yield $F_y = -20$ N and $O_y = +30$ N. F_x, O_x and $|\mathbf{O}|$ are calculated from

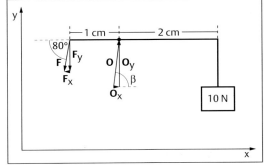

Fig. 5.**5** Determination of the joint force $\mathbf{O}$ of a beam balance loaded on one side by a known weight and on the other by an initially unknown force $\mathbf{F}$, directed at 80° with respect to the horizontal. The method used to obtain $\mathbf{F}$ and $\mathbf{O}$ is identical to that followed in the example given in Fig. 5.**4**. There prove to be only minor differences between $|F_y|$ and $|\mathbf{F}|$ as well as between $|O_y|$ and $|\mathbf{O}|$. In other words, in a set-up as shown here the essential information can be derived from the y-components of the forces; inclusion of the x-components induces only a minor alteration.

$$F_x = F_y/\tan 80° = -3.5 \text{ N}$$

$$O_x = +3.5 \text{ N}$$

$$|\mathbf{O}| = \sqrt{30^2 + 3.5^2} = 30.2 \text{ N}$$

The angle β of $\mathbf{O}$ with the x-axis amounts to

$$\beta = \text{atan} (O_y/O_x)$$
$$\beta = \text{atan} (30.0/3.5) = 83.3°$$

It is obvious that, in this set-up, the difference between the magnitude of the joint force (i. e. 30.2 N) and the magnitude of its y-component (i. e. 30 N) is very small. In other words: the essential information about the magnitude of the joint force can be derived from considering the magnitude of its y-component. Consideration of the x-component results in only a minor, additional change. The direction of O deviates by a small angle (i. e. 6.7°) from the y-direction. It follows that, in cases where the direction of the external force and the equilibrating muscle force almost coincide, the discussion of joint forces may for reasons of simplicity and brevity be limited to the discussion of the large components (in the example discussed here, the y-component) while neglecting the small components.

6   Material Properties of Solid Materials

The mechanical, electrical, magnetic, optical, or chemical properties of materials are determined in standardized experiments. The protocols for such experiments and the description of the material properties are always designed so that the dimensions of the samples under investigation do not influence the result. In other words, the experimentally determined parameters describe the materials as such, for example the properties of the material 'steel' or the properties of the material 'bone'. The properties of structures fabricated from a material, for example the mechanical properties of a frame consisting of steel beams or of a femoral bone consisting of cortical and trabecular bone, must be determined in separate experiments.

A material is designated as homogeneous if its matter is continuously distributed over its whole volume. Any small volume element of a homogeneous material possesses identical physical properties. By contrast, a sample of a material with irregular holes or inclusion of other materials, or impurities, is described as inhomogeneous. A material is designated as isotropic if its internal structure or its elastic properties show no preferred directions. Examples of isotropic materials are rubber or cast iron. In contrast, wood and bone are designated as anisotropic due to the internal alignment of fibers in preferred directions. The material properties of an inhomogeneous material depend on the location from which the sample was cut from a larger block of the material. The material properties of an anisotropic material depend on the orientation in which the sample was cut. Due to the voids between the beams and plates, trabecular bone is inhomogeneous and, due to the alignment of the trabeculae in preferred directions, it is (usually) anisotropic as well. The material properties of a sample of cortical bone will, for example, depend on the site of the bone from where the sample has been cut. In addition, samples cut in a longitudinal or transverse direction from a long bone will also exhibit different properties.

Materials are characterized not by one single but rather by a set of parameters that describe their behavior in different applications and environments. In the context of orthopedic biomechanics, the parameters describing deformation and fracture of a material are of prime importance. For implant materials, the friction and abrasion properties are of importance as well.

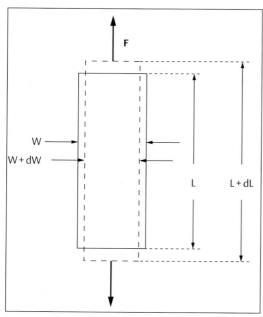

Fig. 6.1   Deformation of a sample of a solid material under the influence of a force **F**. L and W designate the initial length and width of the sample; dL and dW designate the change of length and width. In a tensile test dL is positive and dW negative; in a compression test dL is negative and dW positive.

Elongation and compression

In a tensile test, a beam-shaped sample of a material is subjected to a tensile force **F** (Fig. 6.**1**). In this test, the change dL in the length of the sample is measured in relation to the tensile force. To ensure that the material property to be determined does not depend on the dimensions (cross-sectional area A, length L) of the sample tested, it is not the length change dL in relation to the force F that is reported but rather the strain in relation to the (mechanical) stress (Fig. 6.**2**). The stress σ is defined as the force F divided by the cross-sectional area A of the sample

$$\sigma = F/A$$

Mechanical stress (or simply, stress) is measured in 'newtons per square meter' $[N/m^2]$ or pascals $[Pa]$. The strain ε is defined as the length change dL divided by the initial length L

$$\varepsilon = dL/L$$

As the quotient of two lengths, strain is a dimensionless quantity. For reasons of clarity, however, the dimension of strain is sometimes quoted as $[mm/mm]$ or $[\mu m/\mu m]$.

In qualitative terms, many materials exhibit a similar behavior in a tensile test. Under low values of stress, the strain increases in proportion to the stress. In the region of low stress the dependence of the strain on the stress can be described by a straight line (Fig. 6.2). Above a certain stress value characteristic for the material, the stress-strain graph deviates from a straight line. The quotient of stress and strain in the linear portion of the graph, i.e. the slope of the graph in this region, is termed the 'modulus of elasticity'. The modulus of elasticity is measured in $[N/mm^2]$ or $[Pa]$.

In the linear part of the stress-strain graph Hooke's law is valid

$$\sigma = E \cdot \varepsilon$$

Hooke's law states that the stress is proportional to the strain. A steep slope of the stress-strain graph indicates that a high stress is necessary to effect a specified strain. The modulus of elasticity of such a material has a high numerical value. A shallow slope of the stress-strain graph indicates that a low stress is sufficient to effect a specified strain. The modulus of elasticity of such a material is low. In everyday language, materials with a high modulus of elasticity are termed 'hard' and those with a small one, 'soft'.

Table 6.1 quotes moduli of elasticity of technical materials that are frequently used for construction of implants and, for comparison, the moduli of cortical and trabecular bone. In order to avoid quoting large numbers, the moduli are usually quoted in units of N/mm^2, not in units of N/m^2. The numbers in Table 6.1 illustrate that, compared with metals, cortical bone and polyethylene are soft and trabecular bone is very soft. The numerical values in Table 6.1 are only approximate, because the precise value of the modulus of elasticity depends for metals on the details of the production process, for polyethylene on the degree of polymerization, and for

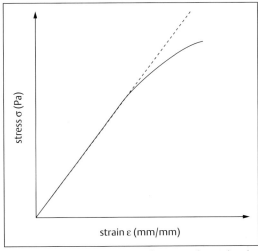

Fig. 6.2 Typical stress-strain diagram of metals. The slope of the graph in its linear part is called the 'modulus of elasticity'. In the region of higher stress the graph deviates from a straight line.

cortical and trabecular bone on the location, the orientation, and the bone density of the sample tested.

In a tensile test it is not only a change in the length of a sample that is observed but also a decrease in the diameter, of the magnitude $|dW|$ (Fig. 6.1). The quotient of the strains in longitudinal and transverse directions

$$\mu = -(dW/W)/(dL/L)$$

is a parameter characteristic for every material and is termed 'Poisson's ratio'. μ usually has values between 0.2 and 0.5.

Instead of being subjected to a tensile force, a material sample may be subjected to a compressive force and the compressive strain dL/L can be plot-

Table 6.1 Moduli of elasticity of materials employed in the construction of implants in relation to the moduli of cortical and trabecular bone

material	modulus of elasticity E [N/mm²]	source
stainless steel	$2 \cdot 10^5$	
titanium alloy	$1 \cdot 10^5$	
polyethylene	$1 \cdot 10^3$	
cortical bone	$18 \cdot 10^3$	Yamada
trabecular bone	90	Yamada

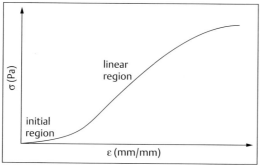

Fig. **6.3** Typical stress-strain diagram of soft tissues. An initial region with large increase in strain under low stress is followed by a region with an (approximately) linear increase of the strain with the stress. In the region of higher stress, the graph deviates again from a straight line.

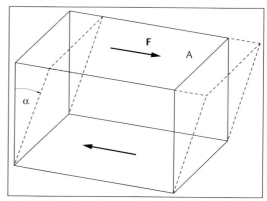

Fig. **6.4** Loading of a sample by a shear force **F** effects no changes in width or length but an angular deformation.

ted in relation to the compressive stress. In such a test, however, it must be ensured that the sample will not bend under the influence of the compressive force. A change in length caused by bending and not by pure compression would not allow direct comparison with the results of a tensile test. Experiments show that for many materials in the region of low stress (i.e. stress much lower than that which would effect destruction of the sample) the dependence of strain and stress in the linear region is virtually identical in tensile and compressive tests. In this region, then, the modulus of elasticity characterizes the deformation of a material under tensile as well as under compressive stress.

Some materials, for example soft tissues, exhibit, in a tensile test a comparatively large increase in their length under low values of stress before a point is reached where the stress increases (approximately) in proportion to the strain. Under further increase of the stress, a disproportionate increase in strain may again be observed (Fig. 6.**3**). In such cases the slope of the stress-strain curve, and thus the modulus of elasticity, depends on the strain. If a modulus of elasticity is quoted, it must be specified at which strain value it has been measured. As guide value, the modulus of elasticity derived from the (approximately) linear portion of the stress-strain curve may be quoted.

Shear

If two parallel and opposite forces of magnitude F act on two sides of a cuboid (Fig. 6.**4**) a shear stress τ is generated

$$\tau = F/A$$

A shear stress does not effect a change in length but rather a change in the shape of the sample. The initially vertical faces of the cuboid are now seen to be tilted. For small angles of tilt it holds that

$$\tau = G \cdot \alpha$$

G is a material constant and is termed the 'shear modulus'. The angle α is measured in radians. It can be shown (the proof is not given here) that the modulus of elasticity E, Poisson's ratio μ and the shear modulus G are related

$$E = 2 \cdot G \cdot (1 + \mu)$$

Thus the deformation of a homogeneous, isotropic material is fully characterized by two of these three material constants.

Elastic, viscoelastic, and plastic deformation

For some materials in a tensile test, if the stress is first increased and subsequently reduced to zero, the stress-strain curves for increasing and for decreasing stress are observed to be superimposed. After completion of the load cycle a sample of such a material is restored to its initial length. This type of deformation (or this material) is termed 'elastic'. If the stress is increased above a certain peak value, characteristic for each material, the stress-strain curves for increasing and decreasing stress are ob-

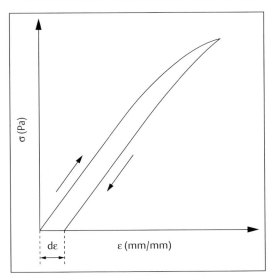

Fig. 6.**5** For some materials the strain under increasing stress is observed to be different to that under decreasing stress. The stress-strain diagram forms a 'hysteresis loop'. If a deformation remains after the end of a load cycle under zero stress, the material (or the deformation) is designated as 'viscoelastic' or 'plastic'.

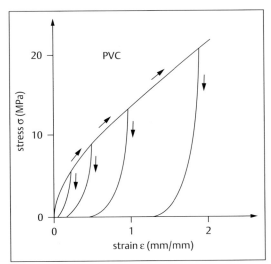

Fig. 6.**6** Viscoelastic or plastic deformation depends on the magnitude of the stress previously exerted upon it. This example shows the plastic deformation of PVC in relation to the maximal value of the stress. (Adapted from: Andrews EH. In: 'The mechanical properties of biological materials'. *Soc Exp Biol Symp No 34*. Cambridge: Cambridge University Press, 1980)

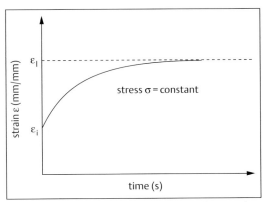

Fig. 6.**7** Under constant stress the strain of a viscoelastic material increases with time. This effect is termed 'creep'.

served to be no longer superimposed; deviations from elastic behavior will then be observed. The description of a deformation or a material as 'elastic' must therefore be supplemented by information on the maximal stress level involved. Most metals, for example, show elastic deformation, provided the maximum stress is not too close to that leading to destruction of the sample.

If tissues of the human body or plastics are subjected to a tensile test, striking deviations from elastic behavior are observed. The stress-strain curve for increasing stress deviates from the curve for decreasing stress; the two curves form a hysteresis loop (Fig. 6.**5**). At the end of the load cycle, i.e. when the load and thus the stress have returned to zero, the sample is not restored to its original

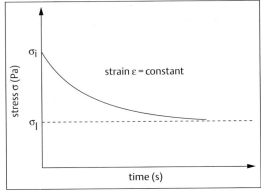

Fig. 6.**8** Under constant strain the stress of a viscoelastic material decreases with time. This effect is termed 'stress relaxation'.

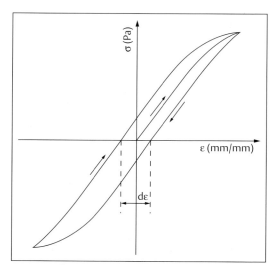

Fig. 6.**9** If a viscoelastic or plastic material is cyclically loaded in tension and compression, the stress-strain graph follows a complete hysteresis loop. The magnitude of the region of deformation dε, observed at zero stress, depends on the mechanical history (maximum values of the tensile and compressive stresses previously exerted).

length but a strain dε remains. If, over time and without any exposure to an external force, this strain dε recedes to zero, the deformation is termed 'viscoelastic'. If, by contrast, the strain dε remains constant, the deformation is termed 'plastic'. As an example of a plastic deformation Fig. 6.6 shows the measured stress-strain curves of the material PVC. In this material, the plastic deformation increases with increasing peak stress.

If a sample of a viscoelastic material is held under constant stress, the initial strain ε_i is observed to increase with time until it reaches a limiting value ε_l (Fig. 6.7). The increase in strain under constant stress is termed 'creep'. The decrease in strain under zero stress after completion of a load cycle, mentioned above, is the reverse event.

If a sample of a viscoelastic material is loaded to a certain strain level and the strain is subsequently kept constant, it is observed that the stress within the material decreases with time from its initial value σ_i to a limiting value σ_l (Fig. 6.**8**). This effect is termed 'stress relaxation'.

If a sample of a viscoelastic or plastic material is cyclically elongated and compressed, the stress-strain curve forms a complete hysteresis loop (Fig. 6.**9**). In addition to the hysteresis loop, Fig. 6.**9** shows the stress-strain curve of the first half of the first loading cycle, which starts at the origin of the

graph. It should be noted that, due to the viscoelastic or plastic properties of the material, the strain at zero stress is indeterminate; it may vary within a certain region dε. The size of this region dε depends on the peak values of the tensile and compressive stresses. If the peak values are increased, the viscoelastic or plastic deformation of the material increases as well. In other words, the deformation seen at zero stress in cyclic loading tests depends on the mechanical history, i.e. the type and magnitude of past loading. Thus, the deformation range dε is not a material property but is dependent on the test conditions.

▨ Hardness

In engineering, three procedures to define the hardness of a material are in use. The Mohs qualitative hardness scale groups mineral materials on a scale from 1 to 10, so that a material of greater hardness will scratch those lower on the scale. The Mohs scale begins with talc (1) and ends with diamond (10). Brinell hardness is defined by measuring the area of the impression of a very hard (virtually non-deformable) sphere pressed against a planar surface of the material under investigation. Thus, Brinell hardness characterizes the plastic deformation of a material. Shore hardness is defined by the depth of impression of a standardized test body (for example pyramid-shaped) under specified loads. Shore hardness thus characterizes the elastic or plastic deformation of a material. The deformation properties of rubber and rubber-like plastics are usually described by their Shore hardness. The hardness of a material according to these tests and the modulus of elasticity of a material are only qualitatively related: the hardness of a material is not equal to the 'hardness' measured in a tensile test (see **Elongation and compression**, above).

In the context of orthopedic biomechanics, Mohs or Brinell hardness is of interest when selecting materials for the construction of artificial joints because hardness influences deformation and wear. Examples are the deformation of a plastic socket loaded by a spherical metal head or the abrasion and wear of small particles of bone cement between the metal head and polyethylene socket of an artificial hip joint. Shore hardness is frequently used to describe the properties of rubber or plastic foams used in the construction of artificial limbs, orthoses, or insoles. The depth of indentation into tissue surfaces by a probe of known shape is employed to characterize the mechanical properties of the tissues. Depth of indentation into the surface of articular cartilage or into the plantar soft tissue provides knowledge on the stiffness of these tissues.

Testing the 'hardness' of a muscle or another organ by palpation for diagnostic purposes is not identical with any of the engineering hardness tests mentioned above, despite a certain similarity to the Shore test. In the clinical context, hardness does not characterize a material but an organ, which may be constructed from a number of different materials. Furthermore, the hardness determined by palpation usually indicates the stress in the organ, for example the state of stress of a muscle. Stress varies according to the level of activation, especially in muscle. Such effects are not encountered in technical materials.

Friction

External friction occurs between solid bodies; this in contrast to internal friction in streaming fluids or gases. We believe external friction to be caused by the interlocking of small irregularities of the contact surfaces, abrasion of small particles from the bodies, and elastic or plastic deformation of impurities (for example, dust) on the surfaces. It is therefore obvious that friction depends critically on the material properties of the bodies, the microscopic geometry of the surfaces, and the presence of impurities or lubricating substances.

The friction force is directed parallel to the contact surface and opposite to the direction of motion or impending motion. Experience shows that, for a given material and surface condition, the friction force depends on the force between the bodies in contact and their relative velocity. We thus discriminate between static and gliding friction. The coefficient of static friction μ_s describes the empirical relationship between the friction force F_f and the component F_n of the force between the contacting bodies, perpendicular ('normal') to the surface

$$F_f = \mu_s \cdot F_n$$

for the case where the bodies are just on the verge of slipping but nonetheless at rest. The coefficient of kinetic friction μ_k describes the empirical relationship between the friction force F_f and the component F_n of the force between the contacting bodies directed perpendicularly to the surface

$$F_f = \mu_k \cdot F_n$$

for the case where the bodies slide at constant speed with respect to each other. The coefficient of

kinetic friction is generally smaller than the coefficient of static friction.

Energy (force times distance) is spent to overcome friction. This energy is to a large extent dissipated as heat. In the biomechanical context, low coefficients of static and kinetic friction between joint surfaces are of extreme importance as large frictional forces would impede movement of highly loaded joints. Wear of contacting surfaces due to friction and, potentially, even heat generation (Bergmann *et al.*, 2001) needs to be considered in the construction of artificial joint replacements.

Fracture

If, in a tensile test, the tensile stress of the sample exceeds a certain limit (characteristic of the material), the sample breaks (Fig. 6.**10**). Materials exhibiting only a small amount of strain before fracture occurs are termed 'brittle'. Examples of brittle materials are glass and bone. Materials that tolerate a larger amount of strain before fracture occurs are termed 'tough'. Examples of tough materials are stainless steel and polyethylene. Materials exhibit-

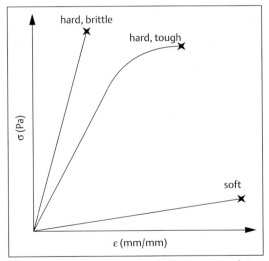

Fig. 6.**10** Stress-strain graph of different materials in a tensile test. The endpoints of the curves represent the points at which rupture of the samples occurred. A steep slope of the initial part of the graph characterizes a hard material; a shallow initial slope characterizes a soft material. Materials tolerating a large strain before fracture occurs are termed 'tough'; materials tolerating only a small amount of strain before fracture occurs are termed 'brittle';

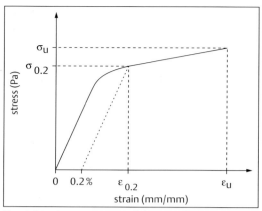

Fig. 6.**11** Determination of the so-called 0.2 % stress and 0.2 % strain from the stress-strain graph. A line, at a distance $\varepsilon = 0.2$ %, is drawn parallel to the initial, linear part of the stress-strain curve. The intersection of this line with the actual stress-strain curve defines stress and strain at the 0.2 % limit.

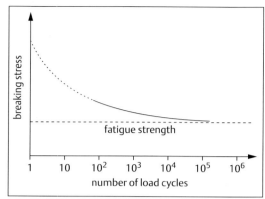

Fig. 6.**12** Under cyclic loading, a decrease in breaking stress (stress where fracture occurs) is observed. This effect is termed 'material fatigue'. The breaking stress at high load cycle numbers approaches a lower limit termed 'fatigue strength'. If the stress level stays below this value, an arbitrary number of load cycles may be endured without fracture occurring.

ing a large amount of deformation at low stress values are designated as 'soft'.

Quantitatively, the fracture properties of a material are characterized by specifying the ultimate stress σ_u and the ultimate strain ε_u at the point of fracture (Fig. 6.**11**). The region of stress and strain where the stress-strain curve deviates notably from a straight line is characterized by 'stress and strain at the 0.2 % limit'. To locate this limit, a straight line is drawn parallel to the linear part of the stress-strain curve, at a distance of $\varepsilon = 0.2$ %. The intersection of this line with the stress-strain curve defines stress and strain at the 0.2 % limit.

The value of the ultimate compressive stress, where compression fracture occurs, can be determined in a compression test. To permit comparison with the ultimate tensile stress established in a tensile test, the material sample must be guaranteed not to bend under load before destruction of the sample is observed. Whether a sample under compressive load exhibits pure compression, or bending in addition to compression, depends on the shape of the sample. A long beam will tend to bend under load, a short, squat column will not. If bending occurs, the distribution of stress within the material differs from a uniform compressive stress, and direct comparison with the ultimate tensile stress will not be appropriate. The ultimate compressive stress determined in a compression test is usually not equal to the ultimate tensile stress determined in a tensile test. In viscoelastic materials, the ultimate stress also depends on the loading rate (i.e. on the load change per unit time) and the duration of loading. Thus, the ultimate

Table 6.2 Ultimate tensile stress and ultimate tensile strain (approximate values) of materials employed in the construction of implants, in relation to ultimate stress and ultimate strain of cortical and trabecular bone

material	ultimate stress [N/mm²]	ultimate strain [%]	source
stainless steel	700	15	
titanium alloy	1200	6	
polyethylene	20	400–800	
cortical bone	150	1.5	Yamada
trabecular bone	2	2.5	Yamada

stresses quoted in Table 6.**2** must be regarded as an approximate guide only.

If a material sample is loaded several times in succession, it is observed that the sample fractures at a stress appreciably lower than the ultimate stress observed in a single loading cycle. The decrease in breaking stress with increasing number of loading cycles is termed 'material fatigue'. Fig. 6.**12** illustrates qualitatively the relationship between breaking stress and the number of load cycles. In virtually all materials the breaking stress decreases as the number of load cycles increases. In many (but not all) materials the breaking stress at high load cycle numbers approaches a lower limit termed 'fatigue strength'. If the stress in a sample stays below this value, an arbitrary number of load cycles may be endured without fracture occurring.

Material fatigue occurs because there is no material without internal faults. During production of a material, it is impossible to rule out irregularities in its crystal lattice, inclusions of other materials, or voids, even of small dimensions. Under load, small fissures tend to originate primarily from such inhomogeneities. Surface irregularities like small scratches or indentations have a similar effect. Under repeated loading the fissures grow in length or several small fissures unite. The microdamage increases until macroscopic failure occurs. In some cases the progressive damage to the sample can be seen when inspecting the fracture surfaces.

When investigated in detail, the fatigue process at high stresses and low load cycles is seen to differ from the fatigue process at low stresses and high cycle numbers. These processes are termed 'high cycle' and 'low cycle' fatigue. It follows that material fatigue, i.e. the relationship between breaking stress and load cycle numbers, cannot be described by one single function. In Fig. 6.**12** this is indicated by dividing the curve into a dashed and a solid portion. In other words, no conclusions on the fatigue behavior between, say, 10^2 and 10^6 cycles can be drawn from the fatigue behavior observed between 1 and 100 cycles (and *vice versa*). Fatigue properties at low and high cycle numbers must be documented separately.

Bone fractures interpreted as fatigue fractures are observed *in vivo* in subjects exposed to an activity with many high load cycles without preparatory training. For example, it is hypothesized that fractures of the tibia or the calcaneus seen in young soldiers after marching over long distances are fatigue fractures of the bone material. Fatigue fractures of lumbar vertebrae also seem possible if the spine undergoes a large number of load cycles within a relatively short time interval at the workplace or in athletic training. In an individual case, however, it is difficult to prove conclusively that a fatigue fracture has occurred, because an inspection of the fractured surfaces is not feasible. In addition, it must be kept in mind that repair processes in living tissues may prevent the accumulation of microdamage. Whether fatigue fractures occur in a living tissue depends on the rate of healing in relation to the time interval over which cyclic loading occurs. Fatigue will be evident only if cyclic loading occurs over a time interval that is too short for any significant repair of microdamage.

Further reading

Textbooks and reference books

Abé H, Hayashi K, Sato M. (eds). *Data book on mechanical properties of living cells, tissues, and organs.* Tokyo: Springer; 1996

Alonso M, Finn E. *Physics.* Addison Wesley, Harlow 1996

Fung YC. *Biomechanics. Mechanical properties of living tissues.* 2nd edition. New York: Springer; 1993

Vincent JFV. *Structural biomaterials.* London: Macmillan Press; 1982

Yamada H. *Strength of Biological Materials.* Baltimore: Williams & Wilkins; 1970

Scientific papers cited in the text or the figures

Andrews EH. 'Fracture'. In: The mechanical properties of biological materials'. *Soc Exp Biology Symposia No 34 p 13–36.* Cambridge: Cambridge Univ Press; 1980

Bergmann G, Graichen F, Rohlmann A, Verdonschot N, van Lenthe GH. 'Frictional heating in total hip implants. Part I. Measurements in patients'. *J Biomechanics* 2001; **34**: 421–428

7 Deformation and Strength of Structures

The term 'structure' designates objects built from one or more materials in a specific architecture. In this context, the term architecture stands for the geometrical shape of the objects and the manner by which the components of the structure are assembled and fixed together. Structures in this sense are a beam made out of wood, a vertebral body composed of an outer shell of cortical bone filled with trabecular bone, or a joint of the human body consisting of bone, cartilage, joint capsule, and ligaments. The mechanical properties of a structure depend on its architecture and on the mechanical properties of its building materials.

The deformation of a structure under load depends on a number of variables:
– *The loading mode.* The structure may be loaded by a compressive or tensile force, by a moment, or by a combination of forces and moments. If the structure is loaded by a force, the deformation is measured in meters [m] or relative units [%] in relation to its initial dimensions. When loaded by a moment where a torsion is observed, the deformation is measured in degrees [°]; if bending is observed, the deflection is usually measured in meters [m].
– *The architecture of the structure.* For example, the deformation in bending or torsion of a beam depends on its length and its cross section. The deformation of a joint depends on the deformation of the bone, the cartilage, and the ligaments crossing the joint.
– *The material properties of the building materials.* In the case of a wooden beam, the deformation depends on the type of wood used (for example, oak or pine). In the case of a joint, the mechanical properties of the building materials bone, cartilage, and ligament tissue come into play. The mechanical properties are characterized by the moduli of elasticity and shear and by the elastic, viscoelastic, or plastic properties.

The strength of a structure is defined as that load that effects a destruction of the structure. Destruction occurs if the tensile, compressive, or shear stress in any one component of the structure exceeds its ultimate value, and the structure (or a part of it) is torn, fractured, or irreversibly deformed. Depending on the loading mode, we distinguish between compressive, tensile, or shear strength of a structure. Strength under tensile or compressive load is designated by the force effecting the destruction and quoted in newtons [N]. Torsional or bending strength is designated by the moment effecting the destruction and designated in newton-meters [Nm].

Tensile, compressive, bending, or torsional strengths of a structure are independent of one another and may assume widely different values. A pile of bricks, for example, has high compressive but very low tensile strength. The compressive strength of cortical bone is higher than its tensile strength. A rope, a muscle, or a ligament has high tensile but only low compressive, torsional, or bending strength.

Deformation and strength of structures may be determined experimentally or by calculation. For experimental determination the testing methods are similar to those employed when determining properties of materials. The structures are set up in a testing machine and loaded by a tensile or compressive force, or by a moment in bending or torsion. The resulting change in shape (deformation) is recorded in relation to the load. If the load is further increased, the load effecting destruction will eventually be found. Alternatively, a deformation can be imposed on the structure and the reaction force (i.e. the resistance to the deformation) or the reaction moment can be recorded. It must be pointed out, however, that interpretation of the results of such experiments differs from interpretation of the results of experiments determining material properties. This is due to the fact that, when testing structures, the architecture as well as the properties of the building materials influence the result. It is obvious that a low-strength structure can be built with high-strength materials. On the other hand, a structure made out of relatively low-strength materials may have a high strength.

For structures composed of one single material and having simple geometrical shapes, formulae are available that allow deformation and strength to be calculated in the case of simple loading modes, provided the material properties are known. Simple geometrical shapes are, for example, beams or tubes with rectangular or circular cross sections. Simple loading modes include, for example, tension or compression or torsion about the axis of such beams. The prerequisite for the validity of these formulae is that the resulting deformations under load remain small. If more than one material is used to build a structure, and, in the case of irregular shapes and simultaneous loading by forces and moments, deformation, stress and strength can be determined by the method of finite elements (FEM).

Experimental determination of deformation and strength

The relationship between deformation and load may vary within broad limits. In the following, this is illustrated by examples of different tissues and organs. A tensile test provides data for deformation and strength under a tensile force. Fig. 7.**1** shows the tensile force of a ligament in relation to its increase in length. At each point of the force-deformation curve, the slope is approximated by the quotient dF/dL. In this expression dL designates the length change observed under a small change dF of the tensile force applied. dF/dL is termed the 'stiffness' of the structure. Stiffness is measured in newtons per meter [N/m] or newtons per millimeter [N/mm]. The numerical value of the stiffness indicates how many newtons are necessary to effect a length change of 1 m or 1 mm respectively.

The shape of the curve shown in Fig. 7.**1** is typical of the behavior of soft tissues under tension. In general the force-deformation graph does not follow a straight line; the slope of the curve, and thus the stiffness, assume different values along the curve. In the example shown, the slope of the curve and hence the stiffness have low values under low forces and higher values under higher forces. In ligaments, this property is due to the collagen fibers becoming more and more aligned in the direction of the force as the tensile force increases.

If the tensile force F exceeds the strength of the structure, a partial or total rupture of the ligament is observed. In the example shown in Fig. 7.**1** the first partial rupture occurred at a tensile force of about 200 N. It is a common finding in ligaments that rupture occurs stepwise, because under a given load not all fiber bundles of the ligament undergo the same deformation. In each bundle the ultimate tensile strain is reached at a different elongation of the whole ligament. In the example shown, complete rupture occurred only after an increase in length of about 3 mm. Between the point where the tensile strength of the ligament was reached and the total rupture, the ligament can still transmit a tensile force, though of lesser magnitude.

Fig. 7.**2** shows the force-deformation graph of human skin. In this example the initial region of high elongation under low forces (region of low stiffness) and the adjoining region with a relatively

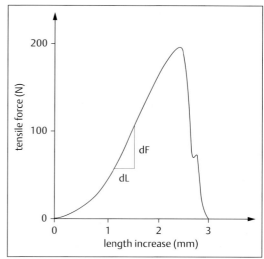

Fig. 7.1 Force-deformation diagram of a ligament under a tensile force. At each point of the curve the stiffness is given by the slope of the curve. The slope is approximated by the quotient dF/dL. The strength is given by the force where rupture occurs. In the example shown, the strength amounts to approximately 200 N. Not all fibers of the ligament rupture at this point. Up to a length increase of 3 mm where complete separation occurs, a decreasing amount of tensile force can still be transmitted. (Adapted from Amiel *et al.*, 1982.)

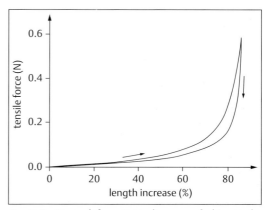

Fig. 7.2 Force-deformation diagram of skin. Under low tensile forces the sample exhibits low stiffness; this region is followed by a region of higher stiffness. The graph forms a hysteresis loop. The deformation is elastic, as the deformation returns to zero as the force returns to zero. (Adapted from Lanir *et al.*, 1974.)

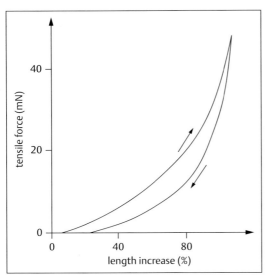

Fig. 7.3 Force-deformation diagram of the passive elongation of a muscle. The graph forms a hysteresis loop. The deformation is viscoelastic or plastic since some deformation remains when the force returns to zero. (Adapted from Sparks and Bohr, 1962.)

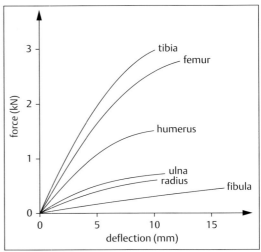

Fig. 7.4 Deflection of human bones under three-point loading. (Adapted from Yamada, 1970.)

low increase of length under higher forces (region of higher stiffness) can be clearly distinguished. The force-deformation graph forms a hysteresis loop. The deformation is elastic because (at the levels of loading shown) no permanent deformation is observed after completion of the load cycle. The force-deformation curve of skin demonstrates that this structure is highly adapted to its physiological function, i.e. enabling large deformations under low forces but only up to a certain limit.

Fig. 7.3 shows the passive force-deformation graph of a muscle *in vitro*. As in the preceding example, the stiffness assumes different values at each point of the graph. The graph forms a hysteresis loop. After completion of the loading cycle, the residual deformation subsequently decreases to zero. This structure is viscoelastic. We expect the force-deformation graph of a muscle measured *in vivo* to assume a different form, because innervation of a muscle will change its stiffness.

Fig. 7.4 illustrates the deflection of bones in a three-point bending experiment. In such an experiment the bone is supported at both ends and loaded in its midsection by a force F. The deflection is measured at the point where force is applied. All curves shown end at the point where fracture occurred. Force-deflection graphs of different bones are given here in one diagram merely to provide an overview. A quantitative comparison of deflection and strength of different bones, for example of fibula and femur, makes little sense, because deflection and bending strength depend on the bone material, the cross-sectional area, and the length of the bones. If, in contrast, effects of implantation-induced temporary immobilization or instrumentation have to be evaluated, conclusions can be drawn by comparing pairs of bones, for example the right and left femur specimen of a subject or of an experimental animal.

Fig. 7.5 shows experimental results for torsional deformation and torsional strength of bones. In this type of experiment, the bone is fixed at one end and a moment about the long axis of the bone is applied at the other. Deformation and torsional strength depend on the bone material, the length, and the cross section of the bone. It is therefore not surprising that large differences with respect to torsional stiffness (slope of the curves), torsional strength and maximal deformation (end point of the curves) of the bones are observed.

Fig. 7.6 depicts the compression of a lumbar vertebral body by a force directed perpendicular to the plane of the vertebral endplates. In this example, the stiffness (slope of the curve) increases with increasing load. The compressive strength of the vertebra shown is approximately 9 kN. After fracture, the ability to support a compressive load is not reduced to zero but is still approximately 5 kN. This is due to the fact that fragments of the trabecular bone may support one another until complete col-

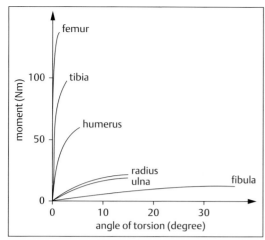

Fig. 7.**5** Torsion of human bones by a moment directed along the long axis of the bones. (Adapted from Yamada, 1970.)

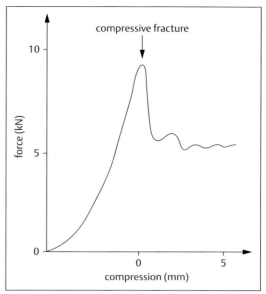

Fig. 7.**6** Compression of a human lumbar vertebral body by a compressive force. In the example shown, the compressive strength amounts to approximately 9 kN. After fracture a load-bearing capacity of approximately 5 kN remains. (Adapted from: Plaue *et al.*, 1973.)

lapse occurs at larger deformations. *In vivo*, the ability to support some compressive force in the long run after occurrence of a compression fracture of a vertebra depends on whether and how fast the fractured bone material can be replaced by new bone.

If a structure contains components made out of viscoelastic or plastic materials, or if the components have some play in their connection so that small relative movements are possible, a permanent deformation is observed after the end of a load cycle. Fig. 7.**7** illustrates this effect using the example of the passive, axial rotation of the cervical spine under the application of an external moment. In the example shown, the range of motion between maximal rotation to the right and to the left is approximately 160°. The angular position of the cervical spine in relation to the moment follows a hysteresis loop. The region of plastic deformation (i.e. the deformation at zero moment) extends from +60° to –60°. In this region the angular position depends on the mechanical history, i.e. on the direction and strength of the previously applied moment.

Following a suggestion by Panjabi, the region of plastic deformation of a structure is occasionally termed the 'neutral zone' in orthopedic and biomechanical literature. Doubt might well be cast on the usefulness of this designation, because the well-established term 'plastic deformation' already describes this effect. In addition, it must be pointed out that the extent of the plastic deformation is not characteristic of the structure under investigation but rather depends on the magnitude of the previously exerted load. If the load is increased or decreased, the 'neutral zone' increases or decreases as well. The so-called neutral zone is thus hardly appropriate for describing biomechanical characteristics of the human locomotor system.

Deforming a structure demands energy (work). Assuming a constant force or a constant moment, deformation energy is defined as force multiplied by change in length or moment multiplied by change in angle. In both cases the dimension of the deformation energy is newton-meters [Nm]. To determine the total energy for a given deformation of a structure, where the force or the moment change as the deformation changes, we imagine the force or moment to be increased from the initial to the final state in very, very small (mathematically: 'infinitesimally' small) increments. The total deformation energy is then obtained by integration and represented by the area below the load-deformation graph.

This is independent of whether the graph follows a straight line or some irregular curve. Fig. 7.**8** shows load-deformation graphs of structures A and B, which have been differently deformed. Structure A exhibits a greater stiffness than structure B. However, the deformation energy, which depends on the shape of the load-deforma-

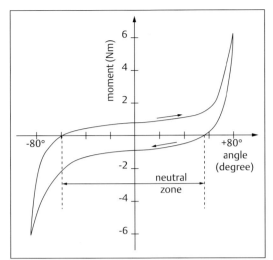

Fig. 7.7 Passive rotation of the cervical spine by an external moment. If rotation is performed to the right and to the left, the moment-deformation graph forms a complete hysteresis loop. The amount of deformation observed at zero moment depends on the magnitude and the direction of the previously exerted moment. The range of plastic deformation is sometimes called the 'neutral zone'. It has to be pointed out that the magnitude of the 'neutral zone' is not characteristic of the structure under investigation because it depends on the experimental set-up, i.e. on the previously exerted moment. (Adapted from McClure *et al.*, 1998.)

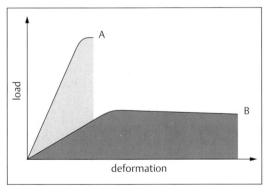

Fig. 7.8 The area under the load-deformation graph is a measure of the deformation energy of the structure. This is valid for the case where the structure is loaded by a force and the deformation is measured in meters as well as where the structure is loaded by a moment and the torsional deformation is measured in radians. In both cases the deformation energy is measured in units of newton meters [Nm]. The diagram illustrates the deformation energies of structures A and B by the areas under the respective curves.

tion graph and on the extent of the deformation, is greater in case B than in case A. Practical use is made of this fact when damping impacts by means of a low-stiffness structure permitting a large deformation so that a large amount of energy can be absorbed.

Deformation and strength of beam-like structures

Structures whose length is large in relation to their cross section are termed 'beams'. If the cross-sectional area has a simple geometrical shape (rectangle, hexagon, circle, tube), and in simple loading modes, the stress distribution in the beam can be deduced theoretically. Examples of simple loading modes are the loading of a beam by a longitudinally directed tensile or compressive force, or by a moment in bending or torsion. If the moduli of elasticity and shear of the material from which the beam has been manufactured are known, the resulting deformation can be calculated from the stress distribution. Since the stresses increase in proportion to the loading force or moment, it is also possible to calculate that magnitude of the load where the stress at some volume element of the beam reaches the value of the ultimate stress. The appertaining load designates the tensile, compressive, or torsional strength of the beam.

In the case of beams with irregularly shaped cross sections or of complex loading modes, the formulae given below allow deformation and strength values to be calculated, at least approximately. For this purpose geometry and loading mode can be sufficiently simplified. The cross section of a long bone can, for example, be approximated by a tube with the diameter of the bone and a wall thickness equal to the mean thickness of the cortical bone. If a structure is loaded by more than one force and/or moment, only the force or moment with the highest magnitude may be taken into account for an initial approximation.

In the following, the procedure used to calculate deformation and strength is illustrated by the examples of a beam of arbitrary cross section under a tensile or compressive force, a beam with rectangular cross section under a bending moment, and a beam with circular cross section under a torsional moment (oriented about its long axis).

Deformation of a beam under tension or compression

If a beam is loaded by a compressive or tensile force directed longitudinally (Fig. 7.**9**) the stress may be taken to assume equal values at each point of the cross sectional area A at some distance from the point of force application. The stress σ has the value

$$\sigma = F/A$$

For the length change dL of the beam of initial length L, we obtain from Hooke's law

$$\sigma = E \cdot dL/L$$
$$dL = \sigma \cdot L/E$$
$$dL = (F \cdot L)/(A \cdot E)$$

The length change is proportional to the initial length L and the force F and inversely proportional to the modulus of elasticity E and the cross-sectional area A.

If the quotient F/A exceeds the value of the ultimate stress of the material, the beam will fracture. It follows that

$$\text{compressive or tensile strength} = \sigma_u \cdot A \; [N]$$

The strength of the beam increases with increasing ultimate stress σ_u and increasing cross-sectional area A. The strength does not depend on the modulus of elasticity E or on the length L of the beam.

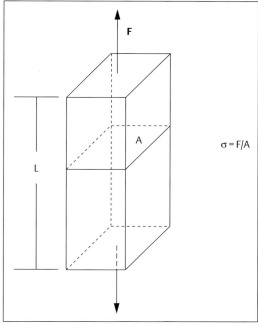

Fig. 7.**9** The tensile stress in a beam loaded by a tensile force **F** assumes equal values on each cross section parallel to A (provided that the cross section is located at some distance from the point of application of the force). Its magnitude is given by σ = F/A. If the stress is known, the length change of the beam can be calculated from Hooke's law. If the ultimate stress is known, the force where fracture occurs can be calculated; this force is called the tensile strength of the beam.

Bending of a beam fixed at one end

If a beam is fixed at one end and loaded at its free end by a force directed perpendicularly to the long axis of the beam, the beam will be bent (Fig. 7.**10**). The material will be elongated on the upper surface of the beam and compressed on the lower surface. The length of the middle layer ('neutral fiber') at the border between regions of compression and elongation will remain unchanged. Inside the beam, tensile and compressive stresses σ_t and σ_c are generated. The stresses have their maximum value at the upper and lower beam surfaces and decrease towards the neutral fiber. At each cross section at a distance L_1 from the point of application of force the tensile and compressive stresses generate a moment which equilibrates the external moment $L_1 \cdot F$.

It can be shown (the proof is not given here) that the deflection f of the beam at its free end is given by (Nelson et al. 1998)

$$f = (F \cdot L^3)/(3 \cdot E \cdot I) \; [m]$$

In this equation, F designates the force, L the length of the beam, E the modulus of elasticity of the beam material; I is called 'moment of inertia' (or 'second moment of area'). The moment of inertia (having nothing to do with the moment of a force) is a geometrical quantity, determined solely by the shape of the cross section of the beam. For a rectangular cross section of width w and height h it holds that

$$I = w \cdot h^3/12 \; [m^4]$$

It is obvious from the above formulae that the length L and the height h of the beam have a great influence on the deflection. The tensile stress at the upper surface of the beam at a distance L_1 from the point of force application is given by

$$\sigma = M/Z \; [N/m^2]$$
$$\sigma = L_1 \cdot F/Z \; [N/m^2]$$

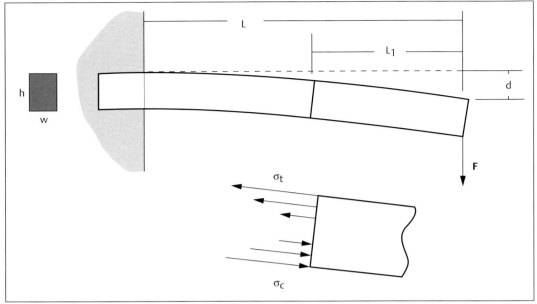

Fig. 7.10 Deflection d of a beam fixed at one end and loaded by a force F at its free end. At each cross section at a distance L_1 from the point of force application, tensile and compressive stresses σ_t and σ_c are generated which balance the external moment $L_1 \cdot F$. The stresses assume their maximum values at the cross section where the beam is fixed. With a given force, the deflection depends on the length, height, and width of the beam and on the modulus of elasticity of its building material. (The distribution of the tensile and compressive stresses over the cross-sectional area of the beam is shown magnified in relation to the rest of the diagram.)

In this formula, M denotes the moment $L_1 \cdot F$. Z is called the 'section modulus'. Like the moment of inertia, Z is a purely geometrical quantity and depends on the shape of the beam's cross section. For a beam with a rectangular cross section it holds that

$$Z = w \cdot h^2/6 \ [m^3]$$

Since the moment of the external force F, and hence the stress on the surface of the beam, increases with increasing distance from the point of application of the force according to $\sigma = M/Z$, it is obvious that the largest value of the stress is to be expected at the location $(L_1 = L)$ where the beam is fixed. If the stress at this location exceeds the ultimate stress of the beam material, the beam will fracture at the fixation. It follows that the bending strength of a unilaterally fixed beam is given by

$$\text{bending strength} = \sigma_u \cdot Z/L \ [N]$$

For a beam with a rectangular cross section it follows that

$$\text{bending strength} = \sigma_u \cdot w \cdot h^2/6 \cdot L \ [N]$$

The formula shows that the bending strength of a beam with a rectangular cross section depends more on the height h than on the width w of the beam. The strength decreases with increasing length L.

Formulae for calculating the moment of inertia I and the section modulus Z for other shapes of cross sections (circle, tube, triangle) are listed in reference books on mechanics. In such books the reader can also find formulae to calculate deflection of beams under other simple loading modes like three-point or four-point bending or uniform distribution of the load along the whole beam. By means of these formulae, deflection and strength can be obtained in the same fashion as in the example set out above.

Torsion of a beam around its long axis

A beam of circular cross section may be fixed at one end and loaded at its free end by a moment directed around its long axis. In order to derive the relationship between the moment, the properties of the beam material, the shape of the beam, and the angle of torsion, we imagine the beam to be divided into a set of thin-walled cylinders (Fig. 7.**11**). The torsion of a cylinder of radius R and wall thickness dR by an angle β effects a shear of the wall of the cylinder by an angle α. The relation between the two angles is

$$\alpha = \beta \cdot R/L$$

On the cross-sectional area of the cylinder the shear stress

$$\tau = G \cdot \alpha \; [N/m^2]$$

is generated. In this formula G denotes the shear modulus. The shear force, given by the product of shear stress τ and cross-sectional area of the cylinder, effects a moment directed opposite to the external moment; the moments of all cylinders together equilibrate the external moment M.

It can be shown (the proof is not given here) that the relation between the angle of torsion β and the external moment is given by

$$\beta = (M \cdot L)/(G \cdot I_p)$$

In this formula M denotes the external moment, L the length of the beam, G the modulus of shear, and I_p the 'polar moment of inertia'. I_p depends only on the geometry of the cross section of the beam. For a beam with a circular cross section and radius R it amounts to

$$I_p = \pi \cdot R^4/2 \; [m^4]$$

The shear stress has its maximum value at the surface of the beam. At each point along the beam the stress has the value

$$\tau = M/Z_p$$

In this formula Z_p denotes the 'polar section modulus'. Z_p depends (like the polar moment of inertia) only on the geometry of the cross section of the beam. For a beam with a circular cross section it amounts to

$$Z_p = \pi \cdot R^3/2 \; [m^3]$$

The torsional strength, i.e. the maximum moment by which the beam can be loaded, is reached when the shear stress at the beam surface assumes its ultimate value τ_u

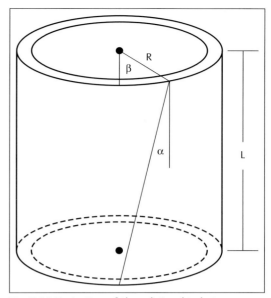

Fig. 7.**11** Derivation of the relationship between moment and torsional deformation of a beam of circular cross section. The beam is imagined to be composed of concentric hollow cylinders. The twist of a hollow cylinder by an angle β corresponds to a shear deformation of the lateral area of the cylinder by an angle α caused by a shear stress τ. τ multiplied by the area gives the appertaining shear force. The external moment equals the sum of the moments exerted by all cylinders, i.e. of the shear forces multiplied by the relevant radii R.

$$\text{torsional strength} = \tau_u \cdot Z_p \; [Nm]$$

Since the shear stress takes equal values along the whole beam between the point of fixation and the point of moment application, no prediction can be made concerning the location at which fracture is to be expected. The location of fracture is determined rather by local deviations from the regular beam geometry or by material inhomogeneities.

Formulae for determining the polar moment of inertia and the polar section modulus for other shapes of cross sections (tubular, rectangle, triangle) are available in reference books of mechanics. Analogous to the example outlined above, these formulae permit the deformation and strength of such beams under torsional loading to be calculated.

Literature

Further reading

Abé H, Hayashi K, Sato M (eds). *Data book on mechanical properties of living cells, tissues, and organs.* Tokyo: Springer; 1996

Alonso M, Finn E. *Physics.* Addison Wesley, Harlow 1996

Gordon JE. *The new science of strong materials, or why you don't fall through the floor.* Baltimore: Penguin Books; 1973

Gross D. *Bruchmechanik.* 2nd ed. Berlin: Springer; 1996

Nelson EW, Best CL, McLean WG. *Engineering mechanics. Statics and dynamics.* 5th ed. McGraw-Hill, New York 1998

Yamada H. *Strength of Biological Materials.* Baltimore: Williams & Wilkins; 1970

Scientific papers cited in the text or the figures

Amiel D, Woo SLY, Harwood FL, Akeson WH. The effect of immobilization on collagen turnover in connective tissue: A biochemical-biomechanical correlation. *Acta Orthop Scand.* 1982; **53**: 325–332

Lanir Y, Fung YC. Two-dimensional mechanical properties of rabbit skin – II. Experimental results. *J Biomechanics.* 1974; **7**: 171–182

McClure P, Siegler S, Nobilini R. Three-dimensional flexibility characteristics of the human cervical spine *in vivo. Spine.* 1998; **23**: 216–223

Plaue R, Gerner HJ, Puhl W. Das Frakturverhalten von Brust- und Lendenwirbelkörpern. 4.Mitteilung: Untersuchung über die Morphologie des Wirbelkompressionsbruches. **Z Orthop.** 1973; **111**: 139–146

Sparks HV, Bohr DF. Effect of stretch on passive tension and contractility of isolated vascular smooth muscle. *Am J Physiol.* 1962; **202**: 835–840

8 Estimation of the Load Transmitted by Joints of the Human Locomotor System by Means of a Biomechanical Model Calculation

Mechanical actions that can have local effects on the tissues include mechanical stress, strain, deformation, and friction. Examples are the pressure on the cartilaginous surface of a joint, the deformation of the trabecular bone beneath a joint surface, and the friction between articulating joint surfaces. Experience shows that excessively high or excessively low mechanical stimuli may have adverse effects in the long run. Mechanical stimuli of moderate magnitude may trigger adaptive processes of the tissues. The benefit derived from this general knowledge, however, is scant, as in most cases of practical interest the limiting values of what exactly constitutes an 'excessively high' or 'excessively low' mechanical stimulus are not known. In addition, detailed knowledge of how adaptive processes are triggered and controlled by mechanical stimuli is widely lacking.

Forces acting in the body, as well as stress and strain on the tissues, can be determined experimentally or by calculation. One example of an experimental procedure is measurement of the stress distribution on the skin of the back or on the sole of the foot. This has been performed to explore the relationship between stress and the development of sores or ulcers. Loads on the hip joint and on spinal implants have been measured by means of artificial joints or implants equipped with force transducers. The aim was to obtain information on joint and implant loading *in vivo* and on adaptive processes in bones. Load on the lumbar spine has been determined from measurement of intradiskal pressure to provide a better understanding of the relation between spinal loading and clinical symptoms. All these experiments have provided new and valuable information. On the other hand, application of experimental methods is limited because some quantities are incapable of measurement and invasive procedures can be applied only in exceptional cases.

If stress or strain on a structure is to be calculated, the loading by forces and moments, and the mechanical properties of the building materials, must be known. While determination of the loading mode already poses considerable problems (as outlined below), the mechanical properties of the tissues of the human locomotor system and their bi-

ological variance are often known only very imprecisely, if at all. For many matters of practical interest it is, however, more important to learn how and in what direction the mechanical influences change with changes in posture or activity, than to know the precise numerical values of stress and strain. For this purpose, deformation of the structures of the locomotor system may be assumed to be small under a given load. Under this assumption, it holds that stress and strain will vary in proportion to the magnitude of the load. If, for example, the distribution of stress on a joint surface (the real aspect of interest) cannot be calculated directly, it is broadly correct to assume that the stress will increase or decrease in proportion to the joint load. Knowledge of the load on a joint thus permits relative comparisons of the magnitude of mechanical actions of local effect.

Because determination of the loading mode constitutes the first step when investigating mechanical influences on tissues, and because conclusions on the change of stress and strain can be drawn from a change in load, determination of the load on muscles, tendons, and joints is a central objective of orthopedic biomechanics. Determination of joint loading would be comparatively simple if a method for measuring muscle forces were available. Unfortunately, this is currently not the case. Electrical signals generated upon the activation of a muscle can be picked up by means of electrodes placed on the surface of the skin, or needle electrodes placed in the volume of a muscle. The signal amplitude of the so-called electromyogram (EMG) and other properties of the EMG-signal do not, however, permit conclusions to be drawn on the magnitude of the muscle force. For this reason joint loading has to be determined mainly from model calculations (save for the rare exceptions mentioned above).

The procedure for calculating joint forces is based on the conditions of mechanical equilibrium. If a system is in mechanical equilibrium, the two conditions (see Chapter 5) permit the determination of one unknown moment and one unknown force. In the case of joint loading these are the moment of a muscle (and, with knowledge of the moment arm, the muscle force) and the force transmitted between the articulating bones. In planar, static, or quasi-static situations, the vectors of external force and muscle force act in the same plane and inertial forces do not exist or are assumed to be negligible. When estimating joint loads in the elbow or the lumbar spine while holding a mass in the hands, for example, these assumptions are usually valid. In the dynamic case, where accelerated movements occur, inertial forces and moments have to be included in the calculation. This is necessary, for example, when the load on the joints of the upper extremity while lifting, or the load on the joints of the lower extremity while walking, are to be determined.

In practically all cases, simplifications have to be introduced, and assumptions on unknown parameters have to be made, before a calculation of forces in the locomotor system can be undertaken. As these calculations treat anatomical structures as simplified models, they are termed 'biomechanical model calculations'. It follows that the validity of the assumptions and simplifications must always be critically reviewed when discussing the results of such calculations. When calculating joint loads, an additional difficulty arises in all cases where more than one muscle crosses a joint; there are then more unknowns than equations available from the equilibrium condition. Additional assumptions have to be made. Either the problem has to be simplified by taking only one muscle into account, or an assumption has to be made that several muscles act as a unit. Different ways of tackling this latter problem are discussed at the end of this chapter.

▨ Calculation of a joint load in the static case, illustrated with the example of the elbow joint

The calculation of the load **O** on the elbow joint when holding a mass in the hand is used here as an example of a biomechanical model calculation in the plane, static case (Fig. 8.**1**). The forearm is held at an angle of 90° with respect to the upper arm. The mass of 10 kg held in the hand exerts a gravitational force of 98.1 N on the hand; this value is rounded up to 100 N in the calculation below. For the time being the weight of the forearm is neglected. To maintain equilibrium the biceps muscle is activated. In relation to the xy-coordinate system shown, both external load and muscle force are parallel to the y-direction; the gravitational force **W** and the muscle force **B** have only y-components. The moment arms of the external force and the muscle force are assumed to be 20 cm and 2 cm, respectively (approximately correct, rounded values).

When writing down the equilibrium condition for the moments, attention has to be paid to using the correct signs. The muscle force **B** effects a rotation in a counterclockwise direction (negative sign); the load **W** effects a rotation in clockwise direction (positive sign)

$$-B \cdot 2 + 100 \cdot 20 = 0 \text{ Ncm}$$

This equation yields for the required force of the biceps muscle

$$B = 1000 \text{ N}$$

In the state of equilibrium the (vector) sum of the forces must equal zero

$$\mathbf{O} + \mathbf{B} + \mathbf{W} = \mathbf{0}$$

The unknown joint force **O** is calculated by summing the y-components of all forces (in this example there are no horizontally directed forces, i.e. no x-components). The y-component of the gravitational force **W** has a negative sign as this force points into the negative y-direction; the biceps muscle force bears a positive sign

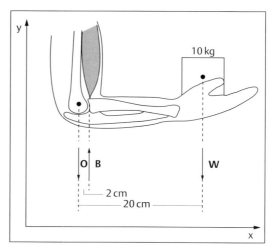

Fig. 8.**1**   Calculation of the load on the elbow joint in static equilibrium. The gravitational force **W** of the mass of 10 kg acts on the hand. The force **B** developed by the biceps muscle and the joint force **O** of the humeroulnar joint are to be determined. The biceps is assumed to be the only active muscle. Rounded values are assumed for the moment arms. The weight of the hand and lower arm is neglected.

$$O + 1000\,N - 100\,N = 0$$
$$O = -900\,N$$

The y-component of the joint force **O** has a magnitude of 900 N. The negative sign means that this force points into the negative y-direction: the humerus is pressed against the ulna with a force of 900 N.

In the example shown in Fig. 8.**1**, equilibrium was established solely by activation of the biceps muscle; antagonistic muscle activation was not taken into account. This is certainly an over simplification because experience shows that agonist *and* antagonistic muscles are usually activated simultaneously for maintaining postures or performing activities. However, consideration of the force **T** of the triceps in addition to the force **B** of the biceps (Fig. 8.**2**), immediately gives rise to the problem that the two equilibrium conditions are insufficient for unequivocal determination of two unknown muscle forces (biceps and triceps) and the unknown joint force. To obtain an unequivocal solution an additional assumption has to be made. In order to explore the extent to which the joint force changes if an antagonist is activated, we assume (arbitrarily) that the force developed by the triceps is small and amounts to 25 % of the force of the biceps

$$T = 0.25\,B$$

To keep the calculation simple, it is further assumed that the force of the triceps is, like the force of the biceps, directed into the positive y-direction. With a moment arm of the triceps of 2 cm (approximate value) and with reference to the sign convention for moments we obtain in the equilibrium of moments

$$-2 \cdot B + 20 \cdot 100 + 2 \cdot T = 0\,Ncm$$
$$-2 \cdot B + 20 \cdot 100 + 2 \cdot 0.25 \cdot B = 0\,Ncm$$

From these two equations we obtain B and T

$$B = 1333.3\,N$$
$$T = 0.25\,B = 333.3\,N$$

In the equilibrium of forces

$$\mathbf{O} + \mathbf{B} + \mathbf{T} + \mathbf{W} = \mathbf{0}$$

we obtain for the y-components of the forces (digits after the decimal point omitted)

$$O + 1333 + 333 - 100 = 0\,N$$
$$O = -1566\,N$$

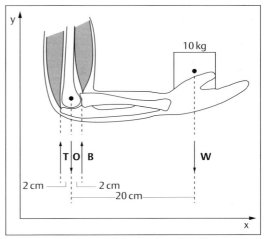

Fig. 8.**2** Calculation of the load on the elbow joint in static equilibrium. The gravitational force **W** of the mass of 10 kg acts on the hand. The force **B** developed by the biceps muscle and the joint force **O** of the humero-ulnar joint are to be determined if, in addition to the agonist (biceps), the antagonist (triceps) is also activated with a force **T**. As in the case shown in Fig. 8.**1**, rounded values are assumed for the moment arms and the weight of hand and lower arm is neglected.

The joint force now amounts to 1566 N. Again, the negative sign indicates that the humerus is pressed against the ulna. It is obvious that the participation of the antagonist increased the joint force by a considerable amount. The force developed by the antagonist was assumed to be 25 % of the force of the agonist; the joint force, however, increased by 74 % (from 900 N to 1566 N). Why nature employs antagonistic muscle activation (and puts up with the accompanying increase in joint loading) is open to speculation. Antagonistic muscle activation may be helpful in stabilizing postures by making them insensitive to small perturbations. If a muscle is forced to effect a movement against strong resistance of the antagonist, very high joint loading is expected to result. This could, for example, occur in spastic patients with over-activation of certain muscles or in elderly persons with Parkinson's disease.

Knowledge of the load on the humeroulnar joint permits the compressive stress on the joint surface to be estimated by applying the formula for the mean pressure p_{mean}. If we assume a projected contact area (i.e. the joint area as seen from the direction of the joint force) between humerus and ulna of 5 cm^2 (equal to $5 \cdot 10^{-4}\,m^2$) and if we insert the joint force of 900 N (the minimum, calculated without antagonistic muscle activation) we obtain

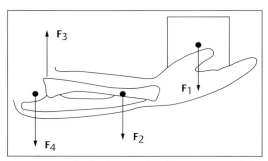

Fig 8.3 Free body diagram for determination of the joint load. The points of application, directions, and magnitudes of all forces, as far as initially known are marked on the free body (imagined to be separated from its environment). Initially, the point of application as well as the direction and magnitude of the gravitational force (weight) F_1 of the mass held in the hand, and of the weight F_2 of hand and lower arm are known. Of the muscle force F_3 the point of application and the direction are known, while the magnitude is unknown. Of the joint force F_4 only the point of application (the center of rotation of the joint) is known. The magnitude of the muscle force is calculated from the equilibrium condition of moments; subsequently the direction and magnitude of the joint force is determined from the equilibrium condition of forces.

$$p_{mean} = 900/5 \cdot 10^{-4} \, N/m^2$$
$$p_{mean} = 1.8 \, MPa$$

In general, the procedure for determining joint forces in a state of static equilibrium can be summarized as follows (Fig. 8.3): magnitudes, directions, and points of application of all forces are marked, in so far as they are known from the outset, on the 'free' body (i.e., imagined to be separated from its environment). This diagram is termed free body diagram. In the case discussed above, the initial knowledge comprised the magnitude, direction, and point of application of the external load F_1 and (in order to complete the description) the gravitational force of forearm and hand F_2. These forces are applied at the center of gravity of the external load and of the forearm, respectively. From the muscle force F_3 only its point of application and its direction are known from anatomical observations. As far as the joint force F_4 is concerned, only its point of application is known: due to the fact that there is only negligible friction between the articulating surfaces, this force is directed through the center of rotation. (The supporting argument for this is that a frictionless joint cannot transmit any moment. If the joint force were not directed through the center of rotation, a moment, and

hence an accelerated rotational movement, would result. Static equilibrium would not exist, in contrast to the assumption.)

In the first step, the moment of the muscle force and (with a known moment arm of the muscle) the magnitude of the muscle force F_3 are determined from the equilibrium condition of moments. In the second step, the magnitude and direction of the joint force F_4 are determined from the equilibrium of forces. The prerequisites for performing this model calculation are: i) assuming only one active muscle, specifically excluding antagonistic muscle activation, ii) assuming a punctiform application of muscle and tendon forces at the bones (instead of an anatomically correct area of force application) and iii) ignoring the elastic tension of other muscles, joint capsules, or ligaments that may traverse the joint in question.

With respect to muscle forces and joint loads, the results obtained at the elbow joint are typical of all joints of the locomotor system:

– The muscle force needed to guarantee equilibrium is, in general, much larger than external forces acting on the body. This is due to the ratio of the moment arm of the external forces compared to the moment arm of the muscle forces. For the long bones of the extremities it holds as a rule that moment arms of external forces are comparable to the length of the bones while moment arms of the muscles are comparable to the diameter of the bones. There is one joint in the body, the temporomandibular joint, where moment arms of external and muscle force are of comparable magnitude.
– The magnitude of the joint load is determined essentially by the muscle force; the external force makes only a small, additional contribution.
– The absolute minimum of the joint force occurs when the agonist muscle alone is activated. Additional activation of an antagonistic muscle increases the joint force disproportionately.
– As the shapes of the articulating bones are in general incongruent, small areas of contact and hence high compressive stresses on these contact areas will result.

The underlying reason for high muscle and joint forces is in the architecture and anatomical function of the muscles (Fig. 8.4). Muscles can produce large tensile forces while the change of muscle length is limited to relatively small values. If the range of motion (ROM) of a joint is large, the muscle must, for geometrical reasons, be positioned close to the joint. Its moment arm dL will then be small. Otherwise, if the muscle were positioned farther away from the joint, the required change in length might exceed the muscle's tolerance limit.

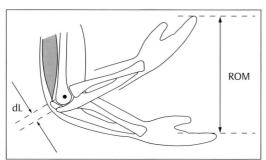

Fig. 8.4 High joint loads are ultimately due to the change in length of muscles being limited to comparatively small amounts. In case of a large range of motion (ROM) of a joint, the muscle must be located close to the axis of rotation so that its length change dL stays below certain limiting values. It follows that the moment arm of the muscle is usually small compared with the moment arms of external forces. Due to the relation of the moment arms, the muscle force will usually be much higher than the external force. Due to the high muscle force the joint force will be high as well.

It follows that (with few exceptions) the moment arms of external forces (or of the body weight) are usually much larger than moment arms of the muscles. The ratio of the moment arms of muscles to external forces requires a large muscle force to guarantee equilibrium. Large muscle forces cause large joint forces. Large joint forces in turn cause high pressure on the articulating surfaces.

Determination of the joint force in the dynamic case, illustrated with the example of the ankle joint

In the dynamic case, when accelerated linear and rotational movements occur, inertial forces and inertial moments have to be taken into account. For the purpose of calculation, the human body is imagined to be divided into segments at the joints. In detail, the following assumptions are made (see, for example, Winter, 1990):

- The mass m of each segment remains constant during the course of the movement.
- The segments are modeled (in simplified terms) as rigid bodies. Thus, during the course of the motion the location of the center of gravity does not change with respect to the anatomical structures (i.e. bones) or to landmarks located at the surface of the segment.
- The moment of inertia I remains constant throughout the course of the movement.

- The joints are frictionless hinge or ball-and-socket joints.
- The linear movement of a segment is represented by the movement of its center of gravity.
- The rotational movement of a segment is represented by the rotation about its center of gravity.

For the examples discussed in this book it is assumed, in addition, that movement takes place in a plane. Numerical data on the location of the centers of mass and the moments of inertia of the body segments can be found, for example, in Pheasant (1986), Jensen (1986) and Chaffin and co-workers (1999).

For a plane movement of a segment of mass m and moment of inertia I about the center of gravity it holds that

$$\sum_1^n R_{ix} = m \cdot a_x$$
$$\sum_1^n R_{iy} + S = m \cdot a_y$$
$$\sum_1^n M_i = J \cdot \alpha$$

The first two equations are known as the scalar equations of plane motion. R_i and M_i are the reaction forces and reaction moments, which are transmitted from the neighboring segments on to the segment under consideration. The moments are regarded as representing pure moments, i. e. moments effected by a force couple. The moments are taken about the center of gravity. The lines of action of the forces R_i pass through the centers of rotation of the joints. The sums are to be extended over all moments and forces from i = 1 to i = n. a_x and a_y are the components of the linear acceleration of the center of gravity; α is the angular acceleration about an axis running through the center of gravity with normal (perpendicular) orientation to the plane of motion. In the equations the effects of inertia (inertial force and moment of inertia) are explicitly specified on the right-hand side of the equations. For this reason, the quantities $m \cdot ax$ and $I \cdot \alpha$ bear positive signs. To formulate the equations as above, the x-axis of the coordinate system is assumed to point into horizontal direction and the y-axis to point upwards. It follows that the gravitational force has only a y-component; this component points into the negative y-direction. $S = -m \cdot g$ is the y-component of the gravitational force.

The reaction forces R_i transmitted from the neighboring segments are not identical to the joint forces but rather represent the net (i.e. the vector sum) force transmitted from one segment to the next. It is shown below that a model of the joint has to be established, in order to calculate joint forces. Such models are derived from the anatomy

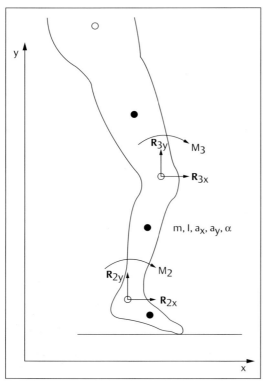

Fig. 8.**5** Reaction forces **R₂** and **R₃** and reaction moments M_2 and M_3 acting distally and proximally on the lower leg segment. The linear acceleration **a** of the center of gravity and the angular acceleration α around the center of gravity are effected by these forces and moments. The solid circle designates the center of gravity of the segment. The open circles represent the centers of rotation. The segment has the mass m and the moment of inertia I related to an axis through the center of gravity and running perpendicular to the plane of motion. In this figure as well as in Figs 8.**6** to 8.**9** the arrows designating the reaction forces **R**$_i$ and the reaction moments M$_i$ are purely symbolic. They indicate that forces and moments are acting, but convey nothing about their magnitude or sense of direction. Magnitudes and directions are obtained as result of the calculation

and specify the directions, points of application, and moment arms relative to the center of rotation for the relevant muscles and tendons of a joint.

Fig. 8.5 illustrates the approach using the example of the lower leg. The leg is imagined to be divided into the three segments foot, lower leg, and upper leg, linked by hinge joints. The reaction force **R₂** with components R_{2x} and R_{2y} and the reaction moment M_2 act on the distal end of the lower leg. The reaction force **R₃** with components R_{3x} and R_{3y} and the moment M_3 act on the proximal end of the

lower leg. The lower leg has the mass m and (relative to the center of gravity) the moment of inertia I. The gravitational force acting on the segment amounts to $S = -m \cdot g$. Under these forces and moments the motion of the lower leg occurs in accordance with the above-stated equations of motion. a_x and a_y are the components of the linear acceleration of the center of gravity; α is the angular acceleration around the center of gravity.

Determination of the forces and moments transmitted from one segment to the next is elaborated below with the example of the ankle joint (Figs. 8.**6** to 8.**9**). The designations are: m = mass of the foot, I = moment of inertia of the foot related to its center of gravity, $m \cdot g$ = gravitational force acting on the foot, a_x and a_y = linear acceleration of the center of gravity of the foot, α = angular acceleration of the foot around its center of gravity, R_{1x} and R_{1y} = components of the reaction force acting distally (on the tip) on the foot, R_{2x} and R_{2y} = components of the reaction force acting proximally on the segment 'foot', M_1 = reaction moment acting distally (this moment is, however, equal to zero because as long as the foot is not glued to the floor, no moment can be transmitted), M_2 = reaction moment acting proximally, L_1 and L_2 = position of the center of rotation of the ankle joint relative to the center of gravity, and L_3 and L_4 = point of application of the reaction force acting from the floor on the foot. (The point of contact between the tip of the foot and the floor actually represents the location of a 'hinge-type joint' between foot and floor.)

To provide clear insight into the calculation and relate it to the determination of the joint force of the elbow joint described above, reaction forces and moments are determined below for three cases:
– Static case: no force between foot and floor. With reference to this case, the relation between joint forces and reaction forces and moments is discussed.
– Dynamic case: accelerated movement of the foot, but no force between foot and floor.
– Dynamic case: accelerated movement of the foot, taking account of a force acting from the floor on the foot.

Case 1: Foot held freely, no motion (Fig. 8.**6**). The force and the moment acting from the floor on the foot and the linear, as well as the angular, accelerations are equal to zero. The gravitational force acts on the foot. With a_x, a_y, R_{1x}, R_{1y}, M_1 and α equal to zero we obtain by insertion into the equations of motion for the forces

$$R_{2x} = 0$$
$$R_{2y} - m \cdot g = 0$$
$$R_{2y} = m \cdot g$$

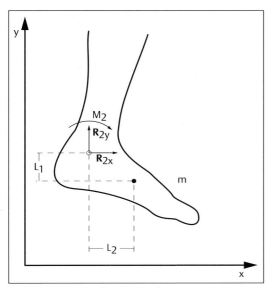

Fig. 8.**6** Reaction force **R**₂ and reaction moment M₂ transmitted from the lower leg onto the freely held, motionless foot. The solid circle designates the center of gravity of the segment. The open circle represents the center of rotation. m designates the mass of the segment. The force **R**₂ is directed through the center of rotation of the joint. L₁ and L₂ are the moment arms of the components of **R**₂ in relation to the center of gravity of the foot.

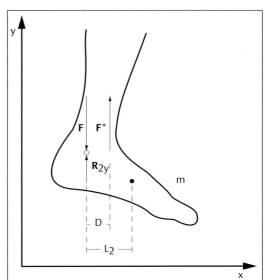

Fig. 8.**7** Biomechanical model designed to determine the load on the ankle joint in the case of the freely held, motionless foot. The reaction moment M₂ (Fig. 8.**6**) is generated by a force couple **F** and **F***. **F*** represents the force of the tendon of the tibialis anterior. The line of action of the tendon is assumed to have a distance D from the center of rotation. Other designations as in Fig. 8.**6**.

and for the moments (moments taken about the center of gravity of the foot, signs according to the sign convention for moments), and with $R_{2y} = m \cdot g$ as determined above

$$M_2 + R_{2y} \cdot L_2 = 0$$
$$M_2 = -m \cdot g \cdot L_2$$

If it is intended merely to calculate the reaction force **R**₂ and the reaction moment M₂ from the lower leg on the foot, the problem is thus solved. For reasons of equilibrium, the force and the moment acting from the foot on the lower leg are opposite but equal to **R**₂ and M₂, i.e. force and moment transmitted from the foot to the lower leg equal −**R**₂ and −M₂. If the motion of the lower leg were to be analyzed, these values would have to be inserted into the equations of motion for the lower leg.

To provide the link between the reaction force and moment between the foot and lower leg and the force on the ankle joint, we start from **R**₂ and M₂ and determine the force between tibia and talus (analogous to the determination of the force acting between humerus and ulna in the case of the elbow joint discussed above). To reach a solution it is nec-

essary to specify which muscle actually provides the moment M₂. An obvious candidate is the tibialis anterior whose tendon effects the dorsiflexion of the foot. We assume that this tendon pulls in the y-direction and at a distance D from the center of rotation (Fig. 8.**7**). The moment $M_2 = -m \cdot g \cdot L_2$, which acts proximally on the foot, is imagined to be generated by a force couple **F** and **F***. The force **F** is exerted at the center of rotation of the tibiotalar joint. **F*** is the tensile force of the tendon of the tibialis anterior; its line of action has a distance D with respect to the center of rotation. **F*** points in the positive, and **F** in the negative y-direction. **F** and **F*** are of equal magnitude.

Expressed by the force couple we write for the moment M₂ (all moments in relation to the center of gravity of the foot)

$$M_2 = -L_2 \cdot |\mathbf{F}| + (L_2 - D) \cdot |\mathbf{F}^*|$$

According to the sign convention for moments, the moment of **F** bears a positive, and the moment of **F*** a negative sign. With

$$M_2 = -m \cdot g \cdot L_2$$

we obtain

$$-m \cdot g \cdot L_2 = -L_2 \cdot |\mathbf{F}| + (L_2 - D) \cdot |\mathbf{F}^*|$$

and with $|\mathbf{F}| = |\mathbf{F}^*|$ it follows that

$$|\mathbf{F}| = |\mathbf{F}^*| = m \cdot g \cdot L_2 / D$$

The forces $\mathbf{R}_2$ and $\mathbf{F}$ act between tibia and talus. The load on the ankle joint is the sum of the forces $\mathbf{F}$ and $\mathbf{R}_{2y}$. The y-component of the load $\mathbf{O}$ is equal to

$$O_y = F + R_{2y}$$
$$O_y = -m \cdot g \cdot L_2 / D + m \cdot g$$

In contrast, the sum of the y-components of all forces acting on the proximal end of the foot segment is equal to

$$F + F^* + R_{2y} = m \cdot g$$
$$R_{2y} = m \cdot g$$

A comparison of these results reveals that $\mathbf{R}_2$ is the net force transmitted from the lower leg segment to the foot segment. In the case discussed here, the force $\mathbf{R}_2$ is directed opposite to the gravitational force of the mass of the foot. (We could have guessed the result for the net force as the foot is freely suspended from the lower leg and only its weight has to be balanced. In contrast, the result for the joint force is not obvious, because it depends on the anatomical architecture of the ankle joint.)

Readers may convince themselves that the result for the joint load of the foot loaded only by gravity and held in equilibrium by activation of the tibialis anterior muscle is exactly analogous to the result obtained above for the elbow joint with gravity acting on the mass held in the hand. If interest had been confined to the load on the ankle joint, it might have been easier to perform a straightforward calculation employing the conditions of equilibrium (as in the case of the elbow) instead of making a detour via reaction forces and moments. If, on the other hand, the movement of the lower leg and the force and moment transmitted from the lower to the upper leg are focuses of interest, knowledge of the reaction force $\mathbf{R}_2$ and the reaction moment M_2 is indispensable. What is not required in this latter case is knowledge of the load (joint force) on the ankle joint.

In addition, the equations show that the load O_y on the ankle joint varies in proportion with the moment M_2. An increase in the moment results in an increased joint load; a decrease results in a decreased joint load. This observation is of general va-

lidity; specifically, it remains valid even if the muscle and/or tendon forces (and their moment arms) generating equilibrium are not known (in other words: if a biomechanical model of the joint is not established). It has to be pointed out, however, that a proportionality between joint loads and transmitted moments is valid only if identical joint positions are compared. If a joint position is changed, the moment arms of the forces may change as well and a comparison of joint loads can no longer be based on the comparison of moments. It is important to keep this restriction in mind when, for reasons of simplification (for example, in ergonomic studies) only the moments of external forces are determined and conclusions on joint loading are based on these moments (with no effort being taken to establish models of the joints).

Case 2: foot with accelerated motion, but not in contact with the floor (Fig. 8.8). The reaction force $\mathbf{R}_1$ and the moment M_1 equal zero as the foot is not in contact with the floor. The linear and angular accelerations are not equal to zero. To determine the proximal reaction force and reaction moment, these accelerations must have been measured, for example from film sequences of the moving foot. By insertion into the equations of motion we obtain

$$R_{2x} = m \cdot a_x$$
$$R_{2y} - m \cdot g = m \cdot a_y$$
$$M_2 + L_1 \cdot R_{2x} + L_2 \cdot R_{2y} = J \cdot \alpha$$

R_{2x} and R_{2y} can be determined from the first two equations; the third equation then permits M_2 to be determined. If the load on the ankle joint were to be determined in this case too, a joint model would have to be established. The muscle or tendon force generating the moment M_2 would then depend on the sense of direction (dorsi- or plantar flexion) of the foot motion. In other words, the model would have to consider either the tibialis anterior or the Achilles tendon and the appertaining moment arms.

Case 3: foot with accelerated motion, at the instant of 'toe off' when walking (Fig. 8.9). In this case the reaction force $\mathbf{R}_1$ is not equal to zero. The components R_{1x} and R_{1y} are required to be available from measurements, for example by means of a force platform (an electronic measuring device recording the forces between foot and floor). A reaction moment M_1 is not transmitted as long as the foot does not stick to the floor (usually not the case). After insertion in the equations of motion we obtain

$$R_{1x} + R_{2x} = m \cdot a_x$$
$$R_{1y} + R_{2y} - m \cdot g = m \cdot a_y$$
$$M_2 + L_1 \cdot R_{2x} - L_3 \cdot R_{1x} + L_2 \cdot R_{2y} - L_4 \cdot R_{1y} = J \cdot \alpha$$

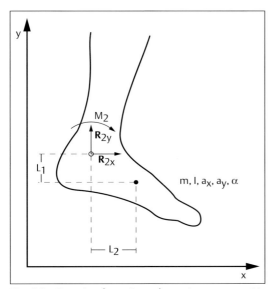

Fig. 8.**8** Reaction force **R**$_2$ and reaction moment M$_2$ transmitted from the lower leg onto the moving foot. **a** designates the linear acceleration of the center of gravity; α designates the angular acceleration around the center of gravity. There is no contact between the foot and the floor, i.e. no forces or moments are transmitted from the floor on to the foot. Other designations as in Fig. 8.**6**.

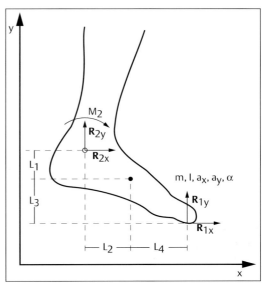

Fig. 8.**9** Reaction force **R**$_2$ and reaction moment M$_2$ transmitted from the lower leg on to the moving foot as well as reaction force **R**$_1$ transmitted from the floor on to the foot. L$_3$ and L$_4$ are the moment arms of the components of the force **R**$_1$ acting at the tip of the foot in relation to the center of gravity of the foot. Other designations as in Fig. 8.**6**.

The moments are, as always, related to the center of gravity of the foot. The minus sign of the moments of the forces R_{1x} and R_{1y} follows from their counterclockwise sense of rotation according to the sign convention for moments. R_{2x} and R_{2y} can be determined from the first two equations; the third equation then permits M$_2$ to be determined.

The case discussed here in detail is the first step taken in determining forces at the knee and hip joint in gait analysis. The moment and the force transmitted from the foot to the lower leg are (for reasons of equilibrium) of equal magnitude and opposite to the moment and force exerted from the lower leg on to the foot. If mass, location of the center of gravity, moment of inertia, and linear as well as rotational acceleration of the lower leg are known, force and moment transmitted from the upper leg to the lower leg can be determined. If points of insertion as well as the directions of muscles and tendons crossing the knee joint are known, the load on the knee joint can be calculated. If measurements and calculations are extended one segment farther into cranial direction, the load on the hip joint can be determined.

Difficulties in determining joint loads in the dynamic case (i.e. with accelerated motion) arise from an inaccurate knowledge of mass, center of gravity, and moment of inertia of the body segments. In reality, segments are not rigid (in contrast to what has been assumed). From sequences of film or video images, the momentary locations of the centers of mass and the centers of rotation (axes of rotation) can be measured only with limited accuracy. The underlying reason is that the location of these centers cannot be measured directly but only via external markers placed on the skin (see, for example, de Leva, 1996). During movements, the markers may perform inadvertent motions due to the deformation of the skin. Determination of acceleration has to be based on the processing of the temporal change of the location of the markers. In practice, this poses considerable instrumental and computational problems. To determine joint loads, the active muscles and their moment arms must be known. If more than one muscle is active at a given instant of time, an approximate solution must be searched for. Alternatively, additional assumptions on the co-activation of several muscles must be put forward in order to find an unequivocal solution (see below).

Determination of joint loads is, of course, not the only aim of gait analysis. As the temporal course of the ground reaction force and of the location (and, derived from this, of the linear and angular velocity and acceleration) of the thigh, the lower leg, and the foot are recorded, a variety of parameters characterizing individual gait is usually inspected. Stride frequency (cadence), duration of the stance phase and stride length are derived from the temporal course and the points of application of the force between foot and floor. Hip, knee, and ankle joint range of motion (ROM) and the relative angular motions of thigh, lower leg, and foot are derived from the temporal course of the measured lower extremity positions. For each joint, the product of the transmitted moment and the angular velocity equals the power. Depending on the positive or negative sign of the power (cf. Chapter 13), this power must be generated or absorbed by the muscles crossing the joint. In the case of one-sided injury or postoperative monitoring, gait parameters of one leg may be compared with those of the other leg. Alternatively, one may try to detect gait abnormalities by comparison with gender- and age-appropriate normal values.

Determination of the joint force if more than one muscle or ligament force has to be taken into account

If more than one single muscle or ligament force has to be taken into account, the two conditions of static or dynamic equilibrium do not suffice to determine all unknowns. In this case we have an 'indeterminate' mechanical system. For an indeterminate system there are usually many possible solutions. Additional information and/or selection criteria are required to choose one such solution.

In principle, indeterminate systems are familiar from everyday life. If, for example, a patient attends a practice run by three therapists, several possible solutions exist for his problem. The patient could be treated by one of the three therapists or he might be referred to another practice or clinic. To arrive at an unequivocal solution, additional information is required. How is the practice organized? Do the therapists always accept patients in turn? What are the patient's symptoms? Do the therapists specialize in specific diagnostic procedures or treatments? Only with such additional information is it possible to predict unequivocally what is going to happen with the patient.

If several muscles are available in the region of a joint that could, in principle, generate the required moment, our locomotor system has to decide which muscle(s) will be activated. Unfortunately, the underlying strategy is not known. Will only that muscle with the largest moment arm be activated? Only the strongest muscle? Only the muscle with the highest resistance to fatigue? Will all muscles be activated? If so, what proportion of the required moment is generated by the individual muscles? How do muscles 'communicate' with one another in order to decide on how to share the required moment?

To reach solutions in biomechanical model calculations despite this (admittedly) substantial gap in our knowledge, different paths are followed. By means of EMG measurements it is possible to document whether or not muscles are active. Using this method, the number of muscles to be taken into account can, at least for some phases of a movement, be reduced to one. Some investigators calibrate the amplitude of the measured EMG signal in individual subjects against the isometric muscle force. These calibration values are then introduced in the model calculation together with correction factors taking account of muscle length change and contraction velocity. Alternatively, various hypotheses on how a set of muscles shares the generation of the required moment have been put forward. The hypotheses are supported by convincing and plausible arguments but with no ultimate proof. These different approaches are outlined below. A competent and critical discussion of this complex problem can be found in Glitsch (1992) and in Glitsch and Baumann (1997).

Reduction of the number of muscles through measurement of muscle activity. If, in principle, several muscles might participate in the generation of the required moment, measuring the muscle activity by EMG may serve to decide in fact whether all these muscles are active in a given phase of the movement under investigation. If only one muscle proves to remain active at certain instants of time or, alternatively, if forces from small muscles are negligible so that only one active muscle remains, the indeterminate system is reduced to a determinate system and an unequivocal solution is feasible. This procedure was applied in the first experiments aimed at determining the load on the joints of the lower extremity from gait analysis. In his pioneering work on the loading of the knee joint when walking, Morrison (1968) assumed that at each phase of the movement either only the flexor or the extensor muscles (treated as one muscle in each case) were active; forces in the ligaments were ignored.

EMG-supported model calculation. EMG-supported model calculations are based on muscle force data derived from electromyographic measurements. For this purpose, a relation between the EMG signal and the muscle forces has first to be established. In a posture where only one single muscle is loaded isometrically, the amplitude of the EMG signal can be calibrated against the moment and (with knowledge of the moment arm) the force of the muscle in an individual test subject. In subsequent postures or movements the EMG signal is recorded; the calibration procedure then yields the muscle force (see, for example, Dolan and Adams, 1998). The difficulty is that only in rare cases is it possible to load a single muscle isometrically in order to perform the required calibration. In each case, correction factors taking account of changes in muscle length or contraction velocity have to be introduced into the model calculation because length change and contraction velocity influence the relation between EMG amplitude and force. (Performing a calibration valid from the very outset for all possible muscle lengths and contraction velocities is a virtual impossibility.) EMG-supported model calculations claim to have the advantage that individual activation patterns can be taken into account. This advantage, however, is not valid for the more deeply located muscles, as their EMG cannot be reliably recorded by surface electrodes.

Alternatively, muscle cross-sectional areas are measured from magnetic resonance (MR) images and the amplitude of the EMG signal, as well as the muscle force, are assumed to be proportional to the cross sectional area (see, for example, Granata and Marras, 1993). Measuring muscle cross sections by MR is not as easy as it may appear on first sight but a difficult problem, because cross sections change with posture; furthermore cross-sectional areas differ *in vitro* and *in vivo* (see, for example, Gatton *et al.*, 1999). The factor by which a given signal amplitude for a given cross section of the muscle can be converted into the muscle force is known only imprecisely and may vary inter-individually. Furthermore, such a factor will probably depend on the muscle length and contraction velocity. Because of these uncertainties EMG-supported model calculations require validation by additional, independent experiments.

Hypotheses on the co-activation of several muscles. Mathematically, the solution of a set of equations containing more unknowns than the number of equations is indeterminate. Introducing additional assumptions or constraints (optimization) allows a unique solution to be enforced. The constraint may imply selection, from the range of pos-

sible solutions, of one single solution for which a specified function ('cost function' or 'objective function') takes an extreme (maximum or minimum) value. It might, for example, be assumed that muscles generate force in such a way that the joint load is minimized. It would follow from this assumption that only the muscles with the largest moment arm were active at any given time while all other muscles with smaller moment arms were inactive. Experience shows that this assumption (sensible though it may seem) is not compatible with physiological observations and EMG measurements.

Alternatively, it can be assumed that the sum of the squares of the muscle stresses or the sum of the muscle stresses raised to the third power will take a minimum value. Muscle stress is defined as the muscle force divided by the cross-sectional area of the muscle. To start with, these assumptions are only mathematical tricks aimed at enforcing an unequivocal solution to the equations of static equilibrium or the equations of motion. To justify the assumptions, sensible, but in no way compelling, arguments are put forward. If the sum of the squares of the muscle stresses takes a minimum value, this will result in the stress being distributed evenly over all muscles in question (the proof of this contention is not presented here). If the sum of the muscle stresses raised to the third power takes a minimum value, this will result in high muscle forces, which may lead to rapid fatigue, being avoided (contention again presented without proof). However, other task-specific strategies for the cooperation of several muscles are conceivable. The activation of muscles in an injured leg, for example, may be quite different from the activation pattern during athletic running.

If a choice between various hypotheses remains after exclusion of the obviously incorrect hypotheses, an attempt can be made to compare the results of model calculations performed under different assumptions with each other or with measured data of joint loading. Such a study has been performed by Glitsch and Baumann (1997) for the lower extremity. The authors showed that results for joint loads obtained under different assumptions exhibited only minor differences. Compared with data on the load of the hip joint measured *in vivo*, the calculations produced relatively high joint loads. For the knee joint, comparison of calculated and measured data was not possible as no experiments *in vivo* with instrumented knee joint replacements had yet been published. According to the authors the (already complex) biomechanical model of the lower extremity needs further refinement.

In conclusion, not being able to decide which objective function to chose for a particular type of motion merely reflects our fragmentary knowledge of the underlying strategy of the neuromuscular control system. There is no doubt that our control system always adheres to a specific strategy (see, for example, Hatze, 1980). In other words, for any intended motion or posture, our control system does not have to solve the mathematically indeterminate problem which muscles, out of a number of potential contributors, to activate in a specific situation. In reality, there exists no indeterminacy problem.

Literature

Text and reference books

Chaffin DB, Andersson GBJ, Martin BJ. *Occupational biomechanics.* 3rd edition. New York: Wiley; 1999

Glitsch U. *Einsatz verschiedener Optimierungsansätze zur komplexen Belastungsanalyse der unteren Extremität.* Dissertation. Köln: Deutsche Sporthochschule; 1992

Pheasant S. *Bodyspace. Anthropometry, Ergonomics and Design.* 1st edition, London: Taylor and Francis; 1986

Winter DA. *Biomechanics and motor control of human movement.* 2nd edition. New York: Wiley; 1990

Scientific papers cited in the text or the figures

de Leva P. Joint center longitudinal positions computed from a selected subset of Chandler's data. *J Biomechanics.* 1996; **29**: 1231–1233

Dolan P, Adams MA. Repetitive lifting tasks fatigue the back muscles and increase the bending moment acting on the lumbar spine. *J Biomechanics.* 1998; **31**: 713–721

Gatton ML, Pearcy MJ, Pettet GJ. Difficulties in estimating muscle forces from muscle cross-sectional area. An example using the psoas major muscle. *Spine* 1999; **24**: 1487–1493

Glitsch U, Baumann W. The three-dimensional determination of internal loads in the lower extremity. *J Biomechanics.* 1997; **30**: 1123–1131

Granata KP, Marras WS. An EMG-assisted model of loads on the lumbar spine during asymmetric trunk exertions. *J Biomechanics.* 1993; **26**: 1429–1438

Hatze H. Neuromusculoskeletal control systems modeling – a critical survey of recent developments. *IEEE Transactions on Automatic Control.* 1980; **AC-25**(3): 375–385

Jensen RK. Body segment mass, radius and radius of gyration proportions of children. *J Biomechanics.* 1986; **19**: 359–368

Morrison JB. *Bioengineering analysis of force actions transmitted by the knee joint.* Biomed Engng. 1968; 3: 164–170

9 Mechanical Aspects of the Hip Joint

Peak values of the load on the hip joint, corresponding to a multiple of the weight of the whole body, occur at every step in the heel-on and toe-off phases. Healthy subjects perform between one hundred thousand and several million steps per year. The hip joint seems to be adapted to this high, repetitive loading. Even in old age the function of the hip joint is only slightly restricted, if at all, in the majority of people. This finding is not inconsistent with the fact that an age-related alteration ('degeneration') of the joint cartilage as well as changes in bone density and trabecular architecture can be regularly observed. Only in a minority of subjects are severe alterations, leading to clinical symptoms and a restriction of joint function, encountered.

If the geometry of the femoral head and acetabulum shows major deviations from the normal shape (as, for example, in dysplastic hips), destruction of the hip joint can be observed, even in young subjects. This experience, together with knowledge of the high load and the high load-cycle numbers, supports the conjecture that primary mechanical factors may cause, or at least exacerbate, the progress of the arthrosis of this joint.

The interest in mechanical aspects of the hip joint has been substantially encouraged by the pioneering work of Pauwels (1980). Following the work of Pauwels, Roesler and Hamacher (1972) and Debrunner (1975) this chapter outlines how to determine the load on the hip joint in the stance phase of slow gait by means of a biomechanical model calculation. Within the framework of this model the question of how the joint load may be influenced by gait technique, walking aids, or surgical interventions is discussed.

Studies determining the stress distribution on the surface of the hip joint by way of calculation or by experiment are reviewed. The procedure followed in the case of the hip joint may also serve as an example on which to base calculations for other joints.

If the measured linear and angular accelerations of the body segments are introduced into a dynamic model calculation, the load on the hip joint during the full gait cycle can be established. Important new information, independent of model calculations, has recently been collected from measurement *in vivo* of the hip joint load by means of instrumented joint replacements.

Load on the hip joint in the stance phase of slow gait

The load on the hip joint is analyzed in the stance phase of slow gait on the basis of the concept that this phase is representative of typical everyday activities. In the stance phase, one foot is on the floor while the other is lifted off the floor with the leg

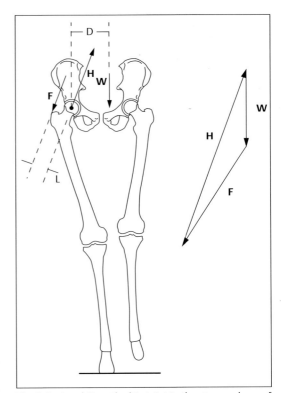

Fig. 9.1 Load **H** on the hip joint in the stance phase of slow gait. The model calculation is based on the condition of equilibrium of the pelvis. The gravitational force **W**, the force of the abductor muscles **F**, and the force **H** transmitted from the femoral head on to the acetabulum act on the pelvis. L denotes the moment arm of the abductor muscles. The forces of other muscles or ligaments crossing the hip joint and contributions from inertial forces of the body segments are disregarded. In equilibrium, the vector sum of **W**, **F**, and **H** equals zero.

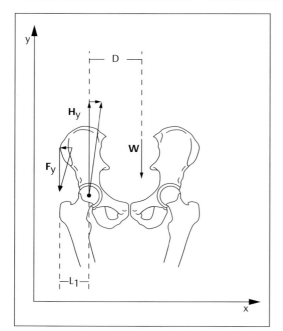

Fig. 9.**2**   Calculation of the y-components **F**$_y$ and **H**$_y$ of the forces **F** and **H** in mechanical equilibrium. D designates the moment arm of the gravitational force **W**$_y$, L$_1$ designates the moment arm of the muscle force **F**$_y$.

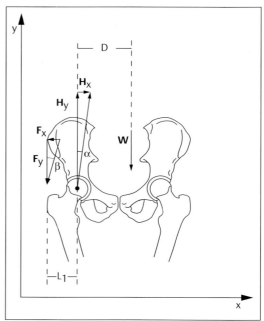

Fig. 9.**3**   With knowledge of the direction of the force **F** (angle β with respect to the y-axis) and knowledge of **F**$_y$, the component **F**$_x$ can be obtained. In equilibrium the component **H**$_x$ of the hip joint load is of equal magnitude and directed opposite to **F**$_x$. From |**H**$_x$| and |**H**$_y$| the angle α of the load vector with respect to the vertical can be calculated. In the stance phase of slow gait the angle α is approximately 10°.

being swung forward through the frontal plane. The designation 'slow' indicates that inertial forces, resulting from slowing down and accelerating the body segments during each step, are negligible.

The model calculation (Fig. 9.**1**) takes into account only forces in the frontal plane. Three forces are assumed to act on the pelvis. **W** is the gravitational force ('weight') of the body mass less the mass of the standing leg. The point of force application is the center of gravity of the body less the standing leg, i.e. the center of gravity of head, arms, trunk, and swinging leg. The gravitational force points vertically downward. **F** is the force of the abductor muscles, which balance the moment of the gravitational force. The vector **F** represents the forces of all muscles that may effect an abduction of the stance leg. **F** closely approximates the force developed by the gluteus medius muscle. The points of force application of **F** are the centers of the insertion areas of the gluteus medius at the iliac bone and at the major trochanter. All additional muscle forces that may be active in stabilizing the hip joint during the stance phase with respect to flexion and extension are disregarded. The hip joint is assumed to be a perfect ball-and-socket joint. In a friction-free ball-and-socket joint the axis of ro-

tation runs through the center of the joint. Thus, the joint force **H** acting from the femoral head on to the acetabulum, runs through the center of the femoral head.

With knowledge of i) the magnitude of **W**, ii) the position of the center of gravity of the body (regardless of the standing leg) and iii) the direction and points of application of the muscle force **F**, the magnitude of **F** can be obtained from the equilibrium condition of moments. The equilibrium condition of forces requires the vector sum of **W**, **F**, and **H** to be equal to zero. As result the direction and magnitude of **H** can be determined unequivocally (Fig. 9.**1**).

To determine **H**, it is advantageous to determine the components **H**$_x$ and **H**$_y$ separately (Figs 9.**2** and 9.**3**). The coordinate system is oriented so that the x-axis points into the horizontal and the y-axis into the vertical direction. Since the gravitational force **W** is vertically, and the muscle force **F** almost vertically, aligned, we expect the load on the hip joint to be determined essentially by the y-components of these forces; the x-components will make only a small, additional contribution.

To obtain an estimate for the gravitational force **W**, we assume the mass of one leg to equal approximately 20% of the body mass. Under this assumption, we obtain for the magnitude of the y-component of the gravitational force

$$|\mathbf{W}_y| = 0.8 \cdot \text{body mass} \cdot \text{gravitational acceleration}$$
$$= 0.8 \cdot m \cdot g$$

In good approximation, the center of gravity of the whole body is positioned above the symphysis (as the architecture of our body is, broadly, right-left symmetrical). The center of gravity of the body regardless of the standing leg is shifted to the side of the swinging leg. For the relationship between the moment arm D of the gravitational force and the moment arm L_1 of the y-component of the muscle force we assume

$$D = 2.0 \cdot L_1$$

Under these assumptions (and in accordance with the sign convention for moments) in the equilibrium of moments we obtain

$$-L_1 \cdot |\mathbf{F}_y| + D \cdot |\mathbf{W}| = 0$$
$$|\mathbf{F}_y| = 2.0 \cdot |\mathbf{W}_y|$$

In the equilibrium of forces it holds for the y-components that

$$H_y + F_y + W_y = 0$$

The addends in this equation (as well as in those that follow) that are derived from the equilibrium condition of forces, are positive or negative numbers. The numbers denote the magnitude and the sense of direction of the forces. (In precise mathematical language, these numbers represent the y-coordinates of the forces. It has, however, become a habit to use the term 'component' synonymously, c.f. Chapter 3 on vector algebra.)

Since both $\mathbf{F}_y$ and $\mathbf{W}_y$ point in the same direction, it follows from the equilibrium condition of moments for the components that

$$F_y = 2.0 \cdot W_y$$

After insertion into the equilibrium condition of forces we obtain

$$H_y = -F_y - W_y$$
$$H_y = -2.0 \cdot W_y - W_y$$
$$H_y = -3.0 \cdot W_y$$

$\mathbf{W}_y$ points in the negative y-direction. As $W_y = -0.8 \cdot m \cdot g$ we obtain by insertion

$$H_y = 2.4 \cdot m \cdot g$$

In other words: the y-component of the force transmitted from the femoral head on to the acetabulum has a magnitude 2.4 times the gravitational force of the whole body. The positive value of H_y indicates that this force points in the positive y-direction; the femoral head exerts a compressive force on the acetabulum.

In equilibrium it follows from the equilibrium condition of forces for the x-components of the muscle force and the joint force (Fig. 9.**3**) that

$$H_x + F_x = 0$$

This equation contains only two addends as the x-component of the gravitational force equals zero. With β as the angle between the vertical and the direction of the force **F** of the abductor muscles, we obtain for the x-component F_x of the muscle force

$$F_x = F_y \cdot \tan\beta$$

and with $F_y = 2.0 \cdot W_y$ we obtain

$$H_x = -F_y \cdot \tan\beta$$
$$H_x = 2.0 \cdot 0.8 \cdot m \cdot g \cdot \tan\beta$$
$$H_x = 1.6 \cdot m \cdot g \cdot \tan\beta$$

Based on anatomical measurements, the angle β is approximately 15°; the tangent of 15° is 0.27. Thus H_x is much smaller than H_y. With knowledge of H_x and H_y the magnitude H of the total joint load can be calculated

$$H = \sqrt{H_x^2 + H_y^2}$$

The angle α between the vector of the hip joint load and the vertical is determined from

$$\tan\alpha = H_x/H_y$$
$$\tan\alpha = 0.27 \cdot 2 \cdot W_y/3 \cdot W_y$$
$$\alpha = 10.2°$$

This shows that, in the stance phase of slow gait, the vector of the hip joint load is not oriented vertically but at an angle of approximately 10° to the vertical.

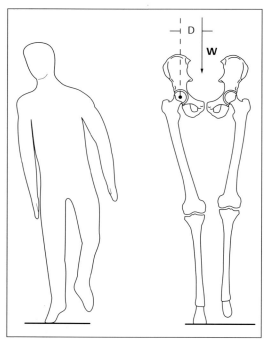

Fig. 9.**4** Effect of the Duchenne limp on the loading of the hip joint. Shifting the body mass to the side of the standing leg decreases the moment arm of the gravitational force **W**. Consequently the muscle force required for equilibrium decreases as well. Due to the decrease in muscle force, the load on the hip joint decreases.

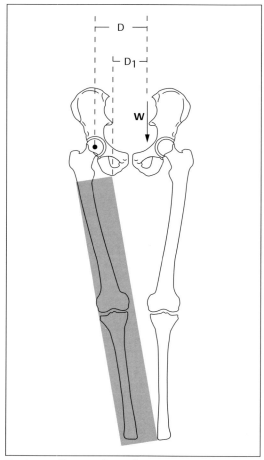

Fig. 9.**5** Influence of an orthosis on the load on the hip joint. The orthosis shifts the center of rotation from the center of the femoral head to the point of support at the tuber ischiadicum. This shift decreases the moment arm of the gravitational force **W** from D to D1. Due to the changed moment arm, the muscle force, and hence the joint load, decrease as well.

Influencing the load on the hip joint by gait technique, walking aids, or surgical interventions

The load on the hip joint can be influenced by changing the moment arm of the gravitational force, by changing the moment arm of the abductor muscle, or by using walking aids.

Gait technique. A gait anomaly termed 'Duchenne limp' is illustrated in Fig. 9.**4**. In this type of gait, the center of gravity of the body is shifted to the side of the standing leg. This shift reduces the moment arm D of the gravitational force. Consequently the force of the abductor muscles required for equilibrium will decrease. This results in a decrease of the load on the hip joint. The Duchenne limp is, however, unsuitable for long-term reduction in load on the hip joint because the accompanying bending of the lumbar spine to the side cannot be tolerated over long periods.

Orthosis. The load on the hip joint can be diminished by employing an orthosis that provides a support at the tuber ischiadicum and below the heel (Fig. 9.**5**). The reduced loading of the hip joint when wearing the orthosis is due to the center of rotation, in effect, being shifted from the center of the femoral head to the location of the support at the tuber ischiadicum. This shortens the moment arm of the body weight from D to D_1 and consequently reduces the muscle force required for the equilibrium of moments. This, in turn, leads to a reduction in joint force. If the orthosis is not correctly fitted by the technician (or is not correctly worn by the patient due to discomfort) so that the support is not provided at the tuber ischiadicum, no unloading of the hip joint will result.

Cane. A cane employed contralaterally effects a decrease of the hip joint force. For reasons of brevity we consider here only the y-component of the joint force, again in the stance phase of slow gait (Fig. 9.**6**). **S** designates the force from the cane on to the hand. S_y is the y-component of this force; it points in the positive y-direction. The assumptions on the magnitude $|W_y|$ and the moment arm D of the gravitational force remain unchanged:

$$|W_y| = 0.8 \cdot m \cdot g$$
$$D = 2.0 \cdot L_1$$

In addition, we assume the moment arm E of the cane to be 4 times the moment arm of the abductor muscle

$$E = 4.0 \cdot L_1$$

With these assumptions we obtain from the equilibrium condition of moments (in accordance with the sign convention for moments)

$$-L_1 \cdot |F_y| + D \cdot |W_y| - E \cdot |S_y| = 0$$
$$|F_y| = 2.0 \cdot |W_y| - 4.0 \cdot |S_y|$$

Using a cane reduces the magnitude of the abductor muscle force by an amount equal to four times the force $|S_y|$ between the cane and the hand. In equilibrium it holds for the y-components of the forces that

$$H_y + F_y + W_y + S_y = 0$$

The addends in this equation are positive or negative numbers that designate the magnitude and sense of direction of the forces (in precise terms, these numbers are the y-coordinates of the force vectors). As W_y and S_y point in opposite directions (W_y being negative and S_y positive), we re-formulate the above result obtained from the equilibrium condition of moments as

$$F_y = 2.0 \cdot W_y + 4.0 \cdot S_y$$

It then follows for H_y that

$$H_y = -F_y - W_y - S_y$$
$$H_y = -2.0 \cdot W_y - 4.0 \cdot S_y - W_y - S_y$$
$$H_y = -3.0 \cdot W_y - 5.0 \cdot S_y$$

and with insertion of $W_y = -0.8 \cdot m \cdot g$

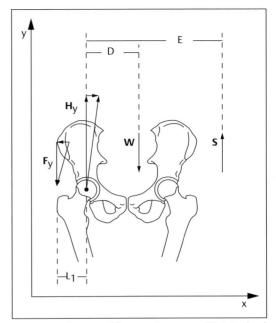

Fig. 9.6 Influence of the use of a cane on hip joint load in the stance phase of slow gait; (only the y-components of the forces are discussed). **S** designates the force from the cane on the hand, E designates the moment arm of the force **S**, other designations as in Fig. 9.2. The moment of the force **S** is opposite to the moment of the gravitational force **W**. The muscle force F_y required for equilibrium is thus reduced; in consequence the hip joint load H_y is reduced.

$$H_y = 2.4 \cdot m \cdot g - 5.0 \cdot S_y$$

Using the cane reduces the y-component of the force on the hip joint by an amount equal to five times the force S_y between cane and hand. The effect can be illustrated with an example. Given a body mass of 60 kg, the gravitational force m·g amounts to 600 N (rounded). The y-component of the force on the hip joint then amounts to

$$H_y = 2.4 \cdot m \cdot g = 2.4 \cdot 600 = 1440 \text{ N}$$

Using a cane and assuming a force of $S_y = +50$ N between hand and cane we obtain

$$H_y = 1440 - 5 \cdot S_y = 1440 - 250 = 1190 \text{ N}$$

Using the cane reduces the joint load by about 20 %. It must be stressed that the reduction in joint load can be achieved only if the cane is used contralaterally to the hip joint in question. Using the cane ipsilaterally would increase the load on the hip joint. Alternatively, a reduction in body mass might be considered in order to decrease the joint load. In principle this is a valid idea as the joint load H_y depends directly on the body mass m. To achieve a reduction in load comparable to that when a cane is used, the body mass must be reduced by approximately 20 %. In many cases this will probably be very difficult to achieve.

Surgical intervention. Surgical interventions can alter the geometry of the bony skeleton and thus change the moment arms of muscles. Fig. 9.**7** shows the example of a varization osteotomy, where a bone wedge is excised from the intertrochanteric region. Geometrically this intervention effects a decrease in the angle between the femoral neck and the femur and lateralization of the major trochanter. Postoperatively the moment arm L_1 of the abductor muscle can be about 15 % larger than the preoperative moment arm L. Due to the larger

moment arm a smaller muscle force is required in equilibrium; due to the smaller muscle force the joint force decreases accordingly.

The surgical intervention has further effects which, however, do not lend themselves readily to quantitative calculations. In addition to the change in moment arm length, the length of the psoas muscle is decreased postoperatively. The reduced elastic tension of this muscle effects a further decrease in the load on the hip joint. For a quantitative statement of this load reduction, the passive stiffness of this muscle is required; this is known only very imprecisely. In addition, the surgical intervention shifts the loaded area of the articular surface of the femoral head. That part of the joint surface which was under the highest pressure preoperatively (see the section below on determination of the stress distribution on the surface of hip joint) is rotated in a clockwise direction into a zone of lower pressure.

Determination of the load on the hip joint by gait analysis

If accelerated linear or rotational motions of the body segments occur, influences of inertial forces and inertial moments must be taken into account when determining the load on the hip joint. To illustrate the effect of inertial forces, we start by discussing a simple example. The posture shown in Fig. 9.**8** is not to be interpreted as the stance phase in slow gait but as the posture assumed when hitting the ground vertically after jumping from a low wall. On landing the velocity of the body mass cranial to the hip joint must be slowed down (decelerated) from its initial value to zero. a designates the magnitude of the acceleration involved. The magnitude of the inertial force $\mathbf{F}_{in}$ amounts to

$$|\mathbf{F}_{in}| = 0.8 \cdot m \cdot a$$

When hitting the ground, the velocity points in the negative y-direction; the acceleration (the change in velocity) points into the positive y-direction. The inertial $\mathbf{F}_{in}$ force is opposite to the acceleration and thus in the negative y-direction, i.e. in the same direction as the gravitational force of the body mass.

The load on the hip joint can now be determined using formulae similar to those in the stance phase of slow gait. The only difference is that instead of the gravitational force $\mathbf{W}_y$ the sum of gravitational and inertial force has to be inserted. This sum is designated by $\mathbf{W}^*$

$$|\mathbf{W}^*| = 0.8 \cdot m \cdot (g + a)$$

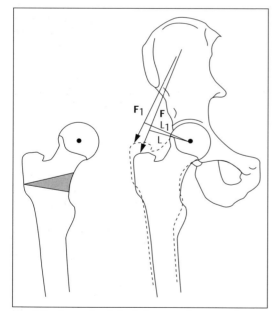

Fig. 9.7   Example of the influence of a surgical intervention on the load on the hip joint. Removal of a wedge between the major and minor trochanter (intertrochanteric varization osteotomy) effects a lateralization of the major trochanter and an increase of the moment arm of the abductor muscles from L to L_1. The muscle force required for equilibrium decreases from the preoperative value $|\mathbf{F}|$ to the postoperative $|\mathbf{F}_1|$. Due to the decrease of the muscle force the hip joint load decreases as well.

For the magnitude of the y-component $\mathbf{H}_y$ of the force on the hip joint we obtain

$$|\mathbf{H}_y| = 2.4 \cdot m \cdot (g + a)$$

In this example the inertial force acts as if the body weight were momentarily increased by an amount equal to $2.4 \cdot m \cdot a$. The numerical value of this increase depends on the magnitude of the acceleration a. If the change from the initial velocity to zero takes place in a short time interval (for example when landing with the legs straight), the acceleration will have a high value. If the change in velocity can be extended over a longer time interval (for example by bending the knees and thus providing a soft impact), the acceleration will assume a lower value.

Following the procedure outlined in Chapter 8, the load on the hip joint when walking or running can be determined in a model calculation if anthropometric data of the test person are known and kinematic (motion-related) as well as kinetic (force-related) data are recorded during the gait cycle. Gait analysis based on model calculations has provided new and important information going substantially beyond the knowledge derived from static analysis of the stance phase in slow gait. Due to the technical and mathematical complexities a comprehensive description of the fundamentals and results of gait analysis is beyond the scope of this book. In what follows, the principle of the procedure is outlined; for details the reader is referred to the original publications. For an overview of recent publications see, for example, Bergmann (1997) and Novacheck (1998).

In the dynamic case, the load on the hip joint can be determined if the body is modeled as a chain of segments linked by hinge or ball-and-socket joints. The segments are: feet, lower legs, upper legs, trunk, arms, and head. The standing leg is modeled as a free body (Fig. 9.**9**). Two approaches to determination of the load on the hip joint are feasible. The ground reaction force $\mathbf{R}_{1F}$ and the linear and angular accelerations of the foot, lower and upper leg segments of the standing leg can be measured. With this knowledge it is possible to determine at each instant in time i) force and moment transmitted from the lower leg to the foot, ii) force and moment transmitted from the upper to the lower leg, and iii) force $\mathbf{R}_{2H}$ and moment M_{2H} transmitted from the trunk to the upper leg. Alternatively, the accelerations of head, trunk, arms, and the swinging leg could be measured and the force $-\mathbf{R}_{2H}$ and the moment $-M_{2H}$ determined. Usually the first approach is followed because the anthropometric data (masses, moments of inertia etc.) of the segments of the lower extremity are known with high-

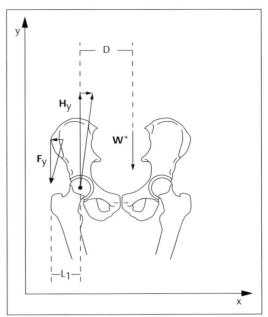

Fig. 9.8 If the body is accelerated in vertical direction, for example during the landing phase after jumping from a low wall, an inertial force acts in addition to the gravitational force. The load on the hip joint can be estimated using the same formulae as in the stance phase of slow gait if the gravitational force **W** is replaced by the force **W***, with **W*** being the sum of gravitational and inertial force. The inertial force, and thus the load on the hip joint, depend on the magnitude of the acceleration.

er precision compared with the respective data for head, arms, and trunk, and because accelerations of only three instead of five segments have to be measured and processed.

In detail, if the first approach is chosen, the input data for a calculation based on the observation of the segment chain foot–lower leg–upper leg are (Winter, 1990):

– mass, location of the center of gravity, moment of inertia in relation to the center of gravity for the foot, lower leg, and upper leg segments. Masses, locations of the centers of gravity, and moments of inertia have been determined in previous studies both *in vitro* or *in vivo*. (See, for example, Pheasant, 1986; Winter, 1990; Chaffin and co-workers, 1999.)

– the temporal course of the linear accelerations of the centers of gravity of the segments and the angular accelerations of the segments in relation to their centers of gravity. The temporal course

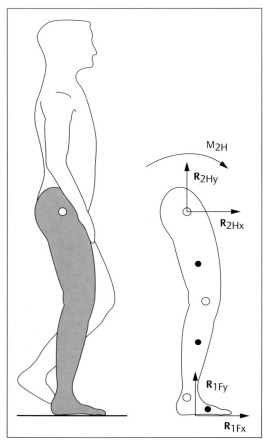

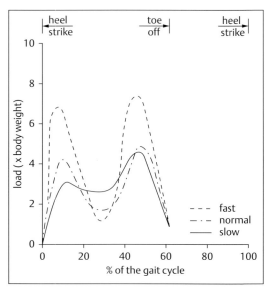

Fig. 9.**10** Load on the hip joint in relation to gait velocity. The interval from 0 % to 100 % designates one full gait cycle. (Adapted from Paul, 1976.)

Fig. 9.**9** Determination of the load on the hip joint from gait analysis. The lower extremity is regarded as a free body. Proximally the reaction force $\mathbf{R}_{2H}$ and the reaction moment M_{2H} and distally the reaction force $\mathbf{R}_{1F}$ act on this body. The lower extremity is subdivided into the segments foot, lower leg, and upper leg, interlinked by hinge joints. The reaction force $\mathbf{R}_{1F}$ as well as the linear and angular accelerations (related to the centers of gravity, solid circles) are measured. From these measured data, together with anthropometric data, $\mathbf{R}_{2H}$ and M_{2H} can be calculated. With knowledge of $\mathbf{R}_{2H}$ and M_{2H} together with a model of the hip joint, describing the geometry of the joint and the lines of action of the relevant muscles, the load on the hip joint can be calculated.

With knowledge of the force $\mathbf{R}_{1F}$ and based on the equations of motion (see Chapter 8) the first step of the calculation determines (at each point in time of the gait cycle) the force and the moment acting proximally on the foot segment. Thus, the force and the moment acting distally on the lower leg segment are known as well. (Force and moment from the foot on to the lower leg are of equal magnitude and opposing direction to the force and moment from the lower leg on to the foot.) The second step of the calculation determines force and moment acting proximally on the lower leg segment. The third step of the calculation determines force $\mathbf{R}_{2H}$ and moment M_{2H} acting proximally on the upper leg segment.

To ascertain the load on the hip joint, the muscle force required to produce the moment M_{2H} must be determined. For this purpose a model of the hip joint is to be established describing the geometry of the joint and the lines of action of the relevant muscles in a realistic fashion. In this model, the moment arms of the muscles are determined from anatomical measurements. If several muscles that might deliver the moment M_{2H} are active at a given instant in time, an unequivocal solution can be obtained only with additional assumptions on the co-activation of these muscles. Alternatively, an attempt can be made to arrive at an approximate solution by considering only one single muscle. In that case it is sensible

of the motion can, for example, be measured from film or video sequences.
- the temporal course of the reaction force $\mathbf{R}_{1F}$ exerted from the floor on to the foot. This is usually measured by means of a force platform (an electronic device for measuring forces) let into the floor.

to choose the muscle with the largest force capacity while disregarding potential contributions from other muscles.

Following the procedure outlined above, Paul (1967, 1976) and Morrison (1968) pioneered the publication of data on the load on the hip joint when walking. Fig. 9.**10** shows the load on the hip joint in relation to the velocity of gait (Paul, 1976). Maximum values of the joint load during heel-strike and toe-off are immediately noted. These peak loads are caused by the deceleration of the body following heel-strike and the acceleration in the toe-off phase. The peak loads rise with increasing gait velocity. At higher gait velocity, peak values of hip joint loading reach up to 8 times body weight.

The peak loading of the hip joint at higher gait velocity suggests that anyone with incipient or advanced osteoporosis should be advised against fast walking, running, or jogging. In these people it can be taken for granted that the trabecular bone below the joint surfaces of the acetabulum and femoral head will exhibit diminished strength. High peak loading of the joint might then lead to overload damage to the joint.

Measurement of the load on the hip joint by instrumented joint replacement

If an artificial hip joint replacement is equipped with force transducers (electronic devices for measuring forces) and the transducer signals are transmitted telemetrically to the outside of the body, the load on the hip joint *in vivo* can be determined directly, free from the numerous restrictions that have to be considered in model calculations. Interpretation of the measured data requires no theoretical assumptions on the co-activation of the muscles crossing the joint. Specifically, antagonistic muscle activity does not have to be excluded. Contributions to the joint load originating from the elastic tension of muscles, tendons or joint capsules are automatically included in the measured results.

Bergmann and co-workers (1989, 1997, 2001) published comprehensive data on the loading of the hip joint, measured by means of instrumented hip joint replacements in a wide range of activities. The outstanding work of these authors provided, for the first time, hip joint load data for postures and movements inaccessible for model calculations. In addition, it allowed comparison of direct measurements of the joint force with the results from model calculations. The outcome is of great significance to future developments in the field of hip joint replacement and to a deeper understanding of bone remodeling in the vicinity of implants. In addition, it allows suggestions of practical importance to the postoperative treatment of patients with artificial hip joints to be made. The development of instrumented joint replacements proved to be a technically demanding problem. As the insertion of such prostheses is not a routine procedure, measurements are confined to a small number of subjects.

Table 9.**1**, extracted from the work of Bergmann (1997), lists the maximum values of the load on the hip joint measured during a number of postures and activities. To simplify comparisons, the load values are quoted in units of body weight; the numbers are rounded to the nearest 100 N. The fact that the load is almost identical with the body weight when a person is standing symmetrically on two legs may seem surprising at first sight. As trunk, head, and arms account for approximately 60 % of the body weight, a simplistic expectation would be of a load of $0.5 \cdot 60 \% = 30 \%$ of the body weight on each hip joint in the symmetrical stance on two legs. In reality the value corresponds to roughly 100 % of body weight, due to the muscle tension still active in relaxed standing and the elastic tension of all tissues (muscles, ligaments, etc.) crossing the joint.

Table 9.**1**   Load on the hip joint, determined by means of instrumented artificial hip joints (after Bergmann, 1997)

activity	load on the hip joint (% of body weight)
two-legged stance	80 %–100 %
slow walking	300 %
quick walking	350 %–400 %
rapid walking	500 %
jogging	500 %
stumbling (peak value)	800 %
walking upstairs	300 %
walking downstairs	500 %
walking with 2 crutches	150 %
cycling (80 watt)	240 %
lifting of the pelvis (supine)	300 %
active lifting of one leg (supine)	150 %

There is satisfactory agreement between the load on the hip joint measured at different gait velocities and the results of model calculations. (This increases confidence in the results of model calculations; precise agreement cannot be expected due to the simplifications made for the purpose of calculation.) Furthermore, the data allow important questions relating to the postoperative rehabilitation of patients with artificial hip joints to be answered. For example, cycling (at a power of 80 watt, i.e. a noticeable exertion) loads the hip joint with 80% of the load observed during slow walking. An orthosis can reduce the load on the hip joint by 30%. (This conforms to the results of the simple model calculation, see above). The work of Bergmann and co-workers also supplies data on hip joint loading in relation to gait style, footwear, and the mechanical properties of the floor, as well as data recorded during gymnastic exercises and exercises performed on muscle training apparatus. For movements performed by patients while lying in bed and during physiotherapeutic exercises, the hip joint load exhibits large interindividual variations. Lifting the leg while lying supine loads the hip joint more than the erect stance on two legs. Thus, if certain limiting values of hip joint loading are not to be exceeded, all activities of the patients must be critically evaluated. It follows from the measurements that, for example, bedridden patients should not lift their pelvis actively for the purpose of pushing a bedpan underneath but should do this only with support from the nursing staff.

Determination of the stress distribution on the surface of the hip joint

Mechanical factors directly influencing the tissues of the joints are the pressure (stress) on the joint surface and the stress within the cartilage and the underlying trabecular bone. Pressure, as well as stress, depend on the direction and magnitude of the force transmitted by the joint. In addition, pressure and stress depend on the shape and fit (congruency) of the articulating bones and on the mechanical properties of bone and cartilage. Knowledge of the stress distribution at the joint surface and within the tissues is not only of academic interest in understanding the function of the locomotor system. With better insight, it is hoped that primary mechanical causes of the destruction of joints may be recognized and helpful suggestions obtained for the construction of artificial joint replacements.

An initial estimate of the magnitude of the pressure on the surface of the hip joint can be achieved by calculating the mean pressure. For this purpose the magnitude and direction of the force **H** on the hip joint must be known. The mean pressure is given by

$$p_{mean} = H/A$$

In this formula, A denotes the projected area of the joint, i.e. the area seen when looking along the direction of the force vector on to the joint (Fig. 9.**11**). If (for reasons of simplification) we disregard the fact that the femoral head is not fully covered by the acetabulum, the area A is a circle with the radius of the femoral head. If the head has a diameter of 5 cm, A amounts approximately to $\pi \cdot 5^2/4 = 20$ cm^2. With a body mass of 60 kg the load on the hip joint in the stance phase of slow gait (see above) amounts to 1500 N (rounded). It follows for the mean pressure that

$$p_{mean} = 1500/20 = 75 \text{ N/cm}^2$$

Under the assumption that the femoral head has a precise spherical shape, being positioned concentrically in the spherical shell of the acetabulum, the articulating area of head and acetabulum can be measured from a radiograph. Fig. 9.**12** shows a graph of the bony contours of head and acetabulum traced from an anterior-posterior radiograph of the hip joint taken while standing. The circular contour of the femoral head is easily recognized. The midpoint of the circle, the projection of the midpoint of the sphere, is the center of rotation of the joint. The contour of the acetabulum starts at the lateral rim of the iliac bone and runs concentrically to the contour of the head. The contour can be followed only over a certain distance in mediocaudal direction; farther medially and caudally it is no longer visible. The ventral rim of the acetabulum can be followed over a certain distance starting from the lateral rim of the iliac bone; the dorsal rim of the acetabulum is usually visible for its whole length. In total, we see the image of an incompletely covered ball-and-socket joint with irregularly formed rims that differ dorsally and ventrally. The gap between the circular contours of head and acetabulum is filled with articular cartilage. The joint surface is located approximately midway between the contours of acetabulum and head.

It is not the whole area where the surfaces of acetabulum and femoral head make contact that can transmit pressure, but only that part of the contact area which is 'seen' when looking along the direction of the load vector on to the joint. In precise terms, pressure is transmitted only by that part of

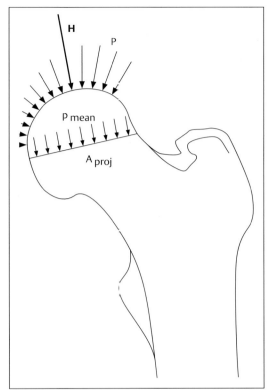

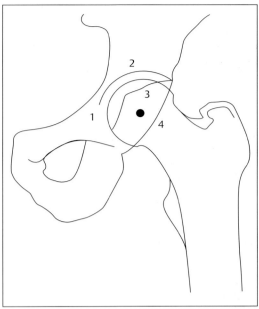

Fig. 9.**12**   Contours of the hip joint visible in an anterior-posterior radiographic view. Solid circle: center of rotation of the joint; 1: contour of the bony femoral head; 2: cranial contour of the bony acetabulum; 3: contour of the ventral rim of the acetabulum; 4: contour of the dorsal rim of the acetabulum. The actual joint surface is located approximately halfway between contours 1 and 2.

Fig. 9.**11**   Estimate of the pressure on the surface of the femoral head by calculation of the mean pressure. The mean pressure is calculated as the quotient of the joint load and the projected joint area A (area seen when looking along the load vector **H** onto the joint). When using this formula, the pressure distribution p on the joint surface is in effect substituted by a uniform pressure p_{mean} over the area A.

the surface of the sphere that is bounded either by the rim of the acetabulum or maximally by a great circle (a mathematical term, the circle with the diameter of the femoral head) in a plane perpendicular to the load vector. The reason for the restriction of the pressure-transmitting (-bearing) surface is due to the fact that joint surfaces can transmit only compressive but not tensile stress. In a spherical joint covered completely by the socket, the bearing surface would correspond to a hemisphere. Due to the irregular shape of the acetabular rim, the bearing surface of the hip joint is smaller than a hemisphere.

Kummer (1968) proposed approximating the bearing surface of the hip joint by a lune (Fig. 9.**13**). The angle of the lune should equal twice the angle between the load vector **H** and a line connecting

the center of the hip joint and the lateral rim of the acetabulum. In an individual case, Kummer's proposal takes account of the direction of the load vector, the radius of the femoral head, and the individual variation of the acetabular extension in a lateral direction. The individual variation of acetabular geometry in ventral and dorsal directions is disregarded in this approximation. It must be pointed out, though, that it is not necessary to search for approximate solutions when determining the contact area between head and acetabulum. Assuming the joint to be of spherical shape, the three-dimensional contact area can be obtained precisely from a measurement of the projection of the acetabular rim. Each point of the acetabular rim seen in a plane radiograph is unequivocally allocated to a point on a sphere concentric with the midpoint of the hip joint.

The type of pressure distribution that can be expected in an incompletely covered ball-and-socket joint is discussed with reference to the model shown in Fig. 9.**14**. In a joint consisting of a hard hemisphere and a hard hemispherical shell sepa-

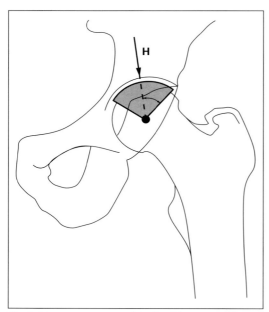

Fig. 9.**13** Approximation of the load-bearing surface of the hip joint by a lune. The angle of the lune is selected as twice the angle (indicated by the arrow) between the point of force application and the lateral corner of the acetabulum.

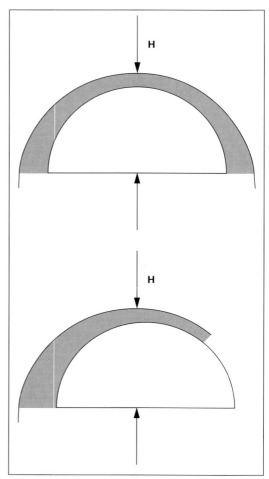

Fig. 9.**14** Model employed to determine the pressure distribution on the surface of a ball-and-socket joint. If the ball is covered by the socket in a symmetrical fashion with respect to the point of application of the force **H** (upper drawing), we expect maximum pressure at the point of force application and zero pressure at the rim of the socket. If the ball is incompletely and asymmetrically covered by the socket (lower drawing) we expect the point of maximum pressure to be shifted away from the point of force application in the direction of the acetabular rim. Over a certain portion of the rim, the pressure does not now equal zero. (Adapted from Brinckmann *et al.*, 1981)

rated from the sphere by an intermediate layer of soft material, the maximum compression of the intermediate layer, and thus the maximum pressure, is expected to occur at the point where the force vector **H** crosses the joint surface. As the articulating surfaces only glide across each other at the rim of the hemisphere, it is reasonable to assume that the pressure falls to zero at the rim. In an incompletely covered joint we expect the location of maximum compression and hence of maximum pressure to be shifted towards the rim of the socket. Due to the left-right asymmetry of the shell and the resulting asymmetry of the counter pressure exerted by the shell on to the head, the head has a tendency to 'slip' sideways out of the shell. This tendency will increase with decreasing coverage of the sphere by the shell. In the limiting case of coverage just up to the point of force application, the loaded sphere would immediately jump out of the shell. (Indeed, dislocation of the femoral head out of the acetabulum is observed in vivo in people with a very small lateral extension of the acetabulum over the femoral head. This is known as luxation of the hip in the case of a dysplastic acetabulum).

The pressure distribution on the surface of the femoral head is determined from the equilibrium condition of forces in the incompletely covered, spherical joint (Fig. 9.**15**). Since friction between the articulating surfaces is virtually zero, force transmission between head and acetabulum can

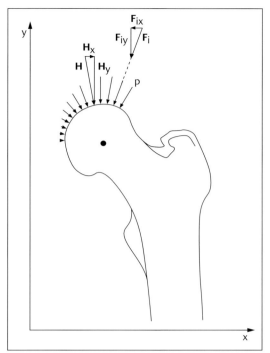

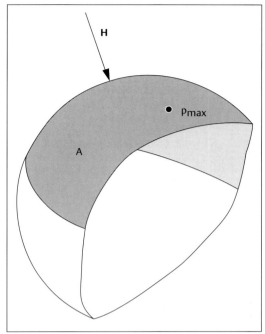

Fig. 9.**15** Equilibrium of forces at the hip joint. The sum of the individual forces **F**$_i$, calculated as a product of the locally effective pressure and the area elements dA$_i$, must be equal to the joint load **H**. Due to the laterally incomplete coverage of the head by the acetabulum, the pressure and thus the forces **F**$_i$ in the region of the lateral acetabular rim must take on high values in order to satisfy the equilibrium condition for the x-components of all forces.

Fig. 9.**16** The loaded area of the femoral head is enclosed by the ventral and dorsal rim of the acetabulum. The point of maximal pressure p$_{max}$ is shifted from the point of application of the load vector **H** in the direction of the lateral rim of the acetabulum. (Adapted from Brinckmann *et al.*, 1981)

only occur perpendicular to the cartilaginous surface. If we imagine the surface area of the head to be subdivided into many small area elements of size dA, the sum of the forces **F**$_i$, defined as the product of local pressure and the appertaining areas dA$_i$, must (in equilibrium) be equal to the hip joint load **H**. For the sums of the x- and y-components it holds that

$$\mathbf{F}_{1x} + \mathbf{F}_{2x} + ... \mathbf{F}_{nx} = \mathbf{H}_x$$
$$\mathbf{F}_{1y} + \mathbf{F}_{2y} + ... \mathbf{F}_{ny} = \mathbf{H}_y$$

To satisfy the equilibrium condition for the y-components, the pressure distribution can vary within wide limits. Even a uniform pressure distribution can satisfy this condition. Satisfying the equilibrium condition for the x-components requires the pressure (and thus the forces) to be much larger laterally than medially from the point of applica-

tion of the vector **H**. Otherwise, because the articulating area between head and acetabulum is smaller laterally than medially, and because the laterally located articulating area is inclined by only a small angle with respect to the x-axis, the summed x-components **F**$_{ix}$ would be too small to balance the component **H**$_x$ of the joint load.

The outcome of this discussion is the model of the hip joint illustrated in Fig. 9.**16**. The joint is a ball-and-socket joint with an irregularly shaped rim of the socket. Only the part A of the articulating surface transmits pressure. The pressure distribution is not uniform. Depending on the location of the rim of the socket with respect to the point of application of the vector **H**, the point of maximum pressure is located somewhere between the rim and the point of force application. While the pressure distribution falls to zero medially from the point, the pressure at the lateral rim of the socket is usually not equal to zero. The maximum pressure value depends on the magnitude of the load vector, the radius of the sphere, and the relative position of the load vector and the rim of the shell.

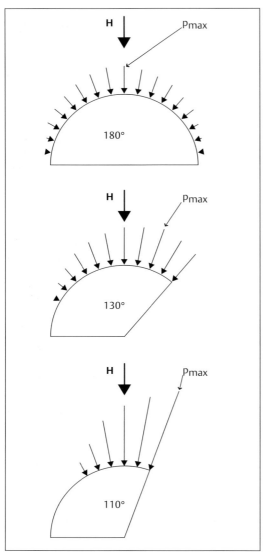

Fig. 9.17 Result of a model calculation of the pressure distribution on the surface of a completely (upper drawing) and an incompletely (middle and lower drawings) covered ball and socket joint. The figure illustrates the magnitude and distribution of the pressure under the identical load **H**. (Adapted from Brinckmann *et al.*, 1980)

For a congruent ball-and-socket joint (or for an initially incongruent joint that becomes congruent under load) we may assume as an initial approxi-

mation that the pressure distribution on the sphere follows a cosine distribution (Greenwald and O'Connor, 1971; Brinckmann *et al.*, 1980, 1981). In a cosine distribution the pressure decreases from a specified point (designated as the pole of the distribution) with the cosine of the angle between the pole and a point on the sphere. Under this model assumption, Brinckmann *et al.*, (1980) calculated the pressure distribution in relation to the coverage of the head by the acetabulum (Fig. 9.**17**). In the case of a sphere covered by the acetabulum over 180° (a form that does not correspond to the form of the human hip joint) the pressure takes its maximum value at the point of application of the force vector **H**. In the case of a sphere covered by 130° (corresponding roughly to the normal shape of human hip joints), the location of the point of maximum pressure is shifted towards the rim of the shell; the value of the maximum pressure is higher than in the case of the symmetrically covered joint. If the sphere is covered only by 110° (a model of a dysplastic acetabulum) the maximum pressure value increases again and the maximum pressure occurs at the rim of the acetabulum.

▨ Measurement of the pressure distribution on the surface of the hip joint

The numerous assumptions and approximations required in the model calculations determining pressure distribution on the hip joint make comparisons with direct experimental data desirable. The results of such experiments, as well as the difficulties encountered in them (also exemplary for other joints) are discussed below with reference to the work of Rushfeldt *et al.* (1981) and Brown and Shaw (1983). Pressure sensitive foils have been developed for measuring pressure distributions over planar surfaces (or surfaces that may be unrolled into planar surfaces). These foils change their color depending on the pressure exerted. Unfortunately the pressure distribution on the hip joint cannot be measured by means of these foils because planar foils cannot be fitted to the spherical femoral head without wrinkling or rippling. In addition, the foils are sensitive to shear forces, so that measurements might be confounded by shear forces occurring on insertion of the head into the socket.

Rushfeldt *et al.* (1981) employed an ultrasound probe for the measurement of the surface geometry and cartilage thickness of human hip joint specimens. These authors found that the cartilaginous surface of the acetabulum deviated by less than

0.15 mm from an ideal spherical shape. The underlying bone surface was not precisely spherical. With respect to its mean value, the thickness of the cartilage exhibited deviations of ± 0.5 mm. Subsequently, pressure distribution was measured, using the head of an artificial hip joint replacement instrumented with miniature pressure transducers. In the dorsoventral direction the measured distribution showed some resemblance to a cosine distribution; in the mediolateral direction, however, the experimental distribution was definitely narrower than a cosine distribution. The extension of the area subject to pressure and the magnitude of the maximum pressure depended very strongly on the diameter of the instrumented artificial joint head. Even when the diameter of the instrumented head was selected as close as possible to that of the anatomic specimen acetabulum, it was not the whole area of the acetabulum that was subjected to pressure. According to the authors, the results of this experiment characterize more closely the pressure between an artificial femoral head and an anatomic acetabulum than the pressure between natural joint components.

Brown and Shaw (1983) instrumented specimens of femoral heads with 24 miniature pressure transducers mounted flush with the cartilaginous surface of the head. The femoral heads were then loaded via the appertaining acetabulum specimens. In the specimens investigated, the maximum of the measured pressure distribution was found within a cone of 30° with respect to the direction of the load vector. The location of the maximum pressure appeared to be shifted at random in a dorsoventral or mediolateral direction. Hypothetically this can be explained by the fact that the experimental set-up of Brown and Shaw permitted motion of the femoral head under load only in the direction of the load vector. Thus, the femoral head was not allowed unrestricted movement with respect to the (fixed) acetabulum. Another problem inherent in instrumented specimens is that the stiffness of the miniature pressure transducers is markedly different from that of trabecular bone and cartilage. We thus have to expect a transducer that has been inserted flush with the joint surface in an unloaded state to project from the surface in a loaded state, because the transducer material (i.e. metal) is stiffer than bone or cartilage. The measurements of Brown and Shaw showed that the pressure distributions under prolonged loading varied over time due to the viscoelastic deformation of cartilage and trabecular bone over time. For the same reason we expect the magnitude of the pressure on the hip joint and the shape of the pressure distribution *in vivo* to vary in relation to the duration of loading.

Pressure on the articular surface as a primary cause of arthrosis of the hip joint

The above discussions show sufficiently clearly that model calculations as well as measurements of the pressure distribution on the surface of the hip joint can only be regarded as an approximation to the anatomic conditions *in vivo*. Nevertheless, it is worthwhile exploring to what extent the theoretical and experimental results may be related to clinical observations from patients with osteoarthrosis of the hip.

Harrison *et al.* (1953) investigated degenerative changes in the cartilage of hip joint specimens. These authors found the first signs of degeneration of the cartilage, interpreted as signs of incipient arthrosis, on those parts of the joint surface that are expected to be subjected to pressure only rarely, if at all. In erect stance, for example, these parts are the mediocaudal surface and laterally that surface not in contact with the acetabulum. The authors concluded that, if the pressure on the cartilage falls below certain limits, degeneration will be triggered (or at least furthered).

Pauwels (1980) hypothesized that arthrosis of the hip joint is caused by excessive pressure on certain parts of the joint surface, specifically in the region of the lateral rim of the acetabulum. Indeed, on radiographs of subjects with a less-than-normal lateral extension of the acetabulum, an increased bone density can regularly be discerned in the region of the lateral aspect of the acetabulum. This increased density, seen even in young subjects, is interpreted as a reaction of the cartilage and the underlying bone to the excessively high mechanical stress. Pauwels showed that such signs of (incipient) joint damage regress after surgical interventions performed to relieve the load on the joint.

Radin *et al.* (1970, 1972) investigated the damping of peak forces using specimens of hip joints. They found that damping is not effected by the cartilage but almost exclusively by the underlying trabecular bone. The authors hypothesize that short episodes of overloading *in vivo* primarily damage the trabecular bone. Once the resulting microfractures are healed, the bone is stiffer. With less damping due to the increased bone stiffness the cartilage is now more subject to mechanical damage by later overloading episodes. According to this hypothesis, arthrosis does not begin in the cartilage but in the bone.

In summary, it has to be admitted that our current knowledge of mechanical aspects of the hip joint does not suffice to clearly favor one of the three above-stated hypotheses on the primary mechanical causes of arthrosis of the hip joint. It is also feasible that excessively high pressure as well as excessively low pressure may be detrimental in the long run. Such a statement is, however, completely meaningless as long as there are no quantitative data on what actually constitutes an 'excessively low' or 'excessively high' articular pressure.

To add to the confusion, a puzzling observation is mentioned. In different positions of the leg in flexion or extension, the direction of the load vector on the hip shows only a small variation in relation to the femoral head. The reason is that almost all relevant muscles run along the direction of the upper leg and thus their force vectors move with the leg. In contrast, with respect to the acetabulum, the line of action of the load vector exhibits a large variation. In flexion of the hip, the load vector is inclined ventrodorsally (i.e. following the direction of the upper leg); in extension it is inclined dorso-ventrally. We conclude that the point of maximum pressure is virtually stationary with respect to the head but shifts from dorsal to ventral with respect to the acetabulum. If the destruction of the joint were due predominantly to mechanical factors, we would then tend to expect signs of mechanical overloading to be visible first in the head and not in the acetabulum. However, this seems not to be the case.

Further reading

Textbooks and review papers

Bergmann G. *In vivo Messung der Belastung von Hüftimplantaten. Wiss. Schriftenreihe Biomechanik* Vol 2. Berlin: Köster; 1997

Chaffin DB, Andersson GBJ, Martin BJ. *Occupational Biomechanics.* 3rd ed. New York: Wiley; 1999

Kassat G. *Biomechanik für Nicht-Biomechaniker. Alltägliche bewegungstechnisch-sportpraktische Aspekte.* Bünde: Fitness Contur; 1993

Kummer B. *Einführung in die Biomechanik des Hüftgelenks.* Berlin: Springer 1985

Novacheck TF. The biomechanics of running. *Gait and Posture.* 1998; **7**: 77–95 [review paper, 83 references]

Pauwels F. *Biomechanics of the locomotor apparatus.* New York: Springer 1980

Pheasant S. *Bodyspace. Anthropometry, Ergonomics and Design.* 1st ed. London: Taylor and Francis; 1986. [Note: Data on mass, center of gravity and moment of inertia of the body segments are contained only in this first edition.]

Winter DA. *Biomechanics and motor control of human movement.* 2nd ed. New York: Wiley; 1990

Original papers cited in the text or in the figures

Bergmann G, Rohlmann A, Graichen F. *In vivo* Messung der Hüftgelenkbelastung. 1.Teil: Krankengymnastik. *Z Orthop.* 1989, **127**: 672– 679

Bergmann G, Kniggendorf H, Graichen F, Rohlmann A. Influence of shoes and heel strike on the loading of the hip joint. *J Biomechanics.* 1995; **28**: 817–827

Bergmann G, Deuretzbacher G, Heller M, Graichen F, Rohlmann A, Strauss J, Duda GN. Hip contact forces and gait patterns from routine activities. *J Biomechanics.* 2001; **34**: 859–871

Bergmann G *et al. Hip 98.* [CD ROM] Berlin: Biomechanics Laboratory of the Free University; 2001

Brinckmann P, Frobin W, Hierholzer E. Belastete Gelenkfläche und Beanspruchung des Hüftgelenks. *Z Orthop.* 1980; **118**: 107–115

Brinckmann P, Frobin W, Hierholzer E. Stress on the articular surface of the hip joint in healthy adults and persons with idiopathic osteoarthrosis of the hip joint. *J Biomechanics.* 1981; **14**: 149–156

Brown TD, Shaw DT. In vitro contact stress distributions in the natural human hip. *J Biomechanics.* 1983; **16**: 373–384

Debrunner HU. Studien zur Biomechanik des Hüftgelenkes I. Ein neues Modell zur Berechnung der Hüftbelastung. *Z Orthop.* 1975; **113**: 377–388

Greenwald AS, O'Connor JJ. The transmission of load through the human hip joint. *J Biomechanics.* 1971; **4**: 507–528

Harrison MHM, Schajowicz F, Trueta J. Osteoarthritis of the hip: a study of the nature and evolution of the disease. *J Bone Jt Surg.* 1953; **35 B**: 598–625

Kummer B. Die Beanspruchung des menschlichen Hüftgelenks. I. Allgemeine Problematik. *Z Anat Entwicklungsgeschichte.* 1968; **127**: 277–285

Morrison JB. Bioengineering analysis of force actions transmitted by the knee joint. *Biomed Engng.* 1968; **3**: 164–170

Paul JP. Forces transmitted by joints in the human body. *Proc Inst Mech Eng.* 1967; **181**: 8–15

Paul JP. Forces transmitted by joints in the human body. *Proc R Soc Lond B.* 1976; **192**: 163–172

Radin EL, Paul IL. Does cartilage compliance reduce skeletal impact loads? The relative force attenuating properties of articular cartilage, synovial fluid periarticular soft tissue and bone. *Arthritis Rheum.* 1970; **13**: 139–144

Radin EL, Paul IL, Tolkoff MJ. Subchondral bone changes in patients with early degenerative joint disease. *Arthritis Rheum.* 1970; **13**: 400–405

Radin EL, Paul IL, Rose RM. Role of mechanical factors in pathogenesis of primary osteoarthritis. *Lancet.* 1972; 519–521

Radin EL, Parker HG, Pugh JW, Steinberg RS, Paul IL, Rose RM. Response of joints to impact loading – III. Relationship between trabecular microfractures and cartilage degeneration. *J Biomechanics.* 1973; **6**: 51–57

Roesler H, Hamacher P. Die biostatische Analyse der Belastung des Hüftgelenks. Teil I und II. *Z Orthop.* 1972; **110**: 67–75 and 186–196

Rushfeldt PD, Mann RW, Harris WH. Improved techniques for measuring in vitro the geometry and pressure distribution in the human acetabulum. Parts I and II. *J Biomechanics.* 1981; **14**: 253–260 and 315–323

10 Mechanical Aspects of the Knee

Features common to all joints, illustrated by the example of the knee joint

Irrespective of the diversity of their outward appearance, the movable joints (diarthroses) of the locomotor system possess a number of common properties with respect to their architecture and mechanical function. These properties can be appropriately demonstrated using the example of the knee joint.

Incongruency of the articulating bones. When examining the architecture of a 'typical' joint, one is immediately aware that the surface shapes of the articulating bones do not match; the articulating surfaces are incongruent. In the knee joint (Fig. 10.**1**) neither the surfaces of femur and tibia nor those of femur and patella match exactly. Indeed, the shapes of the articulating surfaces are grossly divergent. This characteristic is common to virtually all joints of the body; consider, for example, the joints of the hand or foot skeleton, or the vertebral joints. The only exception might be the hip joint, with the match of its spherical head to the spherical shell of the acetabulum. (The academic debate on whether the head and the acetabulum of the hip match precisely, or whether there is an initial incongruency that is transformed into a congruency under load, is not settled.)

Contact of rigid bodies with incongruent surface shapes can occur only at points or along lines. In the joints of the human body, these points develop into contact areas between the articulating bones, due to the deformation of cartilage and bone under load. Nevertheless, the contact areas are usually small, so that pressure on them is accordingly high. In some highly loaded joints, e.g. between femur and tibia and between vertebral bodies, there are soft tissues (menisci, intervertebral disks) between the articulating bones that increase the articulating (pressure-transmitting) area and thus limit the pressure. While this measure partially solves the pressure problem, a new problem arises as the soft tissues tend to be squeezed out of the joint space under high load. In the knee joint, a load produces force components pushing the interposed, soft menisci to the outside (Fig. 10.**2**). Normally, tensile stress within the menisci balances such forces. If the strength of the fibers of the menisci, or the

strength at their insertion to the tibial plateau, is not sufficiently high, the menisci will tear. Tensile stress in the tissue and a tendency to bulge and displace outwards under load is likewise observed in intervertebral disks.

Dimensions of the bones in the vicinity of a joint. In the vicinity of the joints all bones exhibit greater dimensions compared with those in their mid-section. Like all long bones and the vertebral bodies, the femur and tibia exhibit the typical waisted shape. However, the larger surface area

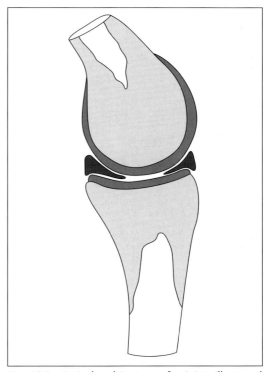

Fig. 10.**1** Typical architecture of a joint, illustrated with the example of the femorotibial joint. Note the increase in bone diameter in the vicinity of the joint, the incongruent shape of the articulating bones, the increase in pressure-transmitting area due to the insertion of soft tissue into the joint space, the coverage of the joint surfaces with cartilage, and the subchondral trabecular bone, located below the articulating surface. (Adapted from Frost, 1973)

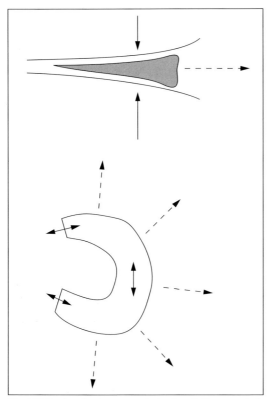

Fig. 10.**2** Load, stress, and strain of the menisci. (Adapted from Frost, 1973)

Fig. 10.**3** Size and localization of the contact area between femur and tibia with and without menisci, related to the angle of flexion of the knee joint. (Adapted from Maquet, 1976)

thus created at the ends of the bones is not utilized as a whole for force transmission. As stated above, due to the incongruency of the articulating surfaces only a fraction of this area is utilized for force transmission.

Architecture of the bones in the vicinity of a joint. In the femur and tibia the thickness of the cortical bone below the articulating cartilage is very low. In the mid-section of both bones the thickness of the cortical bone may well exceed 1 cm. Close to the joint, femur and tibia are filled with trabecular bone; in their mid-portion both bones are practically hollow. These observations are common to other long bones too. (The fact that vertebral bodies are completely filled with trabecular bone may be attributed to their short length.) The thin-layered cortical bone and the trabecular bone below the joint surface are more easily deformable than cortical bone of higher thickness. The resulting deformation under load effectively damps short peak forces. At the same time the pressure-transmitting area is momentarily in-creased; this further reduces the pressure on the joint surface.

Force-transmitting area. All joints appear to tolerate high pressure localized in small areas. While the joint is in motion, the loaded area moves and an alternation occurs between loading and unloading. Fig. 10.**3** shows data on the contact area between femur and tibia measured with and without menisci. As stated above, even with intact menisci the contact area between femur and tibia never extends over the entire tibial plateau. Where menisci are missing, the contact area is decreased by a factor of 3 to 5. Furthermore, the pressure-loaded area is observed to shift with the motion of the joint. With increasing flexion the contact area of the femorotibial joint shifts from ventral to dorsal. In the femoropatellar joint (Fig. 10.**4**), despite the great thickness of its cartilage, the patella never comes into complete contact with the femoral condyles. The shift of the contact area between patella and femur with knee flexion is clearly visible.

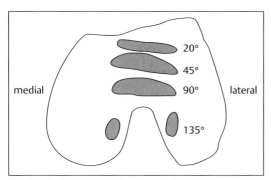

Fig. 10.**4** Size and localization of the contact area between femur and patella. (Adapted from Seedhom *et al.*, 1979)

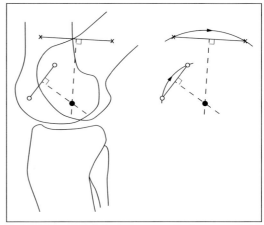

Fig. 10.**5** Protocol for measuring the location of the center of rotation of the knee joint. Two markers are placed on the femur of a knee joint specimen. As the joint is moved while the tibia is held in a fixed position, the markers move on concentric circles around the center of rotation. The center of rotation is given by the point of intersection of the perpendicular bisectors on the lines connecting the locations of the two markers. (The method rests on the assumption that the movement of the joint occurs in a plane.)

Friction properties of joint surfaces. The coefficients of static and sliding friction between cartilage surfaces wetted by synovial fluid are very small. The coefficient of static friction between cartilage surfaces is between 0.005 and 0.02 (Charnley, 1960). By way of comparison, the coefficient of static friction between steel and steel is, approximately, 0.1, and between steel and ice, 0.03. In broad terms, therefore, we may regard the knee joint, as well as all other joints with cartilage surfaces, as friction-free. As high forces are transmitted through the joints, low friction is of extreme importance to their mechanical functioning. If friction in the joints was at any appreciable level, the joints would become virtually immobile and thus useless under high load, due to the high moment exerted by the friction force.

Guidance of the joint motion by ligaments. The integrity of the joints, the guidance of their motion, and the restriction of their range of motion is effected by ligaments. If the ligaments are torn or destroyed, the joints 'fall apart' and the range of motion is no longer controlled. These observations are likewise valid for the cruciate ligaments of the knee as well as, for example, for the ligaments of the hand skeleton or the spinal ligaments. The guidance of motion by the shape of the articulating bones (as seen in the hip joint) or solely by muscles (in the scapulothoracic joint) are exceptions to the general rule.

Axis of rotation. As the articulating surfaces of the bones are incongruent (as stated, the hip joint may be an exception to this rule) and as joint motion is guided by ligaments, no conclusion on the location and orientation of the axis of rotation can be drawn from an inspection of the shape of the articulating surfaces. This holds true for measurements of the three-dimensional shape of joint surfaces from specimens, as well as for measurements of the bony contours of joints visible on radiographs. To predict the course of movement of a joint theoretically, not only the shape of the articulating surfaces but also the thee-dimensional architecture of the ligaments, their mechanical properties, and their elastic pre-tension would have to be known.

Alternatively, the location and direction of the axis of rotation can be measured. Under the assumption that a) the motion is confined to a plane and b) the motion can be described by a pure rotation (see Chapter 4), the center of rotation can be obtained by the procedure illustrated in Fig. 10.**5**. The center of rotation is that point where the axis of rotation crosses the plane of motion. To locate the center of rotation, one of the articulating bones is immobilized and two markers (landmarks) are fixed on the other bone. For investigating joint specimens, metallic markers whose images can be clearly discerned in radiographs are preferred. Investigations *in vivo* are usually based on prominent points of the bones or on markers fixed to the skin of the moving member. Under the assumptions stated above, when the joint is moved the markers move on concentric circles about the center of rotation. The lines connecting the markers in the initial and final position are chords of these circles. The common center of the circles, i.e. the center of rotation, is given by the intersection of the vertical bisectors of the chords. The precision with which the center of rotation is determined experimentally depends on the precision of measurement when locating the landmarks. Precision decreases if the angular range of motion is small, because the construction of the chords, bisectors, and point of intersection will then be less precise due to unavoidable experimental errors.

If a joint is moved in small angular intervals and if the procedure shown in Fig. 10.**5** is performed separately for each of these intervals, the location of the center of motion is found, in most cases, to change with the angular position of the joint. A center of rotation that changes its location in the course of the motion is termed an 'instantaneous' center (likewise, an axis with such a property is termed an 'instantaneous' axis). The fact that the location of a center of rotation varies for different joint positions is not surprising, as the location depends on the articulating areas momentarily in contact and on the momentary alignment and tension of the ligaments.

Motion of the knee joint

Smidt (1973) determined the location of the center of rotation of the knee joint from radiographs taken *in vivo*, following the procedure outlined above (Fig. 10.**6**). The migration of the location of the center of rotation in relation to the angle of flexion is clearly visible. Thus, the knee joint appears to have not a fixed, but rather an instantaneous, center of rotation. A precise knowledge of the location of the instantaneous center of rotation is of practical importance to the construction of artificial knee joint replacements if the cruciate ligaments are preserved during surgery. In this case, guidance of the motion by the joint replacement should resemble as closely as possible the physiologic guidance provided by the cruciate ligaments in the intact knee. Such precise knowledge of the location of the center of rotation is not crucial to other problems, for example to a discussion of the loading of the knee joint in static equilibrium. The migration of the center of rotation may be disregarded, and the center may be assumed to be located above the tibial plateau in the dorsal third of the femoral condyle.

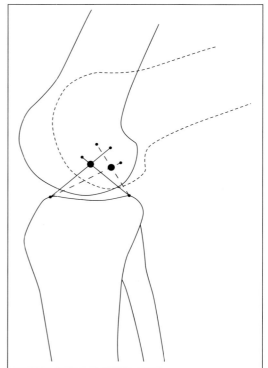

Fig. 10.**7** Description of the motion of the knee joint using the model of a four-bar linkage. The length of the bars is assumed to remain constant during the course of the motion. The location of the instantaneous center of rotation is given by the point of intersection of the two bars representing the cruciate ligaments. As the bending angle changes, the center of rotation moves to another location and the contact area between femur and tibia is shifted along the tibial plateau. (Adapted from Müller, 1982)

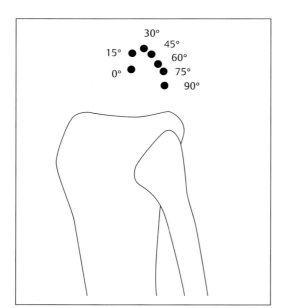

Fig. 10.**6** Results of measurement of the location of the center of rotation of the knee joint in relation to the bending angle *in vivo*. (Adapted from Smidt, 1973)

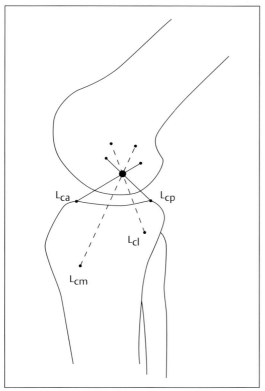

Fig. 10.**8** The collateral ligaments cross close to the intersection of the cruciate ligaments, i.e. the center of rotation of the knee joint. L_{cm} and L_{cl}: ligamentum collaterale tibiale and fibulare, L_{ca} and L_{cp}: ligamentum cruciatum anterius genus and posterius genus. (Adapted from Menschik, 1974)

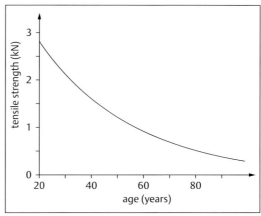

Fig. 10.**9** Mean value of the tensile strength of the anterior cruciate ligament complex related to age. (Adapted from Woo *et al.*, 1991)

Menschik (1974) described the motion of the knee guided by the cruciate ligaments by a surprisingly simple model. If we assume that the length of the cruciate ligaments remains unchanged in the course of the flexion-extension motion, the cruciates guide the motion of the femur relative to the tibia like a four-bar linkage. The four bars of this linkage are formed by the two cruciates and the lines connecting their points of insertion into femur and tibia (Fig. 10.**7**). Under the assumptions of this model, the instantaneous center of rotation is located at the point of intersection of the cruciates (see Chapter 4). The ingenious model devised by Menschik closely describes the migration of the instantaneous center of rotation and the dorsal shift of the femur relative to the tibia during flexion observed *in vivo*. If the path of the collateral ligaments is viewed in addition, these ligaments are found to cross in the general area of the instantaneous cent-

er of rotation (Fig. 10.**8**). Crossing the center of rotation ensures that the length change of the collateral ligaments remains small when flexing or extending the knee.

The migration of the instantaneous center of rotation predicted from the Menschik model is not fully in accordance with the measurements of Smidt. This may be due to the model being oversimplified or due to technical problems encountered with *measurements in vivo* (Kummer, 1982). In contrast to the assumption in the model, the diameters of the two femoral condyles are not equal and some fiber bundles of the cruciate ligaments actually change their length during flexion and extension (van Dijk *et al.*, 1979; Fuss, 1989). Fuss (1989) showed that over the whole range of motion only a fraction of the fibers of the cruciate ligaments is continuously under tension. The fiber bundles under tension guide the motion as described by Menschik and limit the dorsoventral translation of the femur along the tibial plateau. Due to the extended (rather than punctiform) area of insertion of the cruciates, a constant tensile stress of all fiber bundles is impossible for geometrical reasons alone. At the end points of motion, all fibers are under tension. The anterior cruciate ligament limits the motion in extension, and the posterior cruciate ligament limits the motion in flexion. The function of the cruciates in limiting the range of motion of the knee (just as the range of motion of joints is limited in general by ligaments) explains their remarkable tensile strength. Woo *et al.* (Fig. 10.**9**) showed that the tensile strength of the anterior cruciate ligament complex (ligament together with its insertion into the bone) falls from about 3000 N at the age of 20 years to about 500 N at 100 years.

In reality, the motion of the knee joint is not confined to a plane; the description of the knee as a hinge joint is only an approximation. The most striking deviation from plane motion is the so-called 'screw-home' motion. In the last 20° of knee movement before maximum extension is reached, the tibia performs an external rotation in the order of 15° about its longitudinal axis. This rotation is caused by the asymmetry of the femoral condyles in the region in contact with the tibial plateau near full extension. The asymmetry of the shape of the femoral condyles, and thus the screw-home motion, exhibit considerable interindividual differences. Conflicting findings of past studies on the existence and magnitude of the screw-home motion may also be due, in part, to measurement errors (Piazza and Cavanagh, 2000).

A motion in space can be described as a rotation about and a translation along an axis oriented in space, the so-called helical axis (see Chapter B2). The measurement of the orientation and location of this axis as well as the rotation about and the translation along this axis comprehensively describes the spatial motion of the knee joint, composed of flexion-extension, dorsoventral and mediolateral translation of the femur with respect to the tibia, and axial rotation of the tibia. Based on series of stereoradiographs of the knee joint, Blankevoort *et al.* (1990) measured the location and orientation of this axis.

As mentioned above, in healthy subjects knowledge of the location of the axis of rotation of the knee and its migration in the course of extension and flexion is required to understand the physiological function of the joint. Knowledge of the migration of this axis is also of interest for the construction of artificial knee replacements if the cruciate ligaments are to be left intact. In this case, it is of importance for the location and migration of the axis of the implant to resemble as closely as possible the location and migration of the physiological axis. Otherwise, the geometrical balance between length and direction of the cruciates and the surface shapes of femur and tibia would be disturbed. Orthoses for above-knee amputees also employ joints whose axis of rotation migrates in the course of the movement (so-called 'polycentric knees'). Such joints are not intended to imitate the anatomical knee. Rather, the intention is to shift the axis of rotation, during the stance phase, in a dorsal direction so that the vector of the reaction force from the floor on the foot always passes ventrally from this axis. The reaction force then effects an extension moment on the orthosis and the knee remains fully extended up to the stop. (If this were

not the case, the orthosis would flex, resulting in a fall.)

Load on the femorotibial and femoropatellar joint

In the following, loads are determined using a plane model in static equilibrium. In the posture investigated, the trunk is erect and the knees are bent. This posture is assumed, for example, when performing a knee-bend or when climbing stairs. Muscle forces are required to balance the moment of the gravitational force of the body; the joint load depends on these muscle forces. To calculate the joint load, the location of the center of gravity of the body relative to the center of rotation of the knee joint must be known. To find the location of the center of gravity, the following theorem of mechanics is employed: 'In static equilibrium the center of gravity of a body is located above the area of support'. (This statement is justified by the fact that if the center of gravity were not located above the area of support, the body would fall over and, contrary to the assumption, static equilibrium would not exist.) In a posture with a bent knee, only a small area under the forefoot is loaded (Fig. 10.**10**). If the trunk is held erect, the area of support and thus the center of gravity of the body is located dorsally from the knee joint. The moment arm L_1 of the body weight in relation to the center of rotation of the knee is given by the perpendicular distance of the line of action of the gravitational force from the center of rotation. In erect posture of the trunk, the moment arm L_1 is approximately zero in the case of fully extended knees and increases with increasing flexion of the knee.

The tensile force of the patellar tendon must be generated by activation of the quadriceps muscle, in order to balance the moment of force $\mathbf{F}_1$ between floor and foot (Fig. 10.**11**). Force $\mathbf{F}_1$ acts from the floor via the foot on the tibia and is opposite and equal to the gravitational force of the body mass. From the equilibrium condition of moments for force $\mathbf{F}_2$ of the patellar tendon we obtain

$$L_2 \cdot |\mathbf{F}_2| = L_1 \cdot |\mathbf{F}_1|$$
$$|\mathbf{F}_2| = L_1/L_2 \cdot |\mathbf{F}_1|$$

In this model, the gravitational force of the tibia is neglected; in addition it is assumed that, apart from the force of the quadriceps, no other muscle or ligament forces act on the tibia. (In reality, this assumption is not quite correct, as is discussed later.) It can easily be seen that, for larger flexion angles, the quotient L_1/L_2 can assume values well

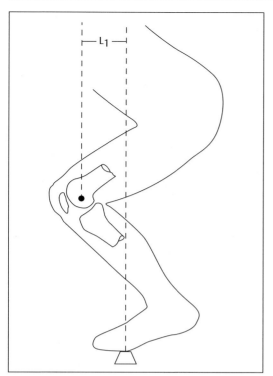

Fig. 10.**10** In static equilibrium the center of gravity of a body is located above the area of support. Consequently, when standing with the knees bent, the center of gravity of the body is located perpendicularly above the capita ossium metatarsalium. With the upper trunk held erect, the moment arm L_1 of the gravitational force increases as the bending angle of the knee joint increases.

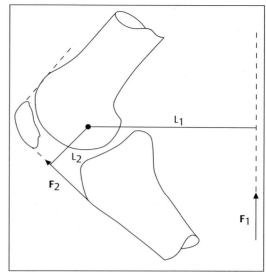

Fig. 10.**11** Determination of force F_2 of the patellar tendon in static equilibrium. L_2, the moment arm of force F_2, is given by the perpendicular distance of the center of rotation of the knee joint from the line of action of force F_2. Force F_1 acts from the floor on to the foot. With the trunk held upright, its moment arm L_1 increases with increasing flexion angle of the knee. In a symmetric knee bend of both legs, the magnitude of F_1 equals 1/2 the gravitational force of the body mass. (The gravitational force of the lower leg and foot is neglected in the model calculation.)

above 1.0 due to the increase of the moment arm L_1. Thus, force F_2 of the patellar tendon may reach values up to several times the gravitational force F_1. In a knee-bend on two legs $|F_1|$ equals $1/2$ body weight. In a knee-bend on one leg, or when climbing stairs, $|F_1|$ equals the gravitational force of the body mass. (Note that, in accordance with previously published work, the method employed to determine knee joint loading, i.e. starting from the force between floor and foot, closely follows the path outlined in Chapter 8.)

The effect of a missing patella is illustrated in Fig. 10.**12**. Without a patella, the moment arm of the tendon tensed by the quadriceps muscle would be equal to L^*. As L^* is smaller than L_2, force F^* of the quadriceps required for equilibrium would have to be correspondingly higher. In consequence, an absence of the patella would require a larger force of the quadriceps and, as shown below, would result in a larger load on the femorotibial joint.

The increase in the moment arm of the patellar tendon by an anterior shift of the tuberositas tibiae (by means of the Maquet-Bandi operation, Fig. 10.**13**) from L_2 initially to L^* postoperatively means that less quadriceps muscle force is required for equilibrium. This in turn relieves the load on the femorotibial and femoropatellar joints. In addition to the change in the moment arm, the anterior shift of the tuberositas tibiae changes the direction of the patellar tendon; this further relieves the load on the femoropatellar joint (Maquet, 1976).

To calculate the force between femur and tibia, the equilibrium of forces on the tibia is considered (Fig. 10.**14**). If we neglect all muscle or ligament forces save the force of the quadriceps, and furthermore neglect the gravitational force of the lower leg and foot, the vector sum of force F_1 from the floor on to the foot, force F_2 of the patellar tendon, and force F_4 between femur and tibia must be zero. It can be seen from the diagram that the magnitude of force F_4 roughly equals the magnitude of force F_2. For larger flexion angles of the knee, the force

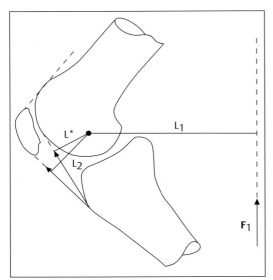

Fig. 10.**12**   In the case of a missing patella the moment arm of the extensor of the knee decreases from L_2 (value with patella) to L^*. Consequently, a higher force in the patellar tendon is required to satisfy the equilibrium condition.

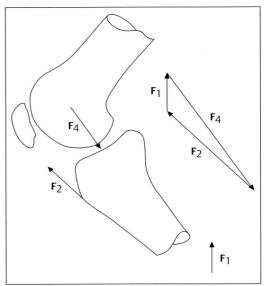

Fig. 10.**14**   Equilibrium of forces at the tibia, if only three forces are assumed to be active: F_1 (force from the floor on to the foot), F_2 (force of the patellar tendon), and F_4 (force exerted by the femur on to the tibia). It can be seen from the diagram that the magnitude of the femorotibial force exceeds that of the force of the patellar tendon. Taking only three forces into account is, however, only a rough approximation, as it is not guaranteed that F_4 is directed perpendicular to the tibial plateau. To satisfy the condition of static equilibrium, additional forces aligned parallel to the tibial plateau are usually required. These forces are resisted by the cruciate ligaments.

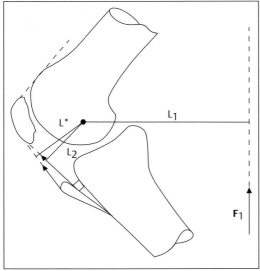

Fig. 10.**13**   Anterior displacement of the insertion point of the patellar tendon, effected by the Maquet-Bandi operation, increases the moment arm of the patellar tendon from L_2 to L^*. Consequently, less force in the patellar tendon is required to satisfy the equilibrium condition.

between femur and tibia, like the force of the patellar tendon, may thus be expected to assume values up to several times body weight.

At this point a severe shortcoming of the oversimplified model becomes apparent. The equilibrium of forces F_1, F_2, and F_4 in Fig. 10.**14** does not guarantee that force F_4 between femur and tibia is directed perpendicular to the tibial plateau. In reality, only a force directed perpendicular to the tibial plateau can be transmitted, due to the theorem of mechanics: 'In equilibrium, only perpendicularly directed forces can be transmitted between frictionless surfaces'. (The supporting argument would be that, in the case where friction is absent, no force component parallel to the contact surface can exist. Otherwise the bodies in contact would be accelerated by this force and, in contrast to the assumption, equilibrium would not exist.) If the force between femur and tibia were not directed perpen-

Fig. 10.**15** Equilibrium of forces at the patella, illustrated with the knee bent at a small angle. The active forces are the force of the patellar tendon F_2, the force of the quadriceps tendon F_3, and the femoropatellar force F_5. The directions of F_2 and F_3 are given by the anatomical directions of the tendons; F_5 is directed perpendicular to the area of contact between femur and patella (this area being approximated by a plane).

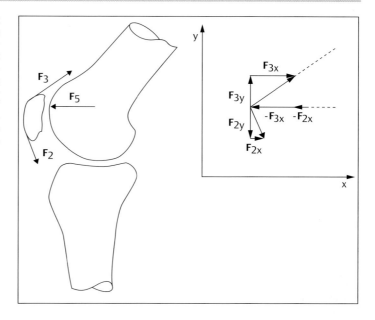

dicular to the tibial plateau in the model shown in Fig. 10.**14**, we would have to conclude that additional, hitherto disregarded, forces are required for equilibrium. As discussed below, these forces are supplied by the cruciate ligaments.

For calculation of the force between femur and patella, the equilibrium of forces at the patella is considered (Fig. 10.**15**). The directions of force F_2 of the patellar tendon and of force F_3 of the quad-

riceps tendon are taken from anatomical measurements. The magnitude of force F_2 of the patellar tendon is determined from the equilibrium condition of moments (see Fig. 10.**11**) from the quotient of the moment arms of the body weight and the tendon force. Since the friction between femur and patella is negligible, force F_5 between femur and patella is directed perpendicular to the area of contact between these bones. The x-axis of the xy-co-

Fig. 10.**16** Equilibrium of forces at the patella illustrated with the knee bent at a large angle. Designations as in Fig. 10.**15**. Compared to the posture with a small bending angle (and still with upright trunk), the magnitude of force F_2 in the patellar tendon increases and the direction of the quadriceps tendon, and hence of F_3, change.

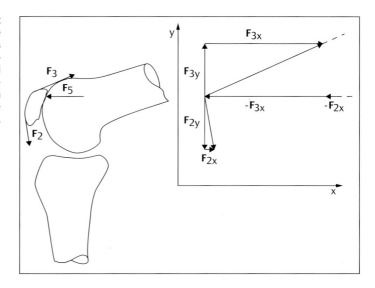

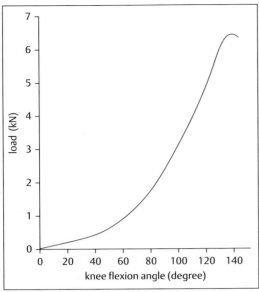

Fig. 10.**17** Load on the femoropatellar joint in relation to the bending angle. The data refer to a body mass of 85 kg and a knee bend on one leg. (Adapted from Reilly and Martens, 1972)

ordinate system is set parallel to the direction of $\mathbf{F}_5$. Equilibrium of the y-components of forces $\mathbf{F}_2$ and $\mathbf{F}_3$ ($\mathbf{F}_5$ has no y-component) results in

$$\mathbf{F}_{3y} = -\mathbf{F}_{2y}$$

As the direction of $\mathbf{F}_3$ is known, we may now construct the x-component of the quadriceps force. In equilibrium it holds for the x-components of forces $\mathbf{F}_2$, $\mathbf{F}_3$, and $\mathbf{F}_5$ that

$$\mathbf{F}_{5x} = -\mathbf{F}_{2x} - \mathbf{F}_{3x}$$

As result, force $\mathbf{F}_5$ (equal to $\mathbf{F}_{5x}$) between femur and patella is known.

Consideration of the equilibrium of forces acting on the patella at larger flexion angles (Fig. 10.**16**) reveals two important changes. 1) The magnitude of force $\mathbf{F}_2$ of the patellar tendon is increased due to the increase of the moment arm of the body weight at larger flexion angles. 2) The angle between the direction of force $\mathbf{F}_3$ of the quadriceps tendon and the x-axis decreases with increasing flexion of the knee joint. If the same calculation as above is performed, the magnitude of $\mathbf{F}_{3x}$ is seen to increase substantially due to the increase of $\mathbf{F}_2$ (and hence $\mathbf{F}_{2y}$) and to the less steep direction of $\mathbf{F}_3$. Con-

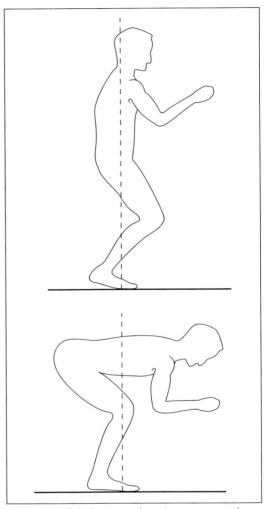

Fig. 10.**18** If the knees are bent in a posture with upright trunk, the center of gravity is located dorsally from the joint. In equilibrium the extensors of the knee must be activated. The trunk can be bent forward so that the center of gravity is located perpendicularly above the center of rotation of the knee. In this posture, neither extensor nor flexor muscle forces are required and the load on the knee joint is minimal.

sequently force $\mathbf{F}_5$ between femur and patella increases as well.

Fig. 10.**17** shows the numerical result of a model calculation of the load of the femoropatellar joint in relation to the flexion angle of the knee. The assumptions are: trunk in erect posture, 85 kg body mass, stance on one leg. The calculation is feasible up to flexion angles of about 150° because at larger

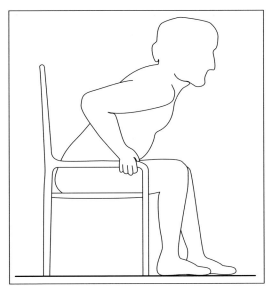

Fig. 10.**19** Forward shift of the trunk, in addition to the support given by the armrests, decreases the force to be generated by the quadriceps muscle and hence the load on the knee joints.

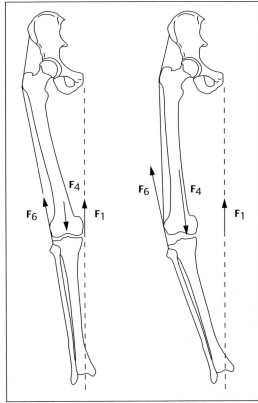

Fig. 10.**20** Equilibrium of forces at the tibia in the frontal plane when standing on one leg. Active forces: force F_1 from the floor on to the foot (equal and opposite to the gravitational force of the body mass), the femorotibial force F_4, and force F_6 designating the combined force of the gluteus maximus muscle and the tensor fasciae latae. The line of action of F_1 passes medially, and the line of action of F_6 laterally, from the knee joint. In varus deformity, the moment arm of force F_1 increases.

angles contact between the upper and lower leg occurs. It can be seen that the load on the femoropatellar joint exhibits a steep increase with the flexion angle of the knee. This finding justifies the advice that persons with decreased bone strength due to osteoporosis should avoid deep knee bends, for example when performing strength training of the quadriceps or when picking up objects from the floor. Subjects with existing patellofemoral pain often exhibit abnormal gait as they tend to avoid larger flexion angles of the knee.

By changing the posture of the trunk, the location of the center of gravity of the body can be shifted with respect to the center of rotation of the knee joint. Specifically, it is possible to bend forward to such an extent that the center of gravity is positioned vertically above the center of rotation (Fig. 10.**18**). In this posture the moment arm of the body weight equals zero, and flexors and extensors of the knee joint are inactive (aside from some minor activation required for stabilizing the posture). Consequently the load on the knee joint is minimal in this posture. The bent-forward posture is not only assumed in certain athletic disciplines but is aimed at, in a similar fashion, by elderly subjects when rising from a chair (Fig. 10.**19**). The forward shift of the center of gravity decreases the moment arm of the body weight and reduces the required

force of the quadriceps muscle. Consequently, the load on the femorotibial, as well as on the femoropatellar, joint is decreased. For the elderly, a higher seat decreases the initial flexion angle of the knee and facilitates the forward bending of the trunk. The support by the hands effectively creates a force directed opposite to the body weight and thus decreases the moment of the body weight with respect to the knee.

In one-legged stance and static equilibrium, the center of gravity of the body is located vertically above the sole of the foot (Fig. 10.**20**). As femur and tibia are not aligned exactly to the vertical, the ground reaction force F_1 (force from the floor on to the foot) creates a moment in the frontal plane with respect to the center of rotation of the knee. This moment must be balanced by a moment of the muscle force F_6. Force F_1 is opposite and equal to the gravitational force of the body mass. The muscle force F_6 represents the force of gluteus maximus and tensor fasciae latae. F_4 designates the force between femur and tibia. In a healthy joint, F_4 is directed on to the center of the knee and aligned perpendicular to the tibial plateau. Thus both tibial condyles bear approximately the same fraction of the load. In varus deformity (displacement of the knee in a lateral direction) the moment arm of the body weight increases. To compensate, the muscle force F_6 must increase as well. If the muscles cannot develop enough force, or if they are not activated strongly enough, the collateral ligament will have to share in balancing the moment. Under tension, the ligament is elongated; in consequence a gap develops in the lateral aspect of the femorotibial joint. Force F_4 (already larger than normal) is then transmitted only via the medial part of the joint. If overload damage occurs in the medial part, the varus deformity will increase and the load on the medial part will increase again.

As with the hip joint, the dynamic load on the knee joint has been determined from gait analysis. Input data for such a calculation are mass, location of the center of gravity, and moment of inertia of the segments 'foot' and 'lower leg', temporal course of the location, velocity and acceleration of these segments, and the force between floor and foot. It is then possible to calculate the reaction force and the reaction moment transmitted from the upper to the lower leg. Employing a model of the knee joint, i.e. with knowledge of the directions and moment arms of all muscles and ligaments involved, then enables the load on the knee joint to be determined.

The foundations of such a calculation were outlined in Chapter 8. Due to the complex architecture of the knee joint there are initially more unknowns than (equilibrium-) equations. Morrison (1968) and Paul (1976) reduced the indeterminate system to a determinate system by representing the forces of several muscles and ligaments by a single force and (based on EMG measurements) by neglecting certain forces in specific phases of the gait cycle. For example, in flexion or extension of the knee only the quadriceps, or only the gastrocnemius, or only the hamstrings were taken into consideration. Fig. 10.**21** shows the results published by Paul (1976) for the load on the femorotibial joint. As in the hip joint, we recognize peak load values during the 'heel on' and 'toe off' phases. When running, both force maxima fuse to one single maximum. The magnitude of the maximum values increases with increasing gait velocity and reaches values of 4 times body weight during fast walking. These results prompt reconsideration of whether it is sensible to recommend running or jogging to elderly persons with diminished bone strength (especially of the trabecular bone below the tibial plateau).

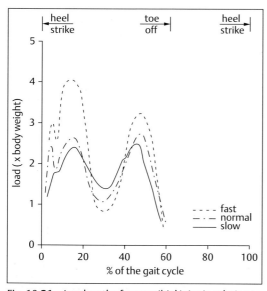

Fig. 10.21 Load on the femorotibial joint in relation to gait velocity as determined from gait analysis. The load is plotted in units of body weight. A full gait cycle corresponds to 100 %; during approximately 60 % of the gait cycle there is contact between the foot and the floor. Peak loads increase with increasing gait velocity. (Adapted from: Paul, 1976)

Pressure distribution in the femoropatellar joint

For a rough estimate of the pressure in the femoropatellar joint, the mean pressure may be calculated. To this end the femoropatellar force is divided by the contact area between patella and femur. For a subject with average body mass and average skeletal dimensions values between 1.5 and 2.5 MPa are obtained, depending on the flexion angle. These figures must, however, be regarded only as reference values, because the pressure-transmitting area of the femoropatellar joint depends on the duration of loading (Hehne *et al.*, 1981, 1982; Ahmed *et al.*, 1983). Under load, the viscoelastic cartilage is deformed and the pressure-transmitting area increases. The pressure will thus be different for short-term and long-term loading.

Several investigators measured the pressure distribution on the femoropatellar joint of specimens by means of pressure-sensitive foils. This measuring method can be applied to the knee (in contrast to other joints with strongly curved surfaces), because the contact area between patella and femur does not deviate appreciably from a plane. To simulate the realistic load *in vivo* on the knee joint specimens in relation to the angle of flexion, the specimens were loaded by a simulated quadriceps force. Hehne *et al.* (1981, 1982) found that the pressure on the articular surface was lower than expected; this was attributed to the noticeable increase in the articulating surface area effected by the load. Huberti and Hayes (1984) reported the pressure distribution in healthy joints to be virtually uniform. In joints with pathological changes due to chondromalacia patellae, a clear-cut non-uniformity of the distributions was observed (Huberti and Hayes 1988).

The femoropatellar joint is one of the few joints where currently available techniques allow actual measurement of the pressure distribution. This offers a unique opportunity to explore the relation between the pressure on the joint surface and the density of the subchondral trabecular bone (located below the articular cartilage). Müller-Gerbl *et al.* (1990) investigated the density of the subchondral bone in specimens of knee joints and documented an increased bone density below those parts of the joint surface that are highly loaded by pressure.

In the context of potential mechanical causes of chondromalacia patellae it is currently under discussion whether an abnormal activity of the muscles crossing the knee joint, alterations of the joint geometry, or peculiarities of the joint motion might result in an asymmetric pressure distribution on the patella. Specifically, it has been conjectured that an 'imbalance' of the forces of the vastus medialis and lateralis muscles might result in a 'wrong' position of the patella and thus in large local peak values of the pressure. This hypothesis is compatible with observations from experiments *in vitro* showing that the retropatellar pressure depends strongly on the direction of the simulated muscle force. The question of whether such an imbalance exists *in vivo* in individual cases, however, cannot be resolved by laboratory experiments. Support for the hypothesis and information on the potential benefit of strength training of parts of the vastus muscle can only be supplied by epidemiologic studies of treatment results.

In addition, experiments *in vitro* show a dependence of the retropatellar pressure distribution on the direction of the patellar tendon. The direction of the tendon relative to the femur is influenced by the axial rotation of the tibia. This is the rationale for the treatment of chondromalacia patellae with orthoses effecting an eversion of the foot. Experience shows that eversion of the foot entails an axial rotation of the tibia. Whether the postulated mechanism is correct can again only be concluded from epidemiologic studies of treatment results.

Loading of the cruciate ligaments

The cruciate ligaments guide the motion of femur and tibia; in addition they limit the range of motion in flexion and extension. To guide the motion, the geometry of the four-bar linkage (i. e. the lengths and insertion points of the cruciate ligaments)

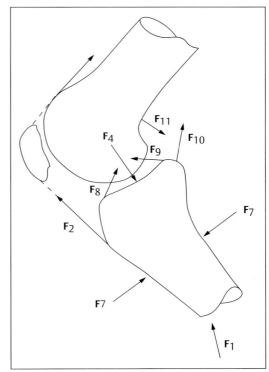

Fig. 10.**22** The force F_4 between femur and tibia is directed perpendicular to the tibial plateau. Forces F_8 and F_9, to be resisted by the cruciate ligaments, depend on force F_2 of the patellar tendon, force F_{10} of the hamstrings, force F_{11} of the gastrocnemius muscle, the ground reaction force F_1 and (potentially) on an additional, dorsoventrally or ventrodorsally directed, external force F_7. When standing, F_1 points vertically upwards; when walking, the direction of F_1 deviates from the vertical.

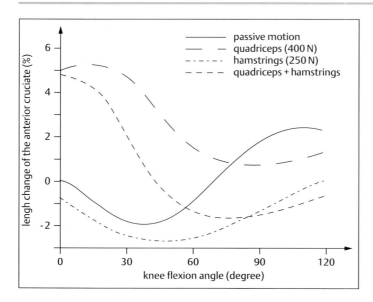

passive motion
quadriceps (400 N)
hamstrings (250 N)
quadriceps + hamstrings

Fig. 10.**23** Change in length of the anterior cruciate ligament in relation to the bending angle of the knee, measured for passive motion and with simulated, isotonic forces of the quadriceps and the hamstrings. (Adapted from Renström *et al.*, 1986)

must be precisely adjusted with respect to the geometry of the articulating surfaces of femur and tibia. An isolated change of only one parameter might obstruct the motion and lead to destruction of the joint. For this reason, when repairing or replacing cruciate ligaments, the surgeon endeavors to restore the original anatomical geometry as accurately as possible.

The cruciate ligaments balance the shear force, in the plane of the tibial plateau, produced by the flexors or extensors or by external forces (Fig. 10.**22**). The shear force depends on the magnitude and direction of the muscle forces, on the co-activation (if present) of flexors and extensors, and on additional, externally exerted forces. For postoperative treatment and rehabilitation after injury to the cruciate ligaments, it is of great importance to know under what circumstances the load on the cruciate ligaments assumes minimum and maximum values. Information on this difficult problem, one of great practical importance, stems to a large extent from experiments with specimens and from biomechanical model calculations.

Renström *et al.* (1986) measured *in vitro* the change in length of the anterior cruciate ligament when passively moving the knee, as well as the change in length when applying a simulated quadriceps or hamstring muscle force. The results (Fig. 10.**23**) showed that the length of the anterior cruciate ligament (and thus its tensile load) depends on the bending angle of the knee. As expected, a simulated force on the quadriceps of 400 N resulted

in an increase in length up to bending angles of 60° and thus in an increase in the tensile force of the ligament. At higher bending angles, the quadriceps force relieved the load on the ligament. This is due to the relative change in the directions of the quadriceps tendon and anterior cruciate ligament at higher bending angles. Compared with passive motion, hamstring activation reduced the load on the anterior cruciate ligament in the whole range of motion. In the region from full extension to 60° of flexion, hamstring activation could not fully compensate the load increase due to the quadriceps force. While the experiment demonstrates the relationship between the load on the anterior cruciate ligament and bending angle and antagonistic activation of quadriceps and hamstrings, it remains uncertain to what extent the simulated muscle forces correctly describe the situation *in vivo*. Fleming *et al.* (1998) succeeded in performing a measurement of the change in length of the anterior cruciate ligament *in vivo*, during training on a bicycle ergometer. Only low strains of the ligament of maximally 2.3 % were recorded. The authors conclude that the exercise investigated does not put the rehabilitation of patients with lesions of the cruciate ligaments at risk.

Employing a biomechanical model of the knee, Zavatsky and O'Connor (1993) and Zavatsky *et al.* (1994) analyzed the loading of the cruciate ligaments during isometric activation of quadriceps and hamstrings. During isometric activation of the extensors or flexors of the knee, an external force

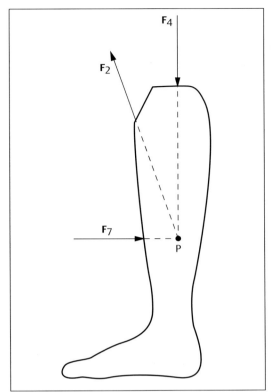

Fig. 10.**24** Equilibrium of forces at the tibia in the case of isometric activation of the quadriceps. Force F_2 of the patellar tendon, force F_4 between femur and patella, and external force F_7 directed perpendicular to the tibia and inhibiting motion of the tibia, are active. If the lines of action of F_2, F_4, and F_7 run though a single point P, the sum of all moments is equal to zero. The cruciate ligaments are not loaded. (Adapted from Zavatsky *et al.*, 1994)

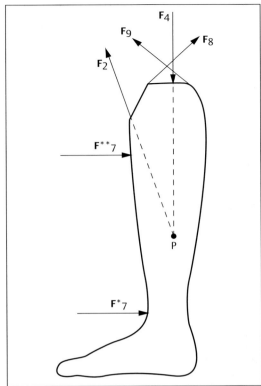

Fig. 10.**25** Equilibrium of forces at the tibia in the case of isometric activation of the quadriceps. If the external force, which hinders extension of the knee, acts distally (F^*_7) or proximally (F^{**}_7) to the point P, where the lines of action of forces F_2 and F_4 cross, either the anterior cruciate (F_8) or the posterior cruciate ligament (F_9) is loaded. (Adapted from Zavatsky *et al.*, 1994)

is required to prevent motion of the tibia. The results published by Zavatsky and colleagues show that the generalized statements 'a ventrally directed force on to the tibia loads the anterior cruciate ligament' and 'a dorsally directed force on the tibia loads the posterior cruciate ligament' are not correct. On the contrary, under isometric activation of the quadriceps, the loading of the cruciate ligaments depends crucially (surprisingly at first sight) on the point of application of the external force applied to inhibit motion of the tibia.

Fig. 10.**24** shows the tibia in a state of equilibrium with isometric activation of the quadriceps. Force F_2 of the patellar tendon, force F_4 directed perpendicular to the tibial plateau between femur and tib-

ia, and force F_7 directed perpendicular to the tibia and inhibiting rotation of the tibia, act on the tibia. If force F_7 is applied at such a location that the lines of action of forces F_2, F_4, and F_7 cross at point P, the sum of the moments of these forces relative to P equals zero (because the moment arms are equal to zero). If the sum of the moments related to one point is zero, and under the assumption that the sum of the forces equals zero, it follows that the sum of the moments equals zero for all other points as well. Thus the equilibrium condition for the moments is met. The magnitude of F_7 depends on the magnitudes of F_2 and F_4, since the sum of the forces in equilibrium must be equal to zero. Additional forces are not required to meet the equilibrium

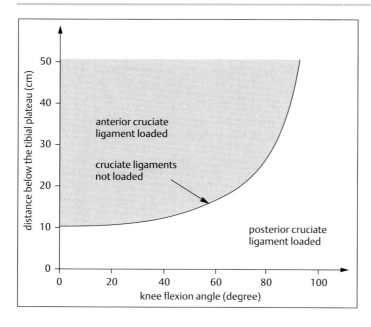

Fig. 10.**26** Point of application of force $\mathbf{F}_7$ in relation to the bending angle of the knee so that the cruciate ligaments remain unloaded on isometric activation of the quadriceps. Deviation of application of the force from the specified point results in a load on the anterior or posterior cruciate ligament. (Adapted from Zavatsky *et al.*, 1994)

conditions. In other words, in the set-up shown, the cruciate ligaments are not loaded.

If, with force $\mathbf{F}_2$ identical to that in Fig. 10.**24**, the external force $\mathbf{F}^*_7$ is applied more distally from the tibial plateau (Fig. 10.**25**), it must be smaller than $\mathbf{F}_7$ because its moment arm in relation to the center of rotation of the knee is larger than the moment arm of $\mathbf{F}_7$, otherwise the equilibrium of moments would not be met. As the magnitude of $\mathbf{F}^*_7$ is now fixed, an additional, fourth force acting in ventrodorsal direction is required to meet the equilibrium of forces. This force is a component of the tensile force $\mathbf{F}_8$ of the anterior cruciate ligament. In other words, the anterior cruciate ligament will be loaded by application of $\mathbf{F}^*_7$. If the motion of the tibia is inhibited by a more proximally acting, external force $\mathbf{F}^{**}_7$, the magnitude of $\mathbf{F}^{**}_7$ must be larger than the magnitude of $\mathbf{F}_7$ due to its smaller moment arm. To balance all forces, an additional force $\mathbf{F}_9$ acting in a dorsoventral direction is now required. In other words, in this situation the posterior cruciate ligament will be loaded.

As the directions of the patellar tendon and the cruciate ligaments vary with the bending angle of the knee, the point of application of force $\mathbf{F}_7$ chosen to prevent loading of the cruciate ligaments will vary as well. Fig. 10.**26** shows the result of a model calculation by Zavatsky *et al.* (1994). It is to be concluded from this diagram that the cruciate ligaments will not be loaded at bending angles between 0° and 50° and with application of force $\mathbf{F}_7$ approximately 10 cm below the tibial plateau. If the point of external force application deviates from this location, either the anterior or the posterior cruciate ligament will be loaded. The results of this model calculation should be interpreted only as a guideline because minor deviations are to be expected for individual knees as their dimensions might deviate from the geometry of the model knee.

Analogous arguments apply in the case of isometric activation of the hamstrings (Fig. 10.**27**). As in the case discussed above, for every flexion angle of the knee (i.e. depending on the direction of force $\mathbf{F}_{10}$ of the hamstrings) there is a point of application of the external force $\mathbf{F}_7$ where the equilibrium of moments is met and the cruciate ligaments are not loaded. Fig. 10.**28** shows the location of this point in relation to the flexion angle of the knee. It is to be concluded from this diagram that, for bending angles between 0° and 10°, force $\mathbf{F}_7$ should be applied approximately 40 cm below the tibial plateau to load the cruciate ligaments only minimally, if at all.

If the loading mode of the lower extremity is changed, the loading of the cruciate ligaments

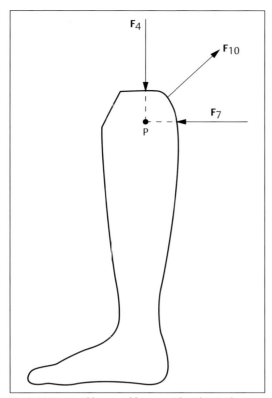

F_4

F_{10}

F_7

P

Fig. 10.27 Equilibrium of forces at the tibia in the case of isometric activation of the hamstrings. Active forces: force F_{10} of the hamstrings, force F_4 between femur and patella, and external force F_7 directed perpendicular to the tibia and inhibiting flexion of the tibia. If the lines of action of F_{10}, F_4, and F_7 run though a single point P, the sum of all moments is equal to zero. The cruciate ligaments are not loaded. (Adapted from Zavatsky *et al.*, 1994)

changes as well. Employing the biomechanical model cited above, O'Connor *et al.* (1990) determined the load of the anterior cruciate ligament when lifting a mass with a bent knee and activation of the quadriceps muscle only. The authors found that activation of the quadriceps muscle loads the anterior cruciate ligament at bending angles between 0° and 85°; at bending angles between 85° and 130° the posterior cruciate ligament is loaded. At an angle of 85° no forces in the cruciate ligaments were required for equilibrium. It must be pointed out that these results are only valid for the case where the quadriceps alone is activated. If the

hamstrings are activated simultaneously, we encounter a different loading mode and thus expect a different loading of the cruciates. The work of O'Connor and colleagues shows that, in postures where the load on the femorotibial and femoropatellar joints assumes maximum values, simultaneous high loading of the cruciate ligaments need not necessarily be expected. The dependence of the loading of the cruciate ligaments on the muscle forces, the external force, and the bending angle of the knee suggest (correctly) that the loading of the cruciate ligaments will be different in different types of rehabilitation exercises (Toutoungi *et al.*, 2000) and, for example, in forward or backward walking, or in forward or backward pedaling on a bicycle ergometer.

Based on the model of the knee joint (O'Connor *et al.*, 1990; O'Connor, 1993), the authors demonstrated that both cruciate ligaments can be unloaded by isometric co-activation of the quadriceps and the hamstrings, though only at a bending angle of about 20° (Fig. 10.**29**). In the whole range of motion of the knee joint, quadriceps, hamstrings, and gastrocnemius can be activated simultaneously in such a fashion that a) the resulting moment about the center of motion of the knee equals zero (so that no movement results) and b) neither cruciate ligament is loaded (Fig. 10.**30**).

Experiments *in vitro* investigating the influence of simulated muscle forces on the load on the cruciate ligaments, and the model calculation discussed above, may account for subjects with a disrupted posterior or anterior cruciate ligament nevertheless exhibiting a normal gait and being otherwise only marginally restricted in their physical activity (see, for example, Jonsson and Kärrholm, 1999). In such cases the functions of restricting the dorsoventral translation of the femur with respect to the tibia, and of limiting the range of motion are obviously taken over by the muscles. Because the direction of the flexors and extensors relative to the tibia changes with the bending angle, the magnitudes of the three muscle forces must be adjusted in relation to the bending angle to fulfill these tasks successfully. If strength training of the knee flexors and extensors is performed with the intention of shielding the cruciate ligaments from excessively high tensile forces, it must be kept in mind that muscle strength alone is not sufficient to meet this aim. In addition, for each bending angle the forces of flexors and extensors must be adjusted relative to each other to effect the desired unloading. Whether a person is really able to adjust the forces of the three muscles exactly in the required proportions as shown in Fig. 10.**30** is not known.

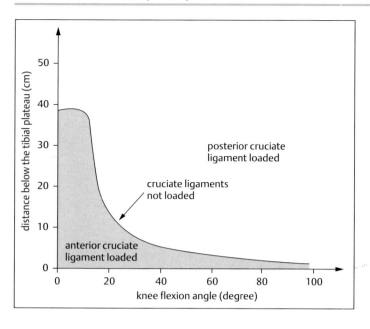

Fig. 10.**28** Point of application of force **F**$_7$ in relation to the bending angle of the knee so that the cruciate ligaments remain unloaded on isometric activation of the hamstrings. Deviation of application of the force from the specified point results in a load on the anterior or posterior cruciate ligament. (Adapted from Zavatsky *et al.*, 1994)

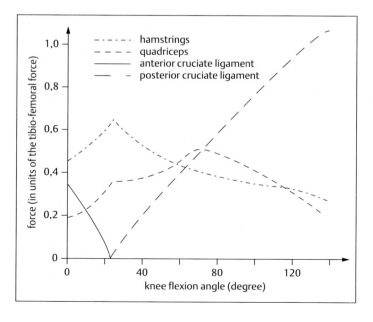

Fig. 10.**29** Load on the anterior and posterior cruciate ligament with isometric, antagonistic activation of quadriceps and hamstrings. Only at a bending angle of 20° is the load on both ligaments equal to zero. At bending angles below 20° the anterior cruciate ligament, and at angles above 20° the posterior cruciate ligament, is loaded. (Adapted from O'Connor, 1993)

Fig. 10.**30** Simultaneous activation of quadriceps, gastrocnemius, and hamstrings, so that the cruciate ligaments are not loaded. The magnitude of the muscle forces required depends on the bending angle of the knee. (Adapted from O'Connor, 1993)

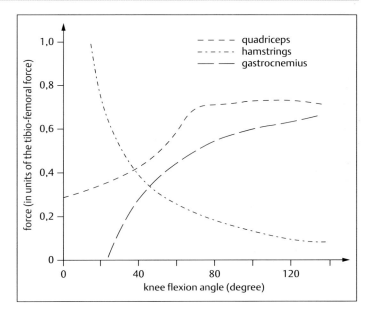

Suggestions for further reading

Textbooks and review papers

Frost HM. *Orthopaedic biomechanics.* Springfield: Thomas; 1973

Maquet PGJ. *Biomechanics of the knee.* Berlin: Springer; 1976

McGinty G, Irrgang JJ, Pezzullo D. Biomechanical considerations for rehabilitation of the knee. *Clinical Biomechanics.* 2000; **15**: 160–166 [review paper, 39 references]

Müller W. *Das Knie. Form, Funktion und ligamentäre Wiederherstellungschirurgie.* Berlin: Springer; 1982

Smith BA, Livesay GA, Woo SLY. Biology and biomechanics of the anterior cruciate ligament. *Clinics in Sports Med.* 1993; **12**: 637–670 [review paper, 104 references]

Original papers cited in the text or in the figures

Ahmed AM, Burke DL, Yu A. In-vitro measurement of static pressure distribution in synovial joints. Part II: retropatellar surface. *J Biomechanical Engineering.* 1983; **105**: 226–236

Blankevoort L, Huiskes R, de Lange A. Helical axes of passive knee joint motions. *J Biomechanics.* 1990; **23**: 1219–1229

Charnley J. The lubrication of animal joints in relation to surgical reconstruction by arthroplasty. *Ann Rheum Dis.* 1960; **19**: 10–19

Fleming BC, Beynnon BD, Renström PA, Peura GD, Nichols CE, Johnson RJ. The strain behavior of the anterior cruciate ligament during bicycling. An *in vivo* study. *Am J Sports Med.* 1998; **26**: 109–118

Fuss FK. Anatomy of the cruciate ligaments and their function in extension and flexion of the human knee joint. *Am J Anatomy.* 1989; **184**: 165–176

Hehne HJ, Ficker E, Jantz W, Mahr D, Schöpf HJ. Eine neue Methode zur Ermittlung lastabhängiger Druck- und Kontaktverläufe an Grenzflächen. *Morphol Med.* 1981; **1**: 95–106

Hehne HJ, Diebolder H, Ficker E, Jantz W. Analoge Druck- und Kontaktflächenmessung des Femoropatellargelenkes mit optisch sensibler Druckmeßfolie. *Z Orthop.* 1982; **120**: 513

Huberti HH, Hayes WC. Patellofemoral contact pressures. The influence of Q-angle and tendofemoral contact. *J Bone Jt Surg.* 1984; **66A**: 715–724

Huberti HH, Hayes WC. Contact pressures in chondromalacia patellae and the effects of capsular reconstructive procedures. *J Orthop Res.* 1988; 6: 499–508

Jonsson H, Kärrholm J. Three-dimensional knee kinematics and stability in patients with a posterior cruciate ligament tear. *J Orthop Res.* 1999; **17**: 185–191

Kummer B. Cinématique du genou. *Acta Orthop Belg.* 1982; **48**: 28–35

Menschik A. Mechanik des Kniegelenks. Teil 1. *Z Orthop.* 1974; **112**: 481–495

Müller-Gerbl M, Putz R, Hodapp N, Schulte E, Wimmer B. Die Darstellung der subchondralen Dichtemuster mittels der CT-Osteoabsorptiometrie (CT-OAM) zur Beurteilung der individuellen Gelenkbeanspruchung am Lebenden. *Z Orthop.* 1990; **128**: 128–133

Morrison JB. Bioengineering analysis of force actions transmitted by the knee joint. *Biomed Engng.* 1968; **3**: 164–170

O'Connor JJ, Shercliff T, FitzPatrick D, Biden E, Goodfellow J. Mechanics of the knee. In Daniel DM et al. (eds). *Knee ligaments. Structure, function, injury and repair,* p. 201–238. New York: Raven Press; 1990

O'Connor JJ, Biden E, Bradley J, FitzPatrick D, Young S, Kershaw C, Daniel DM, Goodfellow J. The muscle stabilized knee. In Daniel DM *et al.* (eds). *Knee ligaments. Structure, function, injury and repair,* p. 239–276. New York: Raven Press; 1990

O'Connor JJ. Can muscle co-contraction protect knee ligaments after injury or repair? *J Bone Joint Surg.* 1993; **75B**: 41–48

Paul JP. Forces transmitted by joints in the human body. *Proc R Soc Lond B* 1976; **192**: 163–172

Piazza SJ, Cavanagh PR. Measurement of the screw-home motion of the knee is sensitive to errors in axis alignment. *J Biomechanics* 2000; **33**: 1029–1034

Reilly DT, Martens M. Experimental analysis of the quadriceps muscle force and patello-femoral joint reaction force for various activities. Acta Orthop Scand. 1972; 43: 126–137

Renström P, Arms SW, Stanwyck TS, Johnson RJ, Pope MH. Strain within the anterior cruciate ligament during hamstring and quadriceps activity. *Am J Sports Med.* 1986; **14**: 83–87

Seedhom BB, Takeda T, Tsubuku M, Wright V. Mechanical factors and patellofemoral osteoarthrosis. Ann Rheum *Dis.* 1979; 38: 307–316

Smidt GL. Biomechanical analysis of knee flexion and extension. *J Biomechanics.* 1973; **6**: 79–92

Toutoungi DE, Lu TW, Leardini A, Catani F, O'Connor JJ. Cruciate ligament forces in the human knee during rehabilitation exercises. *Clinical Biomechanics.* 2000; **15**: 176–187

van Dijk R, Huiskes R, Selvik G. Roentgen stereophotogrammetric methods for the evaluation of the three dimensional kinematic behaviour and cruciate ligament length patterns of the human knee joint. *J Biomechanics.* 1979; **12**: 727–731

Woo SLY, Hollis JM, Adams DJ et al. Tensile properties of the human femur-anterior cruciate ligament-tibia complex: The effects of specimen age and orientation. *Am J Sports Med.* 1991; **19**: 217–225

Zavatsky AB, O'Connor JJ. Ligament forces at the knee during isometric quadriceps contractions. Proc Inst Mech Eng H: J Eng Medicine. 1993; **207**: 7–18

Zavatsky AB, Beard DJ, O'Connor JJ. Cruciate ligament loading during isometric muscle contractions. A theoretical basis for rehabilitation. *Am J Sports Med.* 1994; **22**: 418–423

11 Mechanical Aspects of the Lumbar Spine

Rotational and translational motion of the vertebrae in flexion and extension

The relative motion of neighboring vertebrae can be classified as axial rotation, side bending or flexion-extension. As in virtually all other joints of the body, the motion of the vertebral joint is not guided by the shape of the articulating bones alone but, in effect, by the architecture and material properties of the spinal ligaments and the intervertebral disk. For this reason the pattern of the motion cannot be predicted theoretically but must be recorded experimentally. In order to arrive at a simple description, we describe the flexion-extension motion as a pure, plane rotation. Fig. 11.1 illustrates the procedure used to measure the location of the center of rotation (see also Chapter 4). Two metallic markers are fixed on a specimen of a motion segment (consisting of two vertebrae and intervening disk) and radiographs are taken in two different angular positions of the joint. The center of rotation (the point where the axis of rotation intersects the plane of motion) is given by the intersection of the perpendicular bisectors of the lines connecting the marker locations in the two angular positions. In motion segments with non-degenerated or moderately degenerated disks, the center of rotation is generally found approximately in the center of the disk. The centers of rotation for side bending or axial rotation (rotation about the long axis of the spine) are determined experimentally in a similar fashion. They are also located at the center of the disk. When calculating the load on the spine, the moment arms of external or muscle forces are thus related to the centers of the disks.

A closer look at the relative movement of adjacent vertebrae during flexion and extension reveals that it might be advantageous to describe the sagittal plane motion by a combination of rotational motion and translational motion in a dorsoventral direction. In extension the cranial vertebra rotates and at the same time translates into a dorsal direction with respect to the caudal vertebra; in flexion the converse rotational and translational motion is observed (Fig. 11.2). The coupling (forced combination) between rotation and translation is caused by the shape of the facet joints. In motion segments without degeneration or other pathologic findings, the magnitude

of the dorsoventral shift between full extension and full flexion amounts to approximately 2 mm.

The coupled motion composed of rotation and translation could, in principle, also be described by a pure rotation (see Chapter 4). To describe the motion in this fashion, the center of rotation must be displaced from the center of the disk by a certain distance in a caudal direction. If we assume the caudal vertebra to be fixed, it can easily be imagined that, with a center of rotation located caudally to the center of the disk, the upper vertebra translates in a dorsal direction when a rotation in extension is performed. The translation effect increases with increasing caudal displacement of the center of rotation. The description of the motion by a pure rotation, however, is impractical for two reasons.

- The range of flexion-extension motion of the lumbar vertebral joint is relatively small, amounting to about 12°. In consequence, the construction of the center of rotation, as illustrated in Fig. 11.1 or by means of other algorithms, is

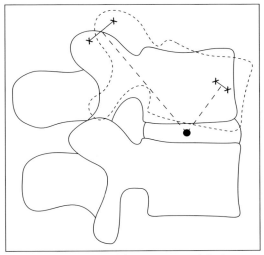

Fig. 11.1 Experimental determination of the location of the center of rotation of a motion segment of the lumbar spine for flexion and extension. Two markers are fixed on the mobile vertebra of the segment. The location of the center of rotation is given by the intersection of the vertical bisectors of the lines connecting the markers in the initial and final state of the motion. Save for maximally degenerated specimens the center of rotation is found approximately at the center of the disk.

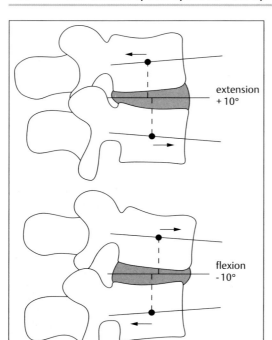

Fig. 11.2 Relative dorsoventral translational motion of the vertebrae, and ventral as well as dorsal radial bulging of the disk in flexion and extension. In flexion, the cranial vertebral body shifts in a ventral direction; in extension the shift occurs in a dorsal direction. In flexion, the radial bulge decreases dorsally and increases ventrally. In extension, the radial bulge increases dorsally and decreases ventrally. (For reasons of clarity, the effects of relative motion and bulge change are depicted in an exaggerated fashion.)

not very precise (Penning *et al.*, 1984). Discrimination between physiologic and pathologic locations of the center of rotation becomes difficult.

– It is possible that a translational motion (however small) might occur in vertebral joints with pathologic alterations while the angular orientation of the vertebrae remained unchanged. If we wanted to describe such a translational motion by a pure rotation, the center of rotation would have to be shifted to infinity. This is awkward as infinity cannot be described by a number (and in graphic illustrations no sheet of paper is large enough to accommodate the location 'infinity').

It is easier to explore the translational and rotational motion separately. With respect to rotation, we do not run into any problems as the angle of rotation suffices for the description. For the translation-

al motion, it must first be agreed in which direction the translational motion is to be specified. With the aim of improving conventional protocols (e.g. Morgan and King, 1957; Bernhardt *et al.*, 1992) Frobin *et al.* (1996) proposed measuring the dorsoventral translational motion along the bisector between the mid planes of the adjacent vertebrae (Fig. 11.2). This definition is symmetric with respect to the two vertebrae. Employing the new protocol, the dorsoventral translational motion can be measured from lateral radiographs of the lumbar spine with an error corresponding to approximately 2% of the depth of the vertebrae. For a vertebra of 35 mm depth this corresponds to a measurement error of 0.7 mm, representing a substantial increase of measurement precision compared with conventional protocols.

The highest precision in the measurement of relative vertebral motion *in vivo* is reached when metallic markers are implanted in the bones and pairs of stereoradiographs are taken. (Stereoradiographs are two radiographs taken from different directions.) The locations of the markers are measured from the films; their three-dimensional coordinates and the parameters of the motion are computed (Selvik, 1989; for application to clinical problems see, for example, Johnsson *et al.*, 1996). Due to its invasive nature, application of the procedure, however, is limited to the postoperative follow-up of small cohorts of patients.

The dorsoventral translational motion has attracted much attention ever since Knutsson (1944) speculated on a correlation between translational motion, deviating from the normal coupling pattern with rotational motion, and clinical symptoms. While a restriction of rotational and translational motion (hypomobility) is not a rare finding, reliably documented cases of excessively large translational motion (hypermobility) seem to be rare (save cases with spondylolysis, i.e. a fracture of the vertebral arch). When this problem is discussed in the medical literature, the term 'instability' is frequently used instead of 'hypermobility'. This is a misleading description as 'unstable' (in contrast to 'stable') characterizes a mechanical state that can be changed completely and irreversibly by a small external perturbation. Such a state does not exist in the lumbar spine, even if the translational motion is observed to be larger than normal.

Calculation of the loading of the lumbar spine: two-dimensional model

In a state of equilibrium, the load on the lumbar spine when holding a mass in the hands can be es-

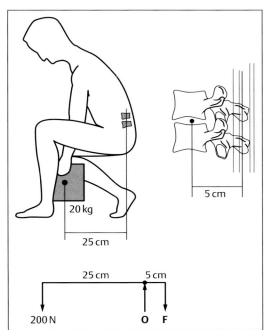

Fig. 11.3 Calculation of the increased load on the lumbar spine, caused by a mass held in the hands. In this example the directions of the gravitational force and of the force of the extensor muscles of the back are assumed to be parallel. The moment arm of the gravitational force is given by the perpendicular distance of the center of gravity of the mass from the center of rotation, located at the center of the disk. This moment arm is assumed to amount to 25 cm. The moment arm of the extensor muscles of the back is given by the distance of the center of the cross-sectional area of these muscles from the center of the disk. This moment arm is estimated to amount to 5 cm.

timated easily if some simplifying assumptions are made. In Fig. 11.3 the mass is located in the sagittal plane. The force of the extensor muscles of the lumbar spine is merged into one single muscle force **F**. The moment arm of the extensor muscles, i.e. the distance from the center of the intervertebral disk to the center of the cross-sectional area of the extensor muscles, is estimated to amount to 5 cm. In addition we assume that the direction of the muscle force at the segment in question points (approximately) in a vertical direction, i.e. parallel to the gravitational force of the mass. With a mass of 20 kg, exerting a gravitational force of 200 N, and a moment arm of 25 cm we obtain the magnitude of the muscle force from the equilibrium condition of moments (signs according to the sign convention for moments)

$$5 \cdot |\mathbf{F}| - 25 \cdot 200 = 0 \text{ Ncm}$$
$$|\mathbf{F}| = 1000 \text{ N}$$

If we count the downwards pointing force components (muscle and gravitational force) as negative, we obtain from the equilibrium condition of forces the component O of the joint load **O**

$$O - 200 + F = 0$$
$$O - 200 - 1000 = 0$$
$$O = +1200 \text{ N}$$

The positive sign of O indicates that **O** is directed oppositely to the muscle and gravitational forces. The joint is loaded by **O** in compression.

If the total load on the lumbar spine is to be estimated in the posture shown in Fig. 11.3, the moment of the body weight cranial to the segment in question has to be taken into consideration, in addition to the moment of the weight held in the hands. To simplify the model calculation and to allow easy adaptation to different postures, the body is subdivided into the segments of head, arms, and trunk (Fig. 11.4). The masses and the locations of the centers of gravity of the segments can be found in reference books (e.g. Pheasant, 1986; Winter, 1990; Chaffin *et al.*, 1999). The moment arms L_2, L_3, and L_4 of the weights of the segments have to be measured, for example, from film or video images. With m_1 as the mass of the handheld mass, m_2, m_3, and m_4 as masses of the segments head, arms, and trunk, g as gravitational acceleration, **F** and L_5 as force and moment arm of the extensors of the back, we obtain in the equilibrium of moments (signs according to the sign convention for moments)

$$-L_1 \cdot m_1 \cdot g - L_2 \cdot m_2 \cdot g - L_3 \cdot m_3 \cdot g - L_4 \cdot m_4 \cdot g + L_5 \cdot |\mathbf{F}| = 0$$

It is again agreed to designate downwards-pointing forces by a negative sign; thus the component F of the muscle force is a negative number. In the equilibrium of forces (or, more precisely, the equilibrium of all vertically directed components) we obtain

$$O - m_1 \cdot g - m_2 \cdot g - m_3 \cdot g - m_4 \cdot g + F = 0$$
$$O = m_1 \cdot g + m_2 \cdot g + m_3 \cdot g + m_4 \cdot g - F$$

It is concluded from this equation that, even without any external load (m_1 = zero), the lumbar spine is loaded by the body weight and in addition by the muscle force required to balance the moment of the weight of head, arms, and trunk in the forward bent posture. This load increases with increased forward bending, i.e. with increased forward dis-

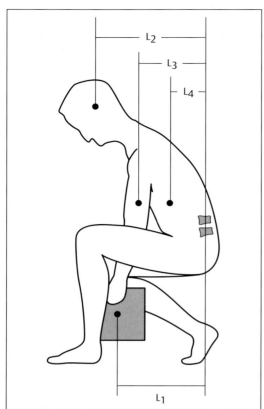

Fig. 11.**4** Total load on segment L4/L5 when holding a mass in the hand. For the purpose of calculation, the body cranial to L4 is imagined to be divided into the segments of trunk, arms, and head, with masses m_2, m_3, and m_4. The solid circles designate the centers of gravity of these segments; L_2, L_3, and L_4 are the moment arms of the gravitational forces. The total load is obtained as the sum of four addends: one contribution from holding the mass (c.f. Fig. 11.**3**) and three contributions from the body segments.

placement of the centers of gravity of the segments.

If an object is not only held or lifted very slowly but noticeably accelerated in the lifting process, inertial forces have to be taken into account. When lifting a mass (Fig. 11.**5**) the accelerations of the mass and the body segments are directed upwards. Thus the inertial force $\mathbf{F}_{in} = -m \cdot \mathbf{a}$ is directed downwards and points in the same direction as the gravitational force. It follows that, when accelerating the object and the body segments (dynamic case), the extensor muscles of the back have to develop a higher force than when simply holding the object (static case). For this reason we expect the load on

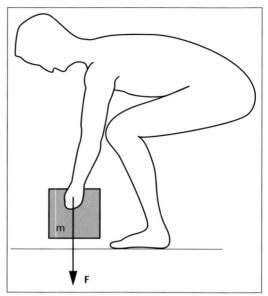

Fig. 11.**5** While holding a mass, the gravitational force **F** acts on the hands. When lifting a mass, the acceleration **a** is directed upwards. The inertial force $\mathbf{F}_{in} = -m \cdot \mathbf{a}$ is directed downwards. When lifting, the sum of gravitational and inertial forces act on the hand. Consequently, the force on the hand is higher when lifting compared to just holding a mass.

the lumbar spine to be higher in the dynamic compared with the static case.

Employing realistic data for the acceleration of objects being lifted obtained from observation of industrial workplaces, Leskinen *et al.* (1983 a, b) calculated that the load on the segment L5/S1 when lifting a mass of 15 kg, by a variety of lifting techniques, amounts to between 5800 and 6600 N. A static calculation, i.e. without inertial forces being taken into consideration, resulted in loads between 3900 and 4600 N. This comparison demonstrates that inertial forces due to anticipated movements (and not only in accident situations) can contribute substantially to spinal loading.

The role of intra-abdominal pressure

Experience shows that many subjects generate a pressure in the abdominal cavity when lifting a heavy object. In the past it was hypothesized that the intra-abdominal pressure relieved the load on the lumbar spine. The reasoning was that the pressure acts in all directions, on the pelvic floor as well as on the diaphragm. This pressure generates a moment opposite to the moment of the object lifted. In consequence, the force of the extensors of the back and the load on the spine ought to be diminished.

The pressurization of the abdominal cavity is effected predominantly by activation of the obliquus internus, obliquus externus and transversus abdominis muscles. Inspection of the direction of pull of the oblique muscles (Fig. 11.**6**) shows that the load-relief mechanism described above cannot be correct. The force of the muscles can be broken down into a component directed circularly with respect to the trunk, and one in the direction of the spine. In equilibrium, the extensors of the back have to deliver an additional force to balance this component of the oblique muscles, to prevent forward bending of the trunk. (This additional activation of the extensors can be verified easily by palpation when voluntarily generating an intra-abdominal pressure.) Consequently, the antagonistic activation of the muscles ventral and dorsal to the spine increases the load on the spine. This increase can, at best, be partially compensated by the extension moment generated by the intra-abdominal pressure; this holds especially for that part of the pressure that is due to the activation of the transversus abdominis muscle. The measurement of spinal loading by means of intradiskal pressure (see below) showed that the spinal load indeed increases when pressure is generated. Complaints by patients about aggravated symptoms when generating intra-abdominal pressure (e. g. when coughing) can be explained by this increase in load.

Various conjectures have been put forward in answer to the question of why intra-abdominal pressure is generated (since it obviously does not unload the spine). It is possible that generation of intra-abdominal pressure is not intentional but merely a by-product of the contraction of the muscles of the trunk. Activation of these muscles serves to stabilize the upper with respect to the lower trunk. Marras *et al.* (1985) showed that, in rapid lifting exercises, peak values of the pressure are reached before peak values of the external moment are observed. This complies with the observation that healthy subjects activate the transversus abdominis muscle before an anticipated activation of the deltoideus muscle and subsequent movement of the arm is made (Hodges and Richardson, 1996). In addition, the above hypothesis is supported by the observation that a high intra-abdominal pressure is usually generated during sit-up exercises. In these exercises the flexion moment due to the pressure is directed opposite to the intended

movement (i. e. extension) of the trunk (McGill, 1995).

Alternatively, it is possible that the intra-abdominal pressure serves to stabilize the form of the

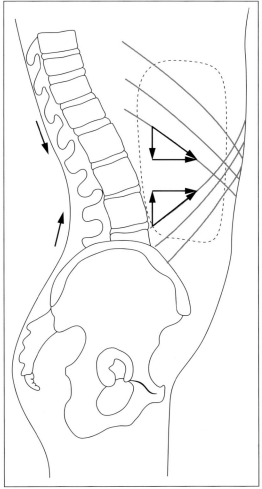

Fig. 11.**6** Intra-abdominal pressure is generated by activation of the obliquus externus and internus muscles. As the forces of these muscles have components in the direction of the spine, the extensors of the back have to be activated to prevent forward bending of the trunk. Due to the antagonistic activation of the muscles ventrally and dorsally to the spine, the load on the spine is increased. It is conjectured that the intra-abdominal pressure increases the stability of the lumbar spine by resisting increase in lordotic curvature. Alternatively, it is possible that intra-abdominal pressure is simply a by-product of the activation of the muscles stabilizing the upper trunk with respect to the lower trunk.

lumbar spine. The pressure generated in the abdominal cavity is usually not very high; peak values of 100 mm Hg (corresponding to 13.3 kPa) are exceeded only when lifting very heavy objects (Davis and Troup, 1964; Stubbs, 1985). The pressure acts, however, on a relatively large area. The dorsally directed force on the lumbar spine may serve to prevent an excessive increase in the lordotic curvature if the spine is under high axial (longitudinally directed) load (Cholewicki et al., 1999). In any event, the intra-abdominal pressure permits the muscles of the trunk to contract while preventing a collapse of the abdominal cavity.

Irrespective of these findings, broad belts are available commercially that promise to relieve the load on the spine in physically demanding workplaces. Experimental and epidemiological studies have demonstrated, however, that wearing such belts neither increases the isometric force of the extensor muscles of the back, nor reduces the rate of injuries to the lumbar spine (McGill, 1993; Reyna et al., 1995; Miyamoto et al., 1999). At most, belts limit the range of motion of the trunk with respect to flexion (Lüssenhop et al., 1996; McGorry and Hsiang, 1999).

Calculation of the loading of the lumbar spine: three-dimensional model

If a calculation of spinal loading is restricted to the erect or forward bent posture and external gravitational forces acting in the sagittal plane, the results will cover only a fraction of postures or loading modes occurring at the workplace or during leisure-time activities. In general, the trunk may be bent sideways or axially rotated. The external force may act on one hand only. The vector of the external force need not necessarily point in the vertical direction but may also point in horizontal direction when pulling or pushing an object.

If the load on the lumbar spine is to be calculated for an arbitrary posture and an arbitrary direction of the vector of the external force, it is obviously no longer permissible to take only one single muscle force of the extensors of the back into consideration. Jäger and colleagues (Jäger, 1987; Jäger and Luttmann, 1993) presented a model that described the muscle architecture of the lumbar spine, ventrally and dorsally, involving eight muscles. Based on the work of Schultz and Andersson (1981), Bean et al. (1988) presented a model taking 10 muscles into account. The area of attachment and spatial direction of the muscles, as well as their variation due to changes in posture (see, for example, McGill et al., 2000), are allowed for in the models, in addition to stature, body mass, and gender, in order to obtain results valid for individual cases.

As there are more unknowns than equilibrium equations available, additional assumptions on the co-activation of the muscles are required (c. f. Chapter 8) in order to arrive at unequivocal solutions for the muscle forces and for the load on the segments of the lumbar spine. Alternatively, attempts are made to eliminate the ambiguity by means of EMG measurements of the back muscles. However, this is a difficult procedure, because the activity of the deeper muscles is inadequately recorded by surface electrodes (Andersson et al., 1996). Despite the necessary simplifications and assumptions, the results of the model calculations provide valuable suggestions for ergonomic improvements at workplaces and for the prevention of overload injuries of the lumbar spine. Numerous workplaces have been analyzed using the model of Jäger and colleagues (see, for example, Jäger et al., 1983, 1991). Lifting an object in an asymmetric posture (i. e. bent sideways) does not necessarily lead to a higher load on the lumbar spine than lifting in the sagittal plane, because the obliques have larger moment arms than the extensors of the back (Dieën and Kingma, 1999). A computer program for calculating the load on the lumbar spine, based on the model of Bean and coworkers (1988), is commercially available (University of Michigan 1995).

Determination of the loading of the lumbar spine from measurements of intradiskal pressure

Using specimens of motion segments of the lumbar spine, Nachemson (1960) explored the relation between an axial compressive force exerted on a motion segment and the pressure in the center of the disk. For this purpose the specimens were loaded in a materials testing machine. The vector of the compressive force was directed perpendicular to the mid plane of the intervertebral disk. The pressure was measured by means of a thin cannula equipped with a pressure transducer (electronic pressure-measuring device) at its tip (Fig. 11.7, upper drawing). Even with no external compressive force a small amount of pressure exists in the disk. This pressure is caused by the elastic tension of the ligaments crossing the vertebral joint. With increasing compressive force, the pressure increases as well; a linear relation between compressive force and pressure is observed (Fig. 11.**7**, lower graph).

By averaging the measurements of the specimens investigated, Nachemson obtained for the pressure p

$$p = (1.5 \pm 0.1) \cdot F/A$$

In this formula F denotes the compressive force and A the cross-sectional area of the disk. Nachemson (1963) showed, in addition, that the factor of proportionality between load and pressure deviates from 1.5 when the angular position (angle of lordosis) of the vertebrae deviates from the position assumed in erect standing. In subsequent investigations *in vivo*, this modification was, however, disregarded when converting the measured pressure into spinal loading.

The calibration 'compressive force versus pressure' derived *in vitro* from specimens was subsequently employed by Nachemson to infer spinal loading *in vivo* from the intradiskal pressure data measured *in vivo*. Via the calibration line a certain magnitude of the compressive force F is assigned to each pressure value p (Fig. 11.**7**, lower graph). For the measurement *in vivo* (Nachemson and Elfström, 1970) a miniature pressure transducer mounted at the tip of a cannula of 2 mm diameter was placed in the L3/L4 disk of volunteers. Disk cross-sectional areas were determined from radiographs. The pressures in different postures and during a variety of activities were recorded and converted into compressive force using the formula given above. Table 11.**1**, extracted from Nachemson's results, lists the spinal load on the segment L3/L4, averaged over the cohort investigated.

According to these measurements, the load on the lumbar spine while standing erect exceeds the weight of the body mass cranial to the segment L3/L4. Approximately 50 % of the body mass is located cranial to segment L3/L4; for a body mass of 60 kg this would correspond to a weight of 300 N. The difference between this and 700 N recorded (see Table 11.**1**) is due to muscle forces required to stabilize the erect posture and to the elastic tension of muscles and ligaments. Nachemson found that, in persons sitting erect on a chair without a backrest, the spine was loaded higher than in the erect stance; for an in-depth discussion of this specific result the reader is referred to Chapter A1. As expected, lying down unloads the spine compared with standing; but even in persons lying supine under application of a tensile force, a compressive force between adjacent vertebrae is still recorded. Lifting a mass results in increased loading of the spine; the magnitude of the measured load agrees satisfactorily with results from model calculations

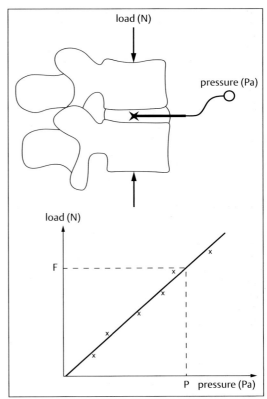

Fig. 11.**7** Calibration of the intradiskal pressure against the load *in vitro* and determination of the load F from the measured intradiskal pressure p *in vivo*. (Adapted from Nachemson, 1960.) Measurements from specimens show a linear relation between load and intradiskal pressure. (The lower diagram shows fictitious points, serving for illustration.) By means of the calibration diagram and with a known cross-sectional area of a disk, the load F [N] *in vivo* can be obtained from the intradiskal pressure p [Pa] measured *in vivo*.

cited above (see the section on calculation of the loading of the lumbar spine: two dimensional model). Isometric activation of the abdominal muscles, i.e. the generation of intra-abdominal pressure, increases the load on the lumbar spine; this complies with the arguments put forward earlier.

Determination of spinal loading from measurements of intradiskal pressure has the advantage that, in contrast to model calculations, no assumptions or simplifications have to be made. On the other hand, there is no guarantee that the posture and motion of the test subjects, as well as the pattern and magnitude of the muscle activation, are

Table 11.1 Mean values of the load on segment L3/L4, determined by measurement of intradiskal pressure; values rounded to full 100 N (extracted from Nachemson, 1985)

activity	load L3/L4
standing, erect	700 N
sitting, erect, without backrest	1000 N
lying supine	300 N
lying, under extension	100 N
lifting 20 kg, trunk bent forward	3400 N
isometric activation of the abdominal muscles	1100 N

not influenced by the instrumentation. Due the invasive nature of the procedure, the application of the method is limited to small cohorts. Although no detrimental after-effects of the placement of the pressure transducer at the center of the L3/L4 disks have been reported, a repetition of intradiskal pressure recordings would nowadays be subject to very strict safety regulations.

Determination of the load on the lumbar spine from measurements of stature change

Since the study by DePuky (1935) it has been known that the stature decreases in the course of a day by 1 to 2 cm due to fluid loss and viscoelastic deformation of the intervertebral disks. Stature decreases most rapidly in the morning immediately after getting out of bed; during the day the rate of loss of stature decreases (Reilly *et al.*, 1984). Due to the lower spinal load during sleep as compared to daytime, the disks imbibe fluid and relaxation of the viscoelastic deformation occurs. As result, stature increases again.

Eklund and Corlett (1984) proposed utilizing the decrease of stature to document spinal loading. As the change of stature during the whole day amounts to less than 20 mm, it is obvious that stature must be measured very precisely when short episodes of spinal loading are to be documented. For this purpose Eklund and Corlett measured stature not while subjects were standing erect but while they were leaning against a frame tilted back by approximately 10° (Fig. 11.**8**). Leaning against the frame permits relaxed standing and relatively good reproduction of the curvature of the spine, especially in the regions of thoracic kyphosis and lumbar lordosis.

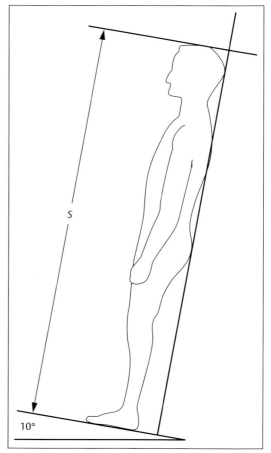

Fig. 11.**8** Set-up for a precision measurement of stature. Stature S is measured with the subject standing while leaning back by about 10°. In addition, the lordosis of the lumbar and cervical spine as well as the kyphosis of the thoracic spine are monitored. (Adapted from Eklund and Corlett, 1984)

In further developing Eklund and Corlett's proposal, Althoff *et al.* (1992) investigated the change of stature when subjecting the spine to quantitatively known additional loads. Fig. 11.**9** shows an example of a measurement. During a pre-test phase of about 40 min the stature of a test subject standing or walking (unloaded) in the laboratory was repeatedly measured at 3 min intervals. An exponential function was fitted to the measured data; this exponential served to predict the temporal course of stature if unloaded standing or walking were continued. During the pre-test phase the stature is seen to have decreased slightly; this decrease is a fraction of that occurring during the whole day.

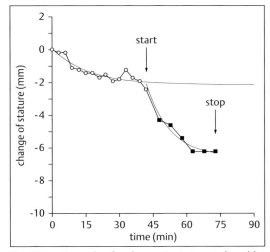

Fig. 11.**9** Example of a change in stature induced by carrying a shoulder load of 30 kg. In the 40 min pre-test phase of standing or slow walking, stature was measured at 3 min intervals (open circles). The loaded phase that followed was interrupted every 5 min by a stature measurement (solid squares). Exponential functions were fitted mathematically to the data points of the pre-test and the test phases. The net change of stature at the end of the test is given by the difference in the fitted functions. In the example shown, the additional load of 30 min duration effected a decrease of stature of approximately 4 mm. (Adapted from Althoff *et al.*, 1993)

Subsequently the test subject was loaded for 30 min by a mass of 30 kg distributed evenly around the trunk. This additional loading was interrupted every 5 min for a stature measurement. Again an exponential function was fitted to the data points. The example shows that the additional load acting over 30 min resulted in a stature decrease of about 4 mm relative to the prediction derived from the unloaded pre-test data.

Althoff and colleagues showed that the stature decrease under static additional load is proportional to the load and inversely proportional to the cross-sectional area of the intervertebral disks. Exposure to whole body vibration had no measurable effect on stature. Sitting in a variety of chairs and in a variety of postures always resulted in an increase of stature. From these observations the authors concluded that sitting unloads the spine compared with standing. At first sight this result appears to be inconsistent with the determination of spinal loading by the measurement of intradiskal pressure. An in-depth discussion of this aspect is presented in Chapter A1.

Determination of spinal loading from measurements of stature change has the advantage that no model assumptions are required. The measurement is not invasive and no measurement apparatus has to be fixed on the subjects under investigation. Apart from the stature measurement itself, observation of the test subjects during the activity under investigation is not necessary. The measurement method seems to be well suited to documenting static loading, for example, additional load due to antagonistic activation of the trunk muscles during activities requiring high concentration. On the other hand, a stature measurement does not furnish quantitative data (in newtons) on spinal loading or unloading. Whether the measurement method is suitable for documenting spinal loading, which exhibits large variations during the period of observation, is not known at present; additional experiments are necessary to clarify this issue.

Recommendations for carrying and lifting

The guidelines and recommendations for lifting and carrying at the workplace, in the household, and during leisure time serve several objectives (see, for example, Waters *et al.*, 1993):

– Subjects are to be protected against exhaustion of the musculature and overexertion of the circulatory system. To this end, maximum values for the frequency of lifts performed are recommended, related to the mass lifted and the posture attained (for example 'trunk bent forward' or 'knees bent'). The recommended limits are based on measurements of cardiac frequency and the energy turnover derived from respiratory gas analysis.

– Accidents are to be avoided. An accident can occur when a subject slips on the floor while carrying an object which would not be difficult to carry under normal circumstances. Uncontrolled movements resulting in high peak loads on the locomotor system may occur while slipping or stumbling. Other potential causes of accidents are missing handles, shifting of loose parts or fluids within a container while lifting or carrying, or obstruction of the view by excessively large objects handled. The recommendations for accident prevention are derived from an analysis of accident reports.

– The lumbar spine is to be protected against overloading. Injuries due to one single overloading episode or to repeated high loads are to be avoided by limiting the maximum mass of the objects handled and by avoiding specific pos-

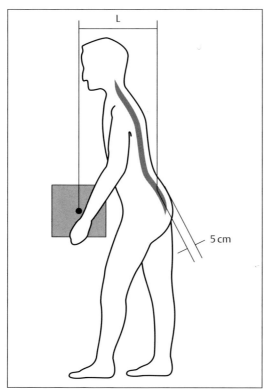

Fig. 11.**10** Since the moment arm of the extensor muscles of the lumbar spine is virtually constant (approximate value 5 cm), the additional load on the lumbar spine in a given posture depends on the magnitude of the mass handled and on its moment arm L. The additional load on the lumbar spine assumes a minimum value when the smallest possible moment arm L of the external load is selected.

tures when lifting and carrying. The recommended limits of the masses are based on epidemiological studies, as well as on a comparison of the results of biomechanical model calculations with the experimentally determined compressive strength of the structures (vertebral bodies, disks) of the lumbar spine. Compliance with the recommendations should guarantee that the lumbar spine can fulfill its function as supporting structure of the trunk in the long term.

For all postures of the trunk, the load on the lumbar spine depends on the moment of the mass being lifted or carried. In order to avoid overload damage, either the mass of the object must be limited or the distance between the center of gravity of the object

and the spine (the moment arm) must be kept as small as possible. Important conclusions for practical applications can already be derived from symmetric, two-dimensional models in the sagittal plane (Fig. 11.**10**). Irrespective of the mass of the object, the load on the lumbar spine will assume its minimum value when the smallest possible moment arm is selected. For this reason it is recommended that objects being lifted or carried should be positioned as close as possible to the spine. If the object is carried ventrally, the minimum magnitude of the moment arm is limited by the abdomen to about 20 cm. A small backward bend of the upper trunk, shifting the common center of gravity of body and object close to the spine, will effect a further reduction of spinal loading.

If the arms hang down and a weight is held in the hands (for example when carrying a suitcase or a stretcher, or when lifting a wheelbarrow), the moment arm in relation to the spine is small. If an object is carried dorsally (for example when lifting a piece of furniture behind the back), the moment arm may well be less than 10 cm. At the same time the moment arm of the abdominal muscles balancing the moment of the weight is substantially larger than that of the extensors of the back. It follows that lifting dorsally may unload the spine in comparison with a ventral lift.

The components of the force transmitted from vertebra to vertebra perpendicular and parallel to the vertebral endplates exhibit characteristic patterns, related to the posture (Fig. 11.**11**). In the erect posture the moment arm L of a mass carried is virtually constant along the lumbar spine (ignoring the curvature of the spine for the time being). The moment of the gravitational force, the required muscle force and the resulting, longitudinally directed force on the spine are thus virtually identical in all segments of the lumbar spine. In this posture, the magnitude of shear forces acting in the plane of the disks is small. This also holds for the segment L5/S1 with the plane of its disk tilted by about 45° to the horizontal. The underlying reason is that by far the largest part of the spinal load stems from the force of the extensor muscles; broadly speaking, the direction of the muscles follows the direction of the spine.

In contrast, in the forward bent posture the moment arm of the weight increases in the craniocaudal direction. Consequently, the additional axial load (directed perpendicular to the endplates) on the lumbar spine increases in a craniocaudal direction as well. To some extent the lumbar spine is adapted to increased loading in the craniocaudal direction, as the compressive strength of the vertebral bodies increases from T12 to L5. In the forward bent posture, the magnitude of the shear

Fig. 11.11 Craniocaudal course of the additional compressive load on the lumbar spine due to holding a mass in the hands. In the erect posture the moment arm, and thus the additional load, is virtually equal for all segments (disregarding the curvature of the spine in the sagittal plane, for the sake of simplicity). In the forward bent posture the moment arm L, and thus the compressive load, increase in the craniocaudal direction. In this posture, loading by the shear force generated by the gravitational force of the mass and acting in the plane of the disks is approximately equal for all segments.

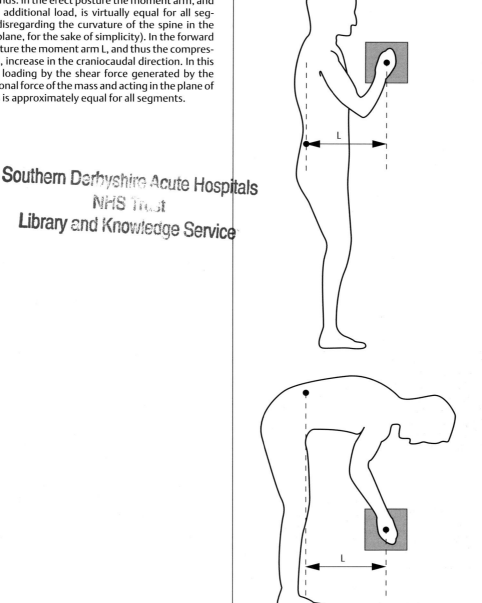

forces acting in the plane of the disks (again ignoring the curvature of the spine) equals the weight of the mass handled in addition to the weight of the body mass located cranially to the segment under consideration. To a large extent, shear forces are balanced by the facet joints and, to a smaller part, by the disks. In all segments of the lumbar spine the shear forces are larger in the forward bent posture than in the erect posture.

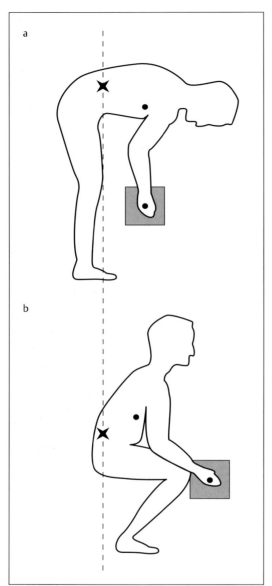

Fig. 11.**12** Comparison of the load on the lumbar spine when lifting a mass with forward bent trunk (**a**) or with the knees bent (**b**). Solid circles: centers of gravity of the body mass cranial to the disk in question. In posture **a** the moment arm of the external load is smaller than in posture **b**. In contrast, the moment arm of the gravitational force of the body mass is greater in posture **a** compared with posture **b**. Depending on the body mass and the mass to be handled, the compressive load on the lumbar spine may assume a maximum in either posture **a** or **b**. In posture **b**, the loading of the knee joints assumes a maximum value.

The rule is generally correct, that, in any given posture, the load on the lumbar spine will assume its minimal value when the moment arm of the object being lifted or carried is selected to be as small as possible. Further recommendations on specific postures to be assumed when lifting or carrying are, however, problematic for a number of reasons:

– Fig. 11.**12** compares lifting with forward bent trunk or with the knees bent, assuming that the dimensions of the object to be lifted do not permit it to be positioned between the knees. In forward bending (a) the moment arm of the object related to the segment L5/S1 is smaller than in posture (b) with the knees bent. In contrast, the moment arm of the body weight is larger in forward bending (a) than in posture (b) with the knees bent. In the borderline case of a very heavy object and very lightweight subject, posture (a) would result in minimal spinal loading and would thus be advantageous; in the case of a heavy subject and a lightweight object, posture (b) would be preferable. If the mass of the subject and the mass of the object are known, it is, of course, possible to decide which of the two postures results in the smaller axial load on the lumbar spine. If the masses are not known, no generally valid advice can be given. In other words: if only one posture were recommended, this might well be the wrong posture in a specific situation (Park and Chaffin, 1974).

– Even if a calculation in the individual case yielded the result that posture (b) loads the lumbar spine less than posture (a), lifting with the knees bent cannot be recommended without reservation to all persons. The reason is that the load on the femorotibial as well as on the patellofemoral joints increases considerably with the bending angle of the knee (see Chapter 10). In elderly subjects with incipient or advanced osteoporosis, a deep bend of the knee may potentially damage the trabecular bone below the tibial plateau.

– In addition, it has to be considered that frequent lifting with the knees bent is energy-consuming and thus very tiring. When straightening up from a knee bend, the center of gravity of the body has to be lifted. For this reason we rarely see bricklayers in the construction industry or planters in the agricultural industry performing a knee bend for each brick or plant handled.

Mechanical properties of lumbar intervertebral disks

Deformation of disks under load

The component of the spinal load directed in the longitudinal direction of the spine is transmitted from vertebra to vertebra virtually only by the disk. As the surfaces of the facet joints in the lumbar spine are oriented approximately perpendicular to the transverse plane, the facet joints normally cannot transmit any part of the axial load. Load transmission via the facet joints occurs in maximal extension or in segments with very low disk height, when bony contact is made between the caudal facet and the lamina of the lower vertebra (El-Bohy *et al.*, 1989).

The component of the spinal load directed parallel to the endplates is transmitted virtually solely by the facet joints. Due to their low stiffness compared with the stiffness of bone, the disks and the ligaments of the vertebral joint transmit only a small fraction of this load. In the case of a fracture of the vertebral arch (spondylolysis) the shear force is resisted only by the disk and the ligaments. A ventral displacement of the cranial vertebra (spondylolisthesis), often progressing in time, is then frequently observed.

The vertebral body and intervertebral disk deform under load (Fig. 11.**13**). The vertebral endplates bulge inwards; the disk bulges outwards. Consequently, the height of the motion segment decreases. Compared with the unloaded state, the incremental inwards bulge of the endplates at the limit of compressive fracture is in the order of 0.5 mm, and the incremental outwards radial bulge of the disks is in the order of 1.0 mm (Brinckmann *et al.*, 1983; Brinckmann and Horst, 1985). If the inwards bulge of an endplate exceeds the limiting value of approximately 0.5 mm, the trabecular bone within the vertebra as well as the endplate may fracture and disk tissue may intrude into the vertebral body. If the radial bulge of the disks becomes too large due to pathologic tissue changes, the nerve tissues may be compromised, especially in the presence of a narrow spinal canal or narrow foramina.

The extent of the ventral and dorsal radial bulge of lumbar disks depends on the angle of lordosis (Fig. 11.**2**). In extension, the bulge is ventrally minimal and dorsally maximal. Conversely, in flexion the radial bulge is dorsally minimal and ventrally maximal (Brinckmann and Porter, 1994). The small bulge occurring ventrally in extension and dorsally in flexion is due to the outer layers of the anulus fibrosus being loaded in tension at the location of the greatest clearance height between the endplates, which hinders the development of bulging. The decrease of the radial bulge ventrally in extension and dorsally in flexion is further promoted by the fact that the cranial vertebra is shifted dorsally in extension and ventrally in flexion in relation to the caudal vertebra. The observations made in specimens concerning the dependence of the radial bulge of the intervertebral disks on the angle of lordosis comply with observations *in vivo* following the injection of contrast media into the spinal canal (see, for example, Inufusa *et al.*, 1996). In addition, they comply with observations made in patients with a narrow spinal canal (lumbar stenosis), who report a decline in their problems when riding a bicycle or when wearing a corset limiting the angle of lordosis (Penning, 1992). In flexion there is more space available than in extension for the spinal cord in the spinal canal as well as for the nerve tissues which pass the foramina.

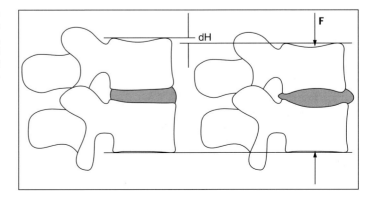

Fig. 11.13 Deformation of the vertebral body and disk under compressive loading. (For reasons of clarity, the inward bending of the endplates and the outward bulging of the disk are shown in an exaggerated fashion.)

Pressure distribution over the vertebral endplates

The distribution of the compressive stress (pressure) over the vertebral endplate is virtually uniform (Fig. 11.**14**). Tensile stress exists only in a small zone of approximately 1 to 2 mm width along the periphery of the intervertebral disk, where the outermost fiber layers of the anulus fibrosus insert

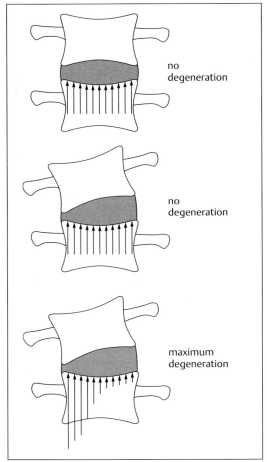

Fig. 11.**14** Pressure distribution at the interface of disk and vertebral body. In non-degenerated or moderately degenerated disks there is uniform pressure over the entire vertebral endplate save for a 1–2 mm wide zone along the periphery, where the outer layer of the anulus fibrosus is under tensile stress. The uniformity of the pressure distribution is not changed under flexion or side bending. In highly degenerated disks the pressure is greater in those regions where the endplates approach each other under flexion or side bending as compared with the opposite region. (Adapted from Horst and Brinckmann, 1981)

(Horst and Brinckmann, 1981; Horst, 1982). The measurements performed by Horst and colleagues disproved previous theoretical considerations, which argued that the pressure below the nucleus should be larger than that below the anulus fibrosus. In a non-degenerated or only slightly degenerated disk, the pressure distribution remains uniform even when the endplates of the adjacent vertebrae are no longer parallel to each other but are tilted in side-bending or flexion. Only in maximally degenerated disks and at the limit of the range of motion is an increased pressure at the location where the endplates approach each other in side-bending, flexion or extension observed. Recent measurements carried out with a miniature pressure probe (Adams *et al.*, 1996) showed deviations from a uniform pressure distribution, depending on the state of degeneration (Fig. 11.**15**) and on the loading history of the specimens tested. (Adams et al., 2000)

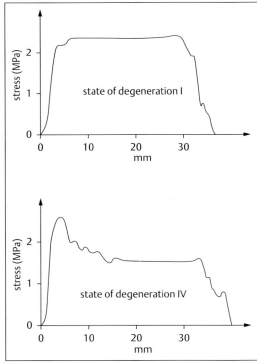

Fig. 11.**15** Vertical component of the compressive stress within the disk, measured over the diameter of the disk. In disks with degeneration grade I (i.e. no degeneration), the stress distribution is virtually uniform. In disks with degeneration grade IV (i.e. maximum degeneration) stress maxima in the region of the periphery of the anulus fibrosus are observed. (Adapted from Adams *et al.*, 1996)

The underlying cause of the uniformity of the pressure distribution can be understood qualitatively if the mechanical properties of disk tissue are considered to lie somewhere between the properties of an ideal fluid and a solid. In contrast to the properties of a solid, no force is required to deform a fluid. Non-degenerated or only slightly degenerated disk tissue can be deformed easily and is able to move (within certain limits) within the disk space. For this reason we observe a virtually uniform distribution of the pressure over the vertebral endplates, irrespective of the geometry of the disk space. The mechanical properties of highly degenerated tissue, or of tissue dehydrated due to long-term loading, resemble more and more those of a solid. There is then more resistance to deformation and less mobility of the tissue within the disk space. If the disk space assumes a wedge shape and the tissue cannot 'sidestep' at those locations where the endplates approach each other, peak values of compressive stress are observed (compare Fig. 11.**14**, lowest diagram).

Intradiskal pressure and mechanical function of the disk

Nachemson (1960) showed in his pioneering study that the relation between load F and pressure p at the center of the disk is described by

$$p = 1.5 \cdot F/A$$

In this formula F denotes the compressive force directed perpendicular to the plane of the disk and A the cross-sectional area of the disk. The factor of proportionality between p and the quotient F/A was observed to be virtually independent of age, degeneration (save for maximum degeneration) and anatomical position (L1/2 to L4/5) of the specimens tested. The numerical value of the experimentally determined factor of proportionality between pressure and the quotient of force and area indicates that the disk cannot simply be regarded as an elastically deformable, intermediate layer between the endplates. If this were the case, a factor of proportionality equal to 1.0 instead of 1.5 would be expected.

In the following, the origin and function of the intradiskal pressure is discussed qualitatively using the model shown in Fig. 11.**16**; for the appertaining formulae see Brinckmann and Grootenboer (1991). The disk tissue contains compounds that have the ability to bind water via an electrochemical process. This ability to bind water is largest under low pressure and decreases with increasing pressure. At night, in the state of low loading, there

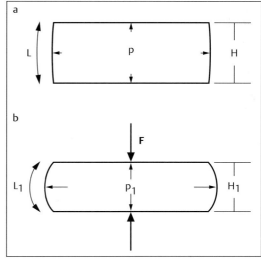

Fig. 11.**16**   Model of an intervertebral disk used to derive the relation between intradiskal pressure and radial disk bulge: incompressible material enclosed between rigid endplates and an outer membrane (i.e. outer layer of the anulus fibrosus) of high tensile strength. H, L, and p designate the height of the disk, the length along the enclosing membrane, and the intradiskal pressure in the case with no external loading (**a**). With external loading (**b**), the disk bulges outwards and the height decreases to the value H_1. The length of the membrane increases from L to L_1. Consequently, the tensile stress of the membrane increases. To fulfill the equilibrium condition of forces, the intradiskal pressure increases and assumes the value p_1.

is a net water uptake by the disk, by diffusion from the surrounding body fluid. The height of the disk increases. Due to the height increase the fibers of the anulus fibrosus are tightened in the longitudinal direction of the spine; the radial bulge of the disk is small (Fig. 11.**16a**). When the fluid-saturated disk is loaded, the intradiskal pressure increases. The pressure acts uniformly in all directions, on both opposing endplates as well as, in a radial direction, on the anulus fibrosus (Fig. 11.**16b**). The anulus bulges outwards and the disk height decreases, due to the shifting of part of the disk tissue into the annular bulge. The outermost fiber layers of the anulus are stretched, resulting in tensile stress acting on the opposing endplates. In consequence, the pressure within the disk must increase in order to balance the resulting tensile force acting at the periphery of the endplates, in addition to the load F. Due to this mechanism, the intradiskal pressure actually rises above the magnitude of the mean pressure F/A.

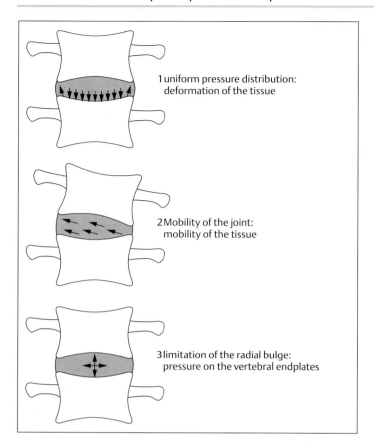

1 uniform pressure distribution: deformation of the tissue

2 Mobility of the joint: mobility of the tissue

3 limitation of the radial bulge: pressure on the vertebral endplates

Fig. 11.**17** Mechanical function of the disk: generation of a uniform distribution of the pressure over the endplates and enabling motion between adjacent vertebral bodies. The intradiskal pressure serves, in effect, to restrict the radial bulge of the disk.

To distribute the pressure uniformly over the surface of the endplates, and to keep the vertebral joint mobile, the disk tissue must be able to shift (at least to a certain extent) within the disk space (Fig. 11.**17**). In this situation, the soft, mobile, highly loaded tissue should not be squeezed out of the disk space. This squeezing out is prevented by the tensile stress in the outer layers of the anulus fibrosus. The tensile stress is, in turn, caused by the intradiskal pressure. The pressure acts in a radial direction and effects the outward bulge of the disk. At the same time the pressure acts on the endplates of the neighboring vertebrae. As the circumferential area of the anulus is smaller than the area of the endplates, the pressure maintains the disk height while limiting the increase of the radial bulge.

The mechanical system of an automobile or bicycle tire is very similar to that of a disk. Inside the tire is pressure; the outer layer of the tire is under tensile stress. Upon pressure increase, the height of the tire increases and its radial bulge decreases. If air is let out of the tire, its height decreases and

its radial bulge increases. The tire model predicts that any loss of disk tissue, caused by disk extrusion, endplate fracture, or surgical intervention, results in a decreased disk height, a decreased intradiskal pressure, and an increased radial bulge. These predictions comply with observations on specimens of the human lumbar spine *in vitro* (Brinckmann and Grootenboer, 1991) and follow-up studies *in vivo* after chemonucleolysis (therapeutic, enzymatic digestion of disk tissue) (Leivseth *et al.*, 1999).

Compressive strength of lumbar vertebrae

Strength is defined as that load which causes irreparable damage to a structure. In principle, bones can be loaded in compression, tension, shear, bending, torsion, or by a combination of these loading modes. For vertebral bodies, the loading mode of

Fig. 11.**18** Results from a study *in vitro* to determine the compressive strength of lumbar vertebrae (T12 to L5). The diagram shows the measured results from individual specimens and the regression line describing the statistical relation between the compressive strength and the product of bone density and endplate area. Both parameters (bone density and endplate area), which influence the compressive strength, were measured by computed tomography (CT). To allow for a comparison of bone density measured on different scanners, the density is quoted in units of the density of a reference substance, in mg/ml K_2HPO_4. (Adapted from: Brinckmann *et al.*, 1989)

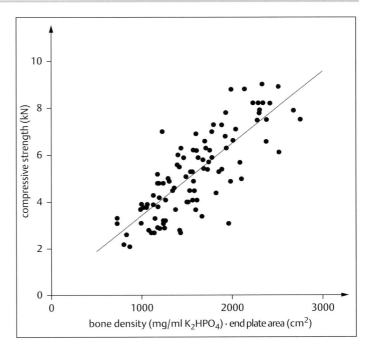

interest is compression by a force directed perpendicular to the endplates. In erect stance, as well as in forward bending, such a force is transmitted to the vertebral bodies via the disks. Only at the limit of extension may a fraction of the load be transmitted by the facet joints and the vertebral arch, but the major part of the load is still given by axial compression. Tensile forces acting on the vertebral body via the ligaments or the disk are, as far as fractures are concerned, of importance only in exceptional situations or accidents. Forces acting in the plane of the disk and moments about the long axis of the spine are resisted by the facet joints. As long as the facet joints do not fracture (which is very rarely the case, save for accidents) shear forces and moments may be neglected when discussing the strength of vertebral bodies. Bending moments are, however, important when discussing the fracture of the vertebral arch (see below).

The compressive strength of lumbar vertebrae can be investigated employing either specimens of isolated vertebrae or specimens of motion segments (two vertebrae with intervening disk). Past experiments, however, need only be considered if the specimens used were not fixed or dehydrated, and if the compressive force was not applied punctiformly to the endplates but via a pressure-distributing, intermediate material layer. The compressive strength of human lumbar vertebrae (T12 to

L5) measured *in vitro* varies between 2 kN and 12 kN. When overloaded, the trabecular bone beneath the endplates fractures first, in the majority of cases. This fracture results in clefts, stepped, or bowl-shaped impressions of the endplates, in part accompanied by intrusion of disk material into the trabecular bone. On overloading, a wedge-like deformation or a decrease in height of the whole vertebra are less frequently observed.

Fig. 11.**18** shows the compressive strength of lumbar vertebrae (T12 to L5) measured *in vitro* in relation to the product of endplate area and bone density, both determined by computed tomography (CT) (Brinckmann *et al.*, 1989). In addition to the data points, the graph shows the regression line representing the statistical dependence of strength on the product of density and area. The data from this experiment show that the compressive strength of vertebrae increases with increasing bone density and increasing dimensions of the vertebral body. If bone density and endplate area are measured *in vivo* by CT, the strength of vertebrae *in vivo* can be predicted from the data shown in Fig. 11.**18** within error limits of ± 1 kN. In the human spine, the strength increases in a craniocaudal direction by approximately 300 N per segment. This increase is caused by the increase in endplate area; the density of the trabecular bone is virtually constant within each individual spine.

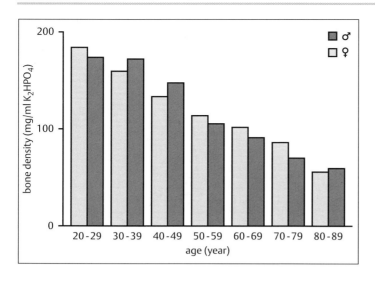

Fig. 11.**19** Density of the trabecular bone within the vertebral bodies of the lumbar spine, shown for male and female subjects by age. (Adapted from Felsenberg *et al.*, 1988)

The scatter of the data about the regression line indicates that compressive strength is influenced (though to a minor extent) by additional factors besides endplate area and bone density. The architecture of the trabecular bone within the vertebral body may play a role here. Up to now, however, the parameter 'architecture' could not be defined quantitatively from radiographs or CT images. Besides CT data, prediction of vertebral strength can also be based on data obtained by dual photon or dual X-ray absorptiometry (DPA, DEXA) or from the ash content of vertebrae. Strength is predicted with virtually equal accuracy when employing any one of these procedures (see, for example, Ebbesen *et al.*, 1999).

The trabecular bone density of lumbar vertebral bodies is age-dependent. Felsenberg *et al.* (1988) published normal values of bone density measured by computed tomography in the age range between 20 and 89 years (Fig. 11.**19**). Bone density assumes its maximum value between 20 and 30 years of age and subsequently decreases monoto-

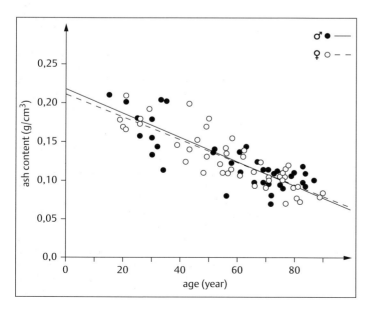

Fig. 11.**20** Ash content of the trabecular bone of vertebra L3, by age. (Adapted from Mosekilde, 1989)

Fig. 11.**21** Compressive strength of lumbar vertebrae (T12 to L5) *in vitro*, in relation to age. The diagram shows the measured results from specimens obtained from male and female subjects (solid circles or crosses respectively) together with the regression line describing the statistical relation between strength and age. On average, compressive strength decreases with age. The data for individual subjects, however, can deviate substantially from the statistical mean. (Adapted from: Biggemann and Brinckmann, 1995)

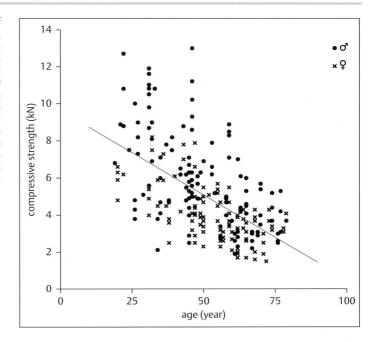

nously with age. There is no significant gender-related difference. With respect to the influence of age and gender, the results of the measurement of the ash content of vertebra L3 by Mosekilde (1989) comply with the CT bone density results published by Felsenberg and colleagues. The ash content (Fig. 11.**20**) exhibits a monotonous decrease with age; here too, there is no gender-related difference. It follows from these measurements that the compressive strength of lumbar vertebrae reaches its maximum value after skeletal maturation and subsequently undergoes a continuous decrease. Men and women are equally subject to the loss of vertebral compressive strength.

Fig. 11.**21** shows a compilation of compressive strength data of human lumbar vertebrae (T12 to L5) *in vitro*, in relation to age and gender. In addition, the diagram contains the regression line describing the statistical relation between strength and age. It can be clearly seen that (for the material investigated) strength decreases on average with age. This decrease is due to the age-related decrease in bone density described above. Yet at any given age, for example at 45 years, the strength data are scattered over a wide range. Age alone does not allow a prediction of vertebral strength in the individual case. Furthermore, it can be recognized that vertebrae of female subjects exhibit lower strength on average than those of male subjects. This is due to the normally smaller dimensions of

vertebrae of female subjects and not to gender-related differences in the material properties of bone. We hypothesize that the difference in strength due to the difference in size accounts for insufficiency fractures in osteoporosis being seen more frequently, and at a younger age, in women than in men.

In addition to the compressive strength, the fatigue strength of lumbar vertebrae has been investigated (Brinckmann et al., 1988). The results show that the probability of a fatigue fracture undergoes a sharp increase if the amplitude of the cyclic load exceeds 50 % of the load, resulting in vertebral fracture in one single loading cycle. The results of this experiment *in vitro*, however, should be regarded only as approximate values. In living subjects, the development of microdamage, eventually leading to fatigue fracture, competes with physiologic repair processes. Experiments *in vitro* demonstrate that, in contrast to traumatic, multiple fractures, fatigue fractures rarely destroy a vertebral body completely. This suggests that the characteristic morphologic alterations in vertebral shape, seen in patients with advanced osteoporosis, are due to fatigue fractures, in the majority of cases.

The results of the strength testing of lumbar vertebrae are of importance for the assessment of the risk of fracture *in vivo*. The maintenance or increase of the compressive strength of lumbar vertebrae can only be effected by the maintenance or in-

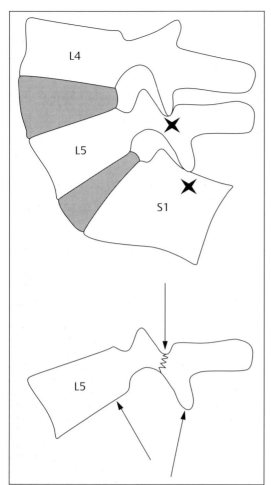

Fig. 11.22 Primary mechanical cause of fracture of the pars interarticularis of the vertebral arch. Bony contact between the processus articularis inferior with the lamina of the caudally adjoining vertebra can occur under simultaneous high axial loading and hyperextension. The vertebral arch is now subjected to three-point bending with the maximum bending moment acting in the pars interarticularis. *In vivo*, fractures are observed in this region; in some patients a progressive, ventrally directed gliding of the cranial vertebra is subsequently observed. (Adapted from Suezawa and Jacob, 1981)

itor bone density. The fracture risk, by contrast, depends on the product of bone density and endplate area. Endplate areas of different subjects may well vary by a factor of 2; assuming equal bone density, strength then varies by a factor of 2 as well. An estimate of the fracture risk based only on a measurement of bone density, as it is often performed in medical screening programs, can thus be expected to be grossly inaccurate. The study of Biggemann *et al.* (1991) showed that a minimum compressive strength of lumbar vertebrae of approximately 2–3 kN is required to resist normal, everyday loading. Virtually all spines with strength of L3 predicted (from CT data) to be lower than 3 kN exhibited single or multiple insufficiency fractures.

Fracture of the vertebral arch

A fracture of the vertebral arch in the pars interarticularis, i.e. between the processus articularis superior and the processus articularis inferior, is not congenital but acquired. The fracture (spondylolysis) may lead to ventral displacement of the vertebral body (spondylolisthesis) and to symptoms and disability requiring treatment. Suezawa and Jacob (1981) explored the loading modes leading to a fracture of the vertebral arch and showed that a shear force directed parallel to the endplates can fracture the arch in the region of the pediculus arcus vertebrae but not in the pars interarticularis. They demonstrated that maximal extension, in combination with high axial loading of the spine, leads to a fracture in the pars interarticularis. In maximal extension (Fig. 11.22) bony contact can occur between the processus articularis inferior and the pars interarticularis of the caudally adjacent vertebra. The center of rotation of the segment is then effectively shifted from the center of the disk to the point of bony contact. In the anterior longitudinal ligament and the ventral part of the disk, tensile stress is created; a compressive force acts at the point of bony contact. The arch is subjected to a bending moment and fracture occurs at the side under tensile stress.

Epidemiological investigations demonstrate that the prevalence of fractures at the pars interarticularis is significantly higher in persons engaged in certain athletic disciplines such as gymnastics, high jump, and pole-vaulting, than in the general population (see for example Blackburne, 1989). It seems that the defect is acquired mainly at a young age. Whether the fracture is caused by one single overload episode or by fatigue due to repeated loadings cannot be determined in retrospect.

crease of the density of the trabecular bone within the vertebral bodies. (Growth of the vertebrae with increase of the area of the endplates is not to be expected beyond skeletal maturity.) It follows that, for purposes of therapy control, it suffices to mon-

Sequence of events: overload injury – low back pain – work loss – disability? A warning

Biomechanical research on the strength of spinal structures (see the foregoing paragraphs and also Chapter A2) has revealed that some components, like vertebral bodies, vertebral arches, and intervertebral disks, are prone to primary mechanical damage in specific, high loading episodes (other than trauma) occurring at the workplace, or in leisure time activities like athletics, or gardening. Such findings *in vitro* appear to support the commonly held belief that physically demanding work is detrimental to the back. It appears intuitively reasonable that single or repeated episodes of mechanical overload may result in damage to spinal tissues, causing back pain, and that further exposure may lead to further damage or at least to lack of recovery so that permanent disability may finally result.

A closer look, based on the available evidence, however, challenges the validity of this chain of events. For an overview on the current scientific literature see for example Burton (1997), Waddell and Burton (2001), and Nordin (2001). The relation between injury, back pain, and the development of disability is, in fact, highly complex and far from being understood. This explains why there is no common agreement on how to cope with the medically and economically important problem of nonspecific low back pain and its consequences with respect to work loss and potential development of permanent disability. (The term 'nonspecific' denotes pain of unknown origin, i.e. not due to known causes like disk prolapse, tumor, etc.)

It is reasonable to assume that we should avoid compressing our vertebrae, fracturing vertebral arches, tearing intervertebral disks, or overstraining spinal ligaments or their insertions into bones. But if damage has occurred (for any reason whatsoever) there is, surprisingly, only a poor correlation between the amount of damage and the intensity of back pain. For example, there are many subjects with compressed vertebrae, protruded or extruded disks, or fractured vertebral arches, who exhibit no clinical symptoms at all. On the other hand, in the majority of cases of even severe back pain, no damage to the spinal tissues can be documented. There are potential explanations; the reader must realize, however, that these speculations must not be mistaken as evidence. Currently available diagnostic tools may still be too crude. Pain cannot be measured and can thus not be compared quantitatively among subjects. Furthermore, pain is certainly influenced by factors other than physiological ones.

There is strong epidemiological evidence that physical demands at the workplace due to handling heavy loads, working in awkward postures, or being exposed to vibration, can be associated with increased reports of back symptoms or aggravation of such symptoms. Contrary to what would be expected in a simple 'cause and effect' chain of events, there is conflicting evidence on the relation between length of exposure and aggravation of symptoms or increased reports of back symptoms. On the other hand, 60–80 % of adults experience low back pain, often persistent or recurrent, at some time, while mechanical risk factors cannot be identified. The prevalence of self-reported back pain among sedentary workers is similar to that among manual workers. Schoolchildren and adolescents report back pain with a prevalence almost as high as among working-age adults. The high prevalence of back pain in the general population not exposed to any (known) risk makes it very difficult to identify mechanical risk factors unequivocally, save for extreme cases.

The high prevalence of back pain in the general population leads to the conjecture that much back pain is work-related only in that people of working age get painful backs. In other words, the subjects in question would probably suffer from back pain whether they were working or not. It would follow that, while reduction of loads handled or avoidance of awkward postures in the course of biomechanics-based ergonomic improvements to the workplace can improve worker comfort (and are thus justifiable), it would not be realistic to expect such improvements to eliminate back pain. One exception is formed by those few workplaces where the workload has been proven to induce measurable damage. Here, ergonomic redesigning is a must, if future damage is to be excluded (though future back pain attacks will probably not be completely avoided).

There is strong evidence that non-biomechanical factors such as job satisfaction, social support at work, or downsizing of a company are associated with increased reporting of low back pain. This suggests that psychosocial advice on the relation of back pain to work, the natural (i.e. generally benign) course of low back pain, fear-avoidance behavior and pain-coping strategies, will be a tool for preventing long-time work loss and a drift into permanent disability.

The high prevalence of back pain in the general population also explains why attempts to identify subjects at risk for low back problems in pre-employment examinations (save for exclusion of serious spinal diseases) have generally failed. For example, neither radiographic inspection, nor strength or endurance tests, can predict the incidence of future back pain episodes. As stated in the literature, the best predictor of future back pain is past episodes of such pain. This statement seems trivial at first sight. A sick subject remains sick as no therapy is available for the very cause of his back pain. Who, then, is surprised at the statistical relation between past and future back pain episodes? The underlying important message is, however, that some subjects appear to have a predisposition to low back pain, while others have not. Hypothetically, the reason may be physiological, psychological, or genetic. Unfortunately, we do not actually know the reason. The question of why some cases of low back pain result in permanent disability while others, under seemingly similar circumstances, do not is strongly influenced by psychosocial factors.

As there seems to be no direct relation between workload and low back pain in most cases, the previously favored treatment of complete load relief until symptoms cease appears not to be appropriate. In fact, most workers continue work or return to work while symptoms are still present. (If nobody returned to work till they were 100 % symptom free, only a minority would ever return to work.) Thus, current strategies aim at an early return to work, assisted by medical treatment and psychosocial support. There is strong evidence that the longer a subject is off work due to low back pain, the lower are the chances of his ever returning to work. After 1–2 years of absence it is unlikely that a subject will return to any form of work, irrespective of further treatment. Again, this finding puts the importance of biomechanical factors in the development of chronic back pain and disability into perspective.

Further reading

Textbooks and review papers

Adams MA, Dolan P. Recent advances in lumbar spinal mechanics and their clinical significance. *Clinical Biomechanics.* 1995; **10**: 3–19

Biggemann M, Brinckmann P. Biomechanics of osteoporotic vertebral fractures. In: Genant H *et al.* (eds). *Vertebral fracture in osteoporosis.* San Francisco: Radiology Research and Education Foundation; 1995

Burton AK. Spine Update. Back injury and work loss. Biomechanical and psychosocial influences. *Spine.* 1997; **22**: 2575–2580 [Review paper, 28 references.]

Chaffin DB, Andersson GBJ, Martin BJ. *Occupational biomechanics.* 3rd ed. New York: Wiley; 1999

Dolan P, Adams MA. Recent advances in lumbar spinal mechanics and their significance for modelling. *Clinical Biomechanics.* 2001; **16 Suppl 1**: S8–S16 [Review paper, 56 references]

Penning L. Functional pathology of lumbar spinal stenosis. *Clinical Biomechanics* 1992; **7**: 3–17 [Review paper, 60 references]

Pheasant S. *Bodyspace. Anthropometry, ergonomics and design.* 1st ed. London: Taylor and Francis; 1986 [NB: Only the first edition of this book contains data on the location of the center of gravity, the mass, and the moment of inertia of the body segments; such data are not contained in later editions of this book.]

Waddell G, Burton AK. Occupational health guidelines for the management of low back pain at work: evidence review. *Occup Med.* 2001; **51**: 124–135 [Review paper, 132 references.]

White AA, Panjabi MM. *Clinical Biomechanics of the spine.* 2nd ed. Philadelphia: Lippincott; 1990

Wiesel SW, Weinstein JN, Herkowitz HN, Dvorak J, Bell GR (eds). *The lumbar spine,* Vol 1–2. 2nd ed. Philadelphia: Saunders; 1996

Winter DA. *Biomechanics and motor control of human movement.* 2nd ed. New York: Wiley; 1990

Scientific papers, cited in the text or in the figures

Adams MA, McNally DS, Dolan P. 'Stress' distributions inside intervertebral discs. *J Bone Jt Surg.* 1996; **78B**: 965–972

Adams MA, May S, Freeman BJC, Morrison HP, Dolan P. Effects of backward bending on lumbar intervertebral discs. Relevance to physical therapy treatments for low back pain. *Spine.* 2000; **25**: 431–437

Althoff I, Brinckmann P, Frobin W, Sandover J, Burton K. An improved method of stature measurement for quantitative determination of spinal loading. Application to sitting postures and whole body vibration. *Spine.* 1992; **17**: 682–693

Althoff I, Brinckmann P, Frobin W, Sandover J, Burton K. *Die Bestimmung der Belastung der Wirbelsäule mit Hilfe einer Präzisionsmessung der Körpergröße. Schriftenreihe der Bundesanstalt für Arbeitsschutz Fb683,* Bremerhaven: Wirtschaftsverlag NW; 1993

Andersson EA, Oddsson LIE, Grundström H, Nilsson J, Thorstensson A. EMG activities of the quadratus lumborum and erector spinae muscles during flexion-relaxation and other motor tasks. *Clinical Biomechanics.* 1996; **11**: 392–400

Bean JC, Chaffin DB, Schultz AB. Biomechanical model calculation of muscle contraction forces. A double linear programming method. *J Biomechanics.* 1988; **21**: 59–66

Bernhardt M, White A III, Panjabi MM, McGowan DP. Lumbar spine instability. In Jayson MIV (ed.): *The lumbar spine and back pain.* p 333–354. 4th Ed. Edinburgh: Churchill Livingstone; 1992

Biggemann M, Hilweg D, Seidel S, Horst M, Brinckmann P. Risk of vertebral insufficiency fractures in relation to compressive strength predicted by quantitative computed tomography. *Eur J Radiol.* 1991; **13**: 6–10

Blackburne JS. Spondylolisthesis in sportsmen. *J R Coll Surg Edinb.* 1989; **34 Suppl**: S12–S14

Brinckmann P, Frobin W, Hierholzer E, Horst M. Deformation of the vertebral end-plate under axial loading of the spine. *Spine.* 1983; **8**: 851–856

Brinckmann P, Horst M. The influence of vertebral body fracture, intradiscal injection, and partial discectomy on the radial bulge and height of human lumbar discs. *Spine.* 1985; **10**: 138–145

Brinckmann P, Biggemann M, Hilweg D. Fatigue fracture of human lumbar vertebrae. *Clinical Biomechanics.* 1988; **3 Suppl 1**: S1–S23

Brinckmann P, Biggemann M, Hilweg D. Prediction of the compressive strength of human lumbar vertebrae. *Clinical Biomechanics*. 1989; **4 Suppl 2**: S1–S27

Brinckmann P, Grootenboer H. Change of disc height, radial disc bulge and intradiscal pressure from discectomy. An in vitro investigation on human lumbar discs. *Spine*. 1991; **16**: 641–646

Brinckmann P, Porter R. A laboratory model of lumbar disc protrusion. Fissure and fragment. *Spine*. 1994; **19**: 228–235

Cholewicki J, Juluru K, McGill SM. Intra-abdominal pressure mechanism for stabilizing the lumbar spine. *J Biomechanics*. 1999; **32**: 13–17

Davis PR, Troup JDG. Pressures in the trunk cavities when pulling, pushing and lifting. *Ergonomics*. 1964; **7**: 465–474

DePuky P. The physiological oscillation of the length of the body. *Acta Orthop Scand*. 1935; **6**: 338–347

Dieën JH van, Kingma I. Total trunk muscle force and spinal compression are lower in asymmetric moments as compared to pure extension moments. *J Biomechanics*. 1999; **32**: 681–687

Ebbesen EN, Thomsen JS, Beck-Nielsen H, Nepper-Rasmussen HJ, Mosekilde L. Lumbar vertebral body compressive strength evaluated by dual energy x-ray absorptiometry, quantitative computed tomography and ashing. *Bone*. 1999; **25**: 713–724

El-Bohy AA, Yang KH, King AA. Experimental verification of facet load transmission by direct measurement of facet lamina contact pressure. *J Biomechanics*. 1989; **22**: 931–941

Eklund JAE, Corlett EN. Shrinkage as a measure of the effect of load on the spine. *Spine*. 1984; **9**: 189–194

Felsenberg D, Kalender WA, Banzer D, Schmilinsky G, Heyse M, Fischer E, Schneider U. Quantitative computertomographische Knochenmineralgehaltsbestimmung. *Fortschr Röntgenstr*. 1988; **148**: 431–436

Frobin W, Brinckmann P, Leivseth G, Biggemann M, Reikerås O. Precision measurement of segmental motion from flexion-extension radiographs of the lumbar spine. *Clinical Biomechanics*. 1996; **11**: 457–465

Hodges PW, Richardson CA. Inefficient muscular stabilization of the lumbar spine associated with low back pain. A motor control evaluation of transversus abdominis. *Spine*. 1996; **21**: 2640–2650

Horst M, Brinckmann P. Measurement of the distribution of axial stress on the endplate of the vertebral body. *Spine*. 1981; **6**: 217–232

Horst M. *Mechanische Beanspruchung der Wirbelkörperdeckplatte. Messung der Verteilung der Normalspannung an der Grenzfläche Bandscheibe-Wirbelkörper. Wirbelsäule in Forschung und Praxis*. Bd. 95. Stuttgart: Hippokrates; 1982

Inufusa A, An HS, Lim TH, Hasegawa T, Haughton VM, Nowicki BH. Anatomic changes of the spinal canal and intervertebral foramen associated with flexion-extension movement. *Spine*. 1996; **21**: 2412–2420

Jäger M, Luttmann A, Laurig W. Biomechanisches Modell des Transports von Müllgroßbehältern über Bordsteinkanten. *Zbl Arbeitsmedizin*. 1983; **33**: 251–259

Jäger M. *Biomechanisches Modell des Menschen zur Analyse und Beurteilung der Belastung der Wirbelsäule bei der Handhabung von Lasten*. Fortschritt-Bericht 17/33. Düsseldorf: VDI Verlag; 1987

Jäger M, Luttmann A, Laurig W. Lumbar load during one-handed bricklaying. *Int J Ind Ergonomics*. 1991; **8**: 261–277

Jäger M, Luttmann A. Entwicklung eines biomechanischen Modells zur Bestimmung der Belastung der Wirbelsäule. *Biomedizinische Technik*. 1993; **38** (Ergänzungsband): 393–394

Johnsson R, Axelson P, Strömqvist B. Mobility provocation of lumbar fusion evaluated by radiostereometric analysis. *Acta Orthop Scand*. 1996; **67** (Suppl): 45–46

Knutsson F. The instability associated with disc degeneration in the lumbar spine. *Acta Radiol*. 1944; **25**: 593–609

Leivseth G, Salvesen R, Hemminghytt S, Brinckmann P, Frobin W. Do human lumbar discs reconstitute after chemonucleolysis? A 7-year follow-up study. *Spine*. 1999; **24**: 342–347

Leskinen TPJ, Stålhammar HR, Kuorinka IAA, Troup JDG. A dynamic analysis of spinal compression with different lifting techniques. *Ergonomics*. 1983a; **26**: 595–604

Leskinen TPJ, Stålhammar HR, Kuorinka IAA, Troup JDG. The effect of inertial factors on spinal stress when lifting. *Engineering in Medicine*. 1983b; **12**: 87–89

Lüssenhop S, Deuretzbacher G, Steuber KU, Rehder U. Zur mechanischen Wirkung von Präventivmiedern (Back Supports) - erste Ergebnisse einer biomechanischen Untersuchung. *Orthop Praxis*. 1996; **32**: 409–412

Marras WS, Joynt RL, King AI. The force-velocity relation and intra-abdominal pressure during lifting activities. *Ergonomics*. 1985; **28**: 603–613

McGill SM. Abdominal belts in industry: A position paper on their assets, liabilities and use. *Am Ind Hyg Assoc*. 1993; **54**: 572–574

McGill SM. The mechanics of torso flexion: situps and standing dynamic flexion manoeuvres. *Clin Biomechanics*. 1995; **10**: 184–192

McGill SM, Hughson RL, Parks K. Changes in lumbar lordosis modify the role of the extensor muscles. *Clin Biomechanics*. 2000; **15**: 777–780

McGorry RW, Hsiang SM. The effect of industrial belts and breathing technique on trunk and pelvic coordination during a lifting task. *Spine*. 1999; **24**: 1124–1130

Miyamoto K, Iinuma N, Maeda M, Wada E, Shimizu K. Effects of abdominal belts on intra-abdominal pressure, intramuscular pressure in the erector spinae muscles and myoelectrical activities of trunk muscles. *Clinical Biomechanics*. 1999; **14**: 79–87

Morgan FP, King T. Primary instability of lumbar vertebrae as a common cause of low back pain. *J Bone Jt Surg*. 1957; **39B**, 6–22

Mosekilde L. Sex differences in age related loss of vertebral trabecular bone mass and structure – biomechanical consequences. *Bone*. 1989; **10**: 425–432

Nachemson A. Lumbar intradiscal pressure. *Acta Orthop Scand*. 1960; **Suppl 43**

Nachemson, A. The influence of spinal movements on the lumbar intradiscal pressure and on the tensile stresses in the annulus fibrosus. *Acta Orthop Scand*. 1963; **33**: 183–207

Nachemson A. Lumbar intradiscal pressure. In: Jayson MIV (ed.). *The lumbar spine and back pain*. 2nd ed. London: Pitman; 1985, 341–358

Nachemson A, Elfström G. Intravital dynamic pressure measurements in lumbar discs. A study of common movements, maneuvers and exercises. *Scand J Rehab Med*. 1970; **Suppl 1**

Nordin M. Backs to work: Some reflections. *Spine*. 2001; **26**: 851–856

Park KS, Chaffin DB. A biomechanical evaluation of two methods of manual lifting. *AIIE Trans*. 1974; **6**: 105–113

Penning L, Wilmink JT, van Woerden HH. Inability to prove instability. A critical appraisal of clinical radiological flexion-extension studies in lumbar disc degeneration. *Diagn Imag clin Med*. 1984; **53**: 186–192

Reilly T, Tyrell A, Troup JDG. Circadian variation in human stature. *Chronobiology Int*. 1984; **1**: 121–126

Reyna JR, Leggett SH, Kenney K, Holmes B, Mooney V. The effect of lumbar belts on isolated lumbar muscle. Strength and dynamic capacity. *Spine.* 1995; **20**: 68–73

Schultz AB, Andersson GBJ. Analysis of loads on the lumbar spine. *Spine.* 1981; **6**: 76–82

Selvik G. Roentgen stereophotogrammetry: A method for the study of the kinematics of the skeletal system. 2nd ed., *Acta Orthop Scand.* 1989; **232**: 1–51

Stubbs DA. Human constraints on manual working capacity: Effects of age on intratruncal pressure. *Ergonomics.* 1985; **28**: 107–114

Suezawa Y, Jacob HAC. *Zur Aetiologie der Spondylolisthesis. Die Wirbelsäule in Forschung und Praxis, Bd 94.* Stuttgart: Hippokrates; 1981

University of Michigan, Center for Ergonomics. *3D Static Strength Prediction Program,* V 3.0 1995. Ann Arbor, MI, USA

Waters TR, Putz-Anderson V, Garg A, Fine LJ. Revised NIOSH equation for the design and evaluation of manual lifting tasks. *Ergonomics.* 1993; **36**: 749–776

12 3Mechanical Aspects of the Shoulder

The upper extremity is designed to fulfill a variety of functions. The chain consisting of thorax, upper arm, lower arm, and hand facilitates movement in a large volume of space. The hand can reach almost any point within a sphere centered at the center of the head with a radius equal to the length of the arm. The wide range of motion and orientation of the hand enables objects to be gripped and manipulated under visual control as well as in regions out of sight (e.g. behind the back). Upper arm, lower arm, and hand can execute quick and forceful as well as fine, very accurately guided, movements. Forces and moments oriented in virtually any direction can be generated. The magnitude of such forces and moments depends critically, however, on the relative position and orientation of the hand with respect to the trunk. Knowledge of this dependence on position and orientation is of practical importance in the design of workplaces or rehabilitation aids, e.g. in the design of the propulsion mechanism of wheelchairs. Basic data on this topic can be found, for example, in Pheasant (1997) or Chaffin *et al.* (1999).

Joints of the shoulder girdle

The shoulder girdle, located at the origin of the linked chain that is the upper extremity, has a complex architecture due to the shape and orientation of the bones, the numerous ligamentous connections, and the variety of insertion areas and force directions of the muscles. The shoulder girdle actually comprises four joints (Fig. 12.1). The clavicle articulates at one end with the sternum (articulatio sternoclavicularis), and at its other end with the scapula (shoulder blade) in the region of the acromion (articulatio acromioclavicularis). With respect to their mechanical function, the sternoclavicular and acromioclavicular joints can be regarded as ball-and-socket joints with their range of motion restricted by ligaments. Within certain limits, both joints permit an angular motion of the clavicle, with respect to the sternum and the scapula, and some rotational motion about the long axis of the clavicle. Apart from its anchor to the sternum, the clavicle is fixed to the thorax by muscles originating from the neck region, the arm, and the thorax.

Fig. 12.**1** Joints of the shoulder girdle; right shoulder, seen from the front. (NB. The scapula and thorax do not form a joint in the anatomical sense. The designation 'articulatio thoracoscapularis' is used to describe the mechanical function of this configuration.)

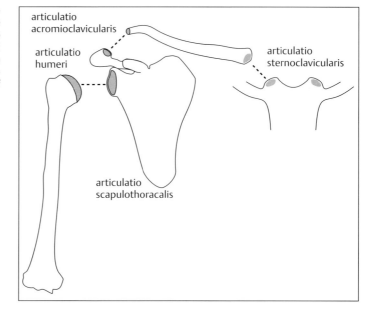

articulatio acromioclavicularis

articulatio humeri

articulatio sternoclavicularis

articulatio scapulothoracalis

The scapula glides on the posterior wall of the thorax. The motion of the scapula can be described as a rotation about its longitudinal axis and/or a displacement on the wall of the thorax. In addition, a tilting of the scapula with respect to the thoracic wall is possible, within a limited range. The scapula articulates with the rest of the skeleton only via the clavicle. Its fixation and guidance on the thoracic wall are effected exclusively by muscles. (The scapula and thorax do not form a joint in the anatomical sense. The designation 'articulatio thoracoscapularis' is used to describe the mechanical function of this configuration.)

The articulating area of the humeral head is spherical. The head articulates with the glenoid cavity of the scapula (articulatio humeri). The glenoid cavity has the shape of a spherical shell. The glenoid cavity and humeral head are not congruent; the radius of the shell is larger than that of the sphere. The articulating area of the glenoid cavity amounts to approximately 6 cm^2 and is thus considerably smaller than that of the humeral head, which is approximately 24 cm^2 (Putz, 1986). Unlike other joints of the skeleton, the glenohumeral joint (shoulder joint) is not stabilized by ligaments but exclusively by muscles arranged around the joint.

The architecture of the shoulder girdle, consisting of sternum, clavicle, and scapula, bears a certain similarity to that of the pelvic girdle. Each of the joints between femur and pelvis, as well as between humerus and scapula, is a ball-and-socket joint. Compared with other joint types (for example, hinge joints) ball-and-socket joints allow for a larger range of motion. Because of the increased range of motion of the glenohumeral joint, the glenoid cavity is consequently not fixed on the thorax but (at least to a certain extent) is able to move synchronously with the humerus (Dempster, 1965). The functional relation of the motions of humerus and scapula is enabled by the joints between scapula and thorax and between scapula and clavicle. In the pelvic girdle there is no counterpart to these joints.

The complex bony architecture of the shoulder girdle is complemented by a complex architecture of the muscles. The muscles can be classified according to their morphology or to their function with respect to movements of the arm (see Tables 12.**1** and 12.**2**). It must be pointed out, however, that parts of individual muscles (e.g. of the deltoid muscle) can have different functions, and functions of specific muscles can depend on the position of the joints.

Table 12.**1** Muscles of the shoulder girdle effecting movement of the arm, in sequence of the location of their insertion (Wirhed, 1997)

Muscles originating at the scapula and inserting at the upper arm	Supraspinatus muscle, teres major muscle, infraspinatus muscle, teres minor muscle, subscapularis muscle, deltoid muscle
Muscles running from the trunk to the scapula	levator scapulae muscle, rhomboid muscle, trapezius muscle, serratus anterior muscle
Muscles running from the trunk to the upper arm	pectoralis major muscle, latissimus dorsi muscle
Muscles originating in the shoulder region and crossing the elbow joint	biceps muscle, triceps muscle

Table 12.**2** Muscles of the shoulder joint, in sequence of their function when moving the arm (Wirhed, 1997)

Flexion	biceps muscle, deltoid muscle, pectoralis major muscle
Extension	deltoid muscle, latissimus dorsi muscle, triceps muscle
Abduction	supraspinatus muscle, deltoid muscle
Adduction	teres major muscle, teres minor muscle, subscapularis muscle, pectoralis major muscle, deltoid muscle
Internal rotation (pronation)	teres major muscle, subscapularis muscle, pectoralis major muscle, latissimus dorsi muscle, deltoid muscle
External rotation (supination)	infraspinatus muscle, teres minor muscle, supraspinatus muscle, deltoid muscle
Motion of the scapula	levator scapulae muscle, rhomboid muscle, trapezius muscle, serratus anterior muscle

Loading of the glenohumeral joint

Due to the complex architecture of the shoulder girdle and the considerable number of muscles involved, two paths are followed in estimating the load on the glenohumeral joint. Either very simple models of the joint are used, or a complex analysis is performed by the method of finite element analysis. Due to the drastic simplifications of the models or the numerous assumptions required in complex analyses we can only expect such investigations to describe the magnitude of the load correctly. In contrast to the case of the hip joint, a validation of the calculated results by means of a direct measurement of the joint load has not been possible up to now.

The glenohumeral joint is loaded even in a posture where the arm hangs down without any load in the hand. The tension of the abductor muscles balances the downward pointing gravitational force of the arm. As the tensile force of the abductors is not perpendicularly aligned, a component of this force points on to the glenoid cavity.

If the arm is raised, the force of the abductor muscles required for equilibrium increases considerably. Fig. 12.**2** shows a simple model for calculation of the load on the glenohumeral joint when the arm is raised to the horizontal, but with no additional load held in the hand (Poppen and Walker, 1978). The gravitational force $\mathbf{F}_1$ acts on the arm; the point of force application is located at the center of gravity of the arm (in the vicinity of the elbow joint). We assume that only the deltoid muscle is activated to generate the moment required for equilibrium. In equilibrium it holds (with reference to the sign convention for moments) that

$$L_2 \cdot |\mathbf{F}_2| - L_1 \cdot |\mathbf{F}_1| = 0$$

By inserting estimated values of 30 cm for L_1, 3 cm for L_2 and 30 N for the gravitational force $|\mathbf{F}_1|$ of the arm (corresponding to 5 % of body weight of a subject with 60 kg body mass) we obtain for the force $\mathbf{F}_2$ of the deltoid muscle

$$|\mathbf{F}_2| = |\mathbf{F}_1| \cdot L_1 / L_2$$
$$|\mathbf{F}_2| = 300 \text{ N}$$

The joint load $\mathbf{O}$ is opposite and equal to the vector sum of muscle force and gravitational force. In the case illustrated here, the angle between the muscle force and the gravitational force amounts to 90°. The magnitude of the joint load is calculated as

$$|\mathbf{O}| = \sqrt{300^2 + 30^2} = 301.5 \text{ N}$$

The force $\mathbf{O}$, from the humeral head on the glenoid cavity, is transmitted to the trunk via the scapulo-thoracic and sternoclavicular joints. The relative fraction of the joint load transmitted via these two paths depends on the position of the upper arm. In the case discussed in Fig. 12.**2** the vector of the joint force is oriented at an angle of

$$\text{atan} (30 \text{ N} / 300 \text{ N}) = 5.7°$$

to the horizontal. Whether or not the line of action of this force points to the glenoid cavity, i.e. whether or not the joint is stable in the posture shown and with activation only of the deltoid muscle, depends on the orientation of the glenoid cavity. If the line of action does not intersect the glenoid cavity, additional muscle forces are required to guarantee the stability of the joint (and our simple model would be invalid).

The additional loading of the joint by a mass held in the hand can be calculated using the model outlined above. The moment arm of the gravitational force of the mass is approximately equal to $2 \cdot L_1$. A mass of 1 kg in the hand would thus require an additional force of the deltoid muscle of $10 \cdot 60/3 = 200$ N. The joint load would then rise to (rounded) $300 + 200 = 500$ N.

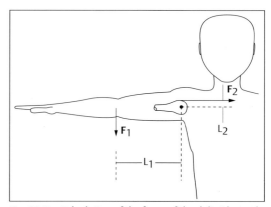

Fig. 12.2   Calculation of the force of the deltoid muscle if the arm is raised to the horizontal (with no additional load in the hand). $\mathbf{F}_1$: gravitational force acting at the center of gravity of the arm; L_1: moment arm of the force $\mathbf{F}_1$ with respect to the center of rotation of the glenohumeral joint; $\mathbf{F}_2$ and L_2: force and moment arm of the deltoid muscle. F_1 amounts to approximately 5 % of the gravitational force of the body mass. L_1 and L_2 are assumed to amount to approximately 30 cm and 3 cm respectively. (Adapted from Poppen and Walker, 1978)

Van der Helm (1994a, b) proposed a detailed model of the shoulder region consisting of the bony elements thorax, sternum, clavicle, scapula, humerus, and 20 muscles, including those muscles running from the shoulder region to the ulna. The geometry of the skeleton, the areas of insertion, and the cross-sectional areas of the muscles were obtained from anatomical studies. The scapulohumeral rhythm (the motion of the scapula accompanying the motion of the humerus) was taken into account as observed in studies *in vivo*. In order to enforce an unequivocal solution for the mechanically indeterminate system, the sum of the squares of the tensile stress generated by muscles was postulated to assume a minimum (see Chapter 8). The maximum tensile stress generated by muscles was assumed to amount to 37 N/cm^2. The calculation yielded muscle and joint forces.

When lifting the upper arm in abduction or anteflexion with a load of 7.5 N in the hand, the load on the sternoclavicular and acromioclavicular joints as well as on the glenohumeral joint assumes, according to van der Helm, maximum values in the abduction or anteflexion region of between 60° and 120°. At 90° of flexion, for example, the load on the sternoclavicular joint amounts to, approximately, 100 N, that on the acromioclavicular joint to 150 N, and the load on the glenohumeral joint to 700 N. Scrutiny of the line of action of the vector of the shoulder load showed that in certain regions of the range of motion of the upper arm, specifically at small abduction or flexion angles, forces of additional muscles (additional to those generating the moment required for equilibrium) are required to guarantee the stability of the joint.

Hughes and An (1996) constructed a model of the glenohumeral joint based on measurements of the cross-sectional areas and moment arms of the muscles of the rotator cuff. In selected postures of the upper and lower arm the maximum moments for internal and external rotation, as well as for adduction and abduction, were measured in a cohort of healthy subjects. With these input data, and a model assumption required to solve the mechanically indeterminate system, muscle forces could be calculated. The results show that internal and external rotation, especially with the upper arm held at 90° of abduction, result in large muscle forces. The supraspinatus tendon (frequently the origin of clinical problems) is subjected to high loading especially in external rotation. The model of Hughes and An may serve to help devise ergonomic improvements of workplaces and to develop guidelines for the rehabilitation of shoulder patients.

Stability of the glenohumeral joint

The issue of 'stability' or 'instability' of joints can be discussed using the example of the glenohumeral joint. A configuration is 'stable', in the mechanical sense, if it returns to its initial state after a small, external perturbation. In contrast, a configuration is termed 'unstable' if a small perturbation suffices to effect a complete change of the configuration. An example of a mechanically stable configuration is the placement of a sphere in a flat hollow. If the sphere is gently kicked, some movement can be observed but the sphere will eventually return to the deepest point of the hollow. An example of a mechanically unstable configuration is the placement of a sphere on top of a hill. If this sphere is kicked, it will roll downhill and never return to its initial location. In this case the final state is completely different from the initial state.

With respect to joints of the human body, the terms stability and instability are occasionally used in an imprecise manner. The term 'instability' is used in some cases where, in reality, only an increased range of motion is observed. An increased relative motion of neighboring vertebrae of the lumbar spine is, for example, termed 'instability of the spine.' The correct designation would be 'hypermobility', because the articulating bones can always return to their initial position. Likewise, the glenohumeral joint is occasionally described as 'unstable', while the humeral head, in reality, is only slightly displaced from the center of the glenoid cavity. A true instability of joints is encountered only in those cases where the articulating bones cannot return to their initial anatomical position after application of an external force or execution of a certain movement.

A true instability of the glenohumeral joint exists if some minor activation of muscle forces, or a small external force, suffices to dislocate the humeral head from the glenoid cavity. An analogous event is the luxation of the femoral head in the case of a dysplastic acetabulum (an acetabulum providing only insufficient, laterally extended coverage of the femoral head). The luxation of the humeral head from the glenoid cavity can occur during apparently insignificant movements, e. g. when putting on a coat, or when turning over in bed. Some athletic disciplines requiring forceful motions of the arm above the head (e.g. javelin throwing) exhibit an increased risk for luxation of the glenohumeral joint (Blevins, 1997). Depending on whether the humeral head dislocated in a caudal, ventral, or dorsal direction from the glenoid cavity, the luxation is designated as 'subglenoidal', 'subcoracoidal', or 'subspinal'. In some cases a combi-

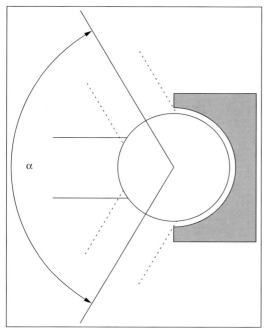

Fig. 12.**3** Due to the impingement of the bone at the base of the sphere on the rim of the socket, the range of rotational motion of the ball-and-socket joint is smaller than 360° minus the enclosure of the ball by the socket. In the example of a ball-and-socket joint with half the ball (i. e. 180°) covered by the socket, the range of motion α is substantially smaller than 180°. To increase the range of motion the diameter of the bone at the base of the sphere must reduce or, alternatively, the amount that the ball is enclosed by the socket must decrease.

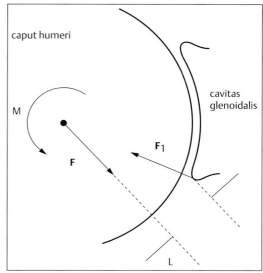

Fig. 12.**4** If the line of action of the force vector **F** does not intersect the glenoid cavity, a moment of the magnitude L · |**F**| with respect to the rim of the cavity results. This moment tends to rotate the head out of the cavity. The force **F**₁ acting from the rim of the cavity on to the head, directed perpendicular to the surface of the head, cannot guarantee equilibrium. A luxation of the head can be prevented only by additional muscle forces that result in the net force vector from the head to the cavity pointing on to the articulating surface of the cavity.

nation of these is observed (multidirectional instability). Subcoracoidal luxation has the highest prevalence; subglenoidal or subspinal luxations are seen less frequently (Saha, 1971).

The risk of instability is the price paid for the extremely large range of motion of the glenohumeral joint. To provide a large range of motion, the glenohumeral joint is laid out as a ball-and-socket joint. A ball-and-socket joint permits angular motion in a large range and simultaneous rotational motion about the long axis of the bone (Fig. 12.**3**). To guarantee that the ball is not displaced from the socket when the joint is loaded from varying directions, the socket must enclose the ball to a certain extent. The more that the socket encloses the ball, the lower is the risk of luxation.

Increasing enclosure of the ball by the socket, however, decreases the range of motion of the joint. The range of motion of ball-and-socket joints

in the human body is ultimately restricted by bony contact of the articulating bone with the rim of the socket. In the example shown in Fig. 12.**3** the socket encloses the ball by 180°. Due to the contact mentioned above, the range of angular motion α is considerably smaller than 180°. A smaller diameter of the bone at the base of the ball would increase the range of motion. Alternatively, a decreased enclosure of the ball by the socket would produce a similar result.

However, the diameter of the bone at the base of the sphere cannot be decreased beyond certain limits because its strength might become inappropriately low. The alternative solution, where the glenohumeral joint has a shallow socket, avoids this (Fig. 12.**4**). But now, if the socket encloses only a fraction of the sphere, the risk of the joint becoming unstable increases. In the absence of additional safety measures, the humeral head glides out of the glenoid cavity when the line of action of the force **F** exerted from the head on to the cavity does not intersect the articulating surface of the cavity. In the example shown in Fig. 12.**4**, the force **F** exerts

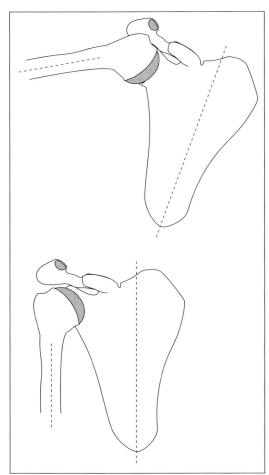

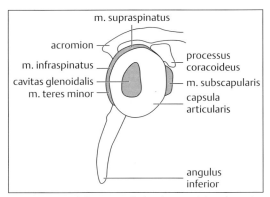

Fig. 12.**6** Stabilization of the humeral head in the glenoid cavity by the muscles forming the so-called rotator cuff. View on to the glenoid cavity of the right shoulder from the right side. (Adapted from van der Helm, 1994a)

Fig. 12.**5** Rotation of the scapula during abduction of the upper arm, shown in the plane of the scapula (right shoulder, seen from the front). The rotational motion of the upper arm is larger than the rotational motion of the scapula. The functionally related motion of the scapula and upper arm is called the 'scapulohumeral rhythm'.

a moment in relation to the point of contact at the lower rim of the cavity of

$$M = -L \cdot |\mathbf{F}|$$

(the minus sign results from the sign convention for moments). This moment tends to rotate the head out of the cavity. Due to the negligibly small friction, the force $\mathbf{F}_1$ acting from the glenoid cavity on to the humeral head is directed perpendicular to the surface of the humeral head and cannot satisfy the condition of equilibrium by itself. Addition-

al, stabilizing forces of muscles or tendons are required in this situation.

The risk of the glenohumeral joint becoming unstable is reduced by allowing the scapula not only to shift on the rib cage, but also to rotate when the upper arm is lifted. The rotation of the scapula follows the abduction of the upper arm (Fig. 12.**5**). If the arm is abducted by more than 30°, the ratio of the rotational movements of upper arm and scapula, observed in a plane fitted to the scapula, varies between 5:4 (Poppen and Walker, 1976) and 3:1 (Högfors *et al.*, 1987). This functionally related movement of the upper arm and scapula is called the 'scapulohumeral rhythm'. The scapulohumeral rhythm is readily reproducible in the individual case and appears to be virtually independent of the loading of the shoulder (Högfors *et al.*, 1991). The combined rotation of upper arm and glenoid cavity ensures that the vector of the force exerted from the humeral head intersects the articulating surface of the cavity, even when the arm is raised very high, thus avoiding an unstable configuration of the glenohumeral joint.

In addition, the glenohumeral joint is stabilized by activation of the muscles crossing the joint. Their tendons merge partially with the joint capsule and form the so-called 'rotator cuff' (Fig. 12.**6**). When the muscles are activated, a component of the muscle and tendon forces directed on to the center of the glenoid cavity acts on the humeral head. Dysfunction of a muscle or traumatic rupture of a tendon may result in instability of the joint. The hypothetical stabilizing function of the muscles of the rotator cuff is substantiated by EMG measurements (Kronberg *et al.*, 1990; Kronberg and Broström, 1995). These measurements show that agonistic and antagonistic muscles are recruited simultaneously for virtually all movements of the upper arm. However, the EMG data do not permit conclusions to be drawn on the muscle forces generated.

Further reading

Textbooks and review papers

Chaffin DB, Andersson GBJ, Martin BJ. *Occupational biomechanics.* 3rd ed. New York: Wiley; 1999

Halder AM, Itoi E, An KN. Anatomy and biomechanics of the shoulder. *Orthop Clin North Am.* 2000; **31**: 159–176 [review paper, 106 references]

Pheasant S. *Bodyspace. Anthropometry, ergonomics and the design of work.* 2nd ed. London: Taylor & Francis; 1997

Perry J. Anatomy and biomechanics of the shoulder in throwing, swimming, gymnastics and tennis. *Clinics in Sports Med.* 1983; **2**: 247–270 [review paper, 61 references]

Refior HJ, Plitz W, Jäger M, Hackenbroch MH (eds). *Biomechanik der gesunden und kranken Schulter.* Stuttgart: Thieme; 1985

Rockwood, CA, Matsen FA (eds). *The shoulder.* 2nd ed. Philadelphia: Saunders 1999

Wirhed R. *Sport-Anatomie und Bewegungslehre.* 2nd Ed. Stuttgart: Schattauer; 1997

Scientific papers, cited in the text or legends

Blevins FT. Rotator cuff pathology in athletes. *Sports Med.* 1997; **24**: 205–220

Dempster WT. Mechanism of shoulder movement. *Arch Phys Med Rehab.* 1965; **46**: 49–70

Högfors C, Sigholm G, Herberts P. Biomechanical model of the human shoulder. I. Elements. *J Biomechanics.* 1987; **20**: 157–166

Högfors C, Peterson B, Sigholm G, Herberts P. Biomechanical model of the human shoulder joint. II. The shoulder rhythm. *J Biomechanics.* 1991; **24**: 699–709

Hughes RE, An KN. Force analysis of rotator cuff muscles. *Clin Orthop Rel Res.* 1996; **330**: 75–83

Kronberg M, Nemeth G, Broström LA. Muscle activity and coordination in the normal shoulder. An electromyographic study. *Clin Orthop Rel Res.* 1990; **257**: 76–85

Kronberg M, Broström LA. Electromyographic recordings in shoulder muscles during eccentric movements. *Clin Orthop Rel Res.* 1995; **314**: 143–151

Poppen NK, Walker PS. Normal and abnormal motion of the shoulder. *J Bone Jt Surg.* 1976; **58A**: 195–201

Poppen NK, Walker PS. Forces at the glenohumeral joint in abduction. *Clin Orthop Rel Res.* 1978; **135**: 165–170

Putz R. Biomechanik des Schultergürtels. *Manuelle Medizin.* 1986; **24**: 1–7

Saha AK. Dynamic stability of the glenohumeral joint. *Acta Orthop Scand.* 1971; **42**: 491–505

van der Helm FCT. Analysis of the kinematic and dynamic behavior of the shoulder mechanism. *J Biomechanics.* 1994a; **27**: 527–550

van der Helm FCT. A finite element musculoskeletal model of the shoulder mechanism. *J Biomechanics.* 1994b; **27**: 551–569

13   Structure and Function of Skeletal Muscle

Muscles are biological machines that convert chemical energy, derived from the reaction between food substrate and oxygen, into mechanical work and heat. Muscle strength can be defined as the ability of skeletal muscles to develop force in order to initiate, decelerate, or prevent movement. One single factor, i. e. force alone, is not, however, sufficient to perform and to control movements, to stabilize posture, or to prevent injuries to the musculoskeletal system. Therefore, for optimum control and performance of the musculoskeletal system, muscle endurance and muscle coordination are required, in addition to force. Muscular endurance can be defined as the ability to maintain a specified force for a given period of time. However, this definition of endurance is not universally applicable, as endurance varies with the type of mechanical work performed.

Skeletal muscle morphology

Skeletal muscle represents the largest organ of the body. It accounts for approximately 40 % of the total body weight and is organized into hundreds of separate entities, or body muscles, each of which has a specific task in enabling the great variety of movements that are essential to normal life. Each muscle is composed of a great number of subunits, muscle fibers, that are arranged in parallel and normally extend from one tendon to another (Fig. 13.1). Muscle fibers are cable-like structures composed of tightly packed subunits, myofibrils, that fill up most of the volume of the fibers. The myofibrils are composed of sarcomeres arranged in series. The sarcomeres, defined as the basic units of the myofibrils, are responsible for force generation and shortening of myofibrils. The basic unit is formed by two contractile proteins, or myofilaments, the myosin (thick) and actin (thin) filaments. Actin filaments are anchored at each end to the Z-disks. A sarcomere is defined as that part of a myofibril enclosed between the Z-disks. When a muscle is in a relaxed state there is some overlap between the myosin and actin filaments.

The basic units generate force by the interaction of actin and myosin filaments (Huxley, 1957, 1973, 1988; Huxley and Peachy, 1961). Cross-bridges are structures forming part of the thick (myosin) filaments of the sarcomere. They attach to the back-bone of these filaments in such a way as to enable them to attach to sites on the thin (actin) filaments in their vicinity. The cross-bridges are functionally identical and act independently. The probability of attaching to an actin filament is influenced by local biochemical conditions, e. g. calcium ion concentration. At any given time during activity of a muscle, some cross-bridges are attached to the thin filaments but others are detached or moving towards new attachment sites.

When attachment of actin and myosin filaments occurs, attached cross-bridges undergo structural deformation. Force is generated and the thin (actin) filament is pulled along the thick (myosin) filament. The myofilaments slide in relation to each other; the overlap between the filaments increases and at the same time the muscle fibers, or the muscle, shorten (Fig. 13.2). According to the theory of contraction, the length of the myosin filaments is assumed to be constant and not to contribute to the shortening of the sarcomere. Therefore, the shortening of a sarcomere is assumed to occur only via the sliding of the filaments relative to each other. The total shortening of the myofibril is the sum of the length changes occurring in the sarcomeres arranged in series. Supposing we have two myofibrils, one consisting of 10 sarcomeres and the other of 5 sarcomeres arranged in series. It follows that the amount of shortening of the former will be twice the shortening of the latter.

It is assumed that active muscle force originates exclusively from cross-bridges. As a consequence, active force generated at any given time is dependent on the number of parallel cross-bridges attached to the thin (actin) filaments. Because of the series arrangement of sarcomeres within a myofibril, the force generated by one unit has to be maintained and transmitted to the next unit. Therefore, the force of the whole structure is equal to the force of one unit, i. e. the force of one sarcomere. If the force developed in one half of a sarcomere is to be transmitted to the other Z-disk of a sarcomere, the force in the other half of a sarcomere has to be equal in magnitude (Huijing, 1983) (Fig. 13.3). It follows that an equal number of active cross-bridges in both parts of the sarcomere should be attached. If the number of active cross-bridges is low, the developed force is low. If the number of active cross-bridges increases, the force developed will increase as well.

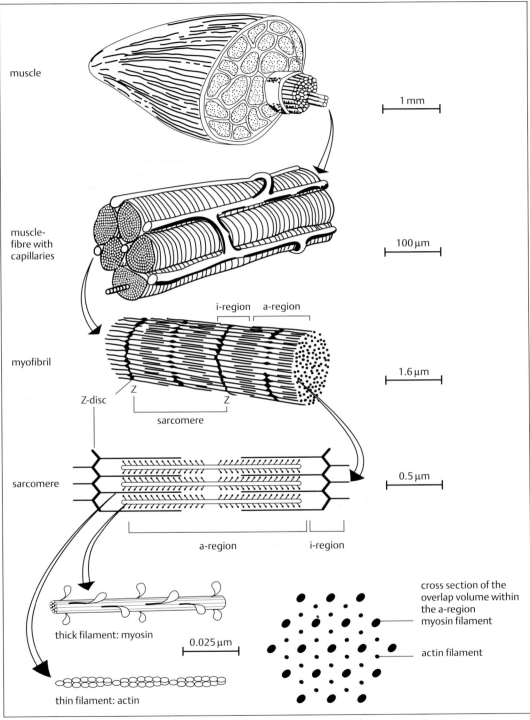

muscle

1 mm

muscle-
fibre with
capillaries

100 µm

i-region   a-region

myofibril

1.6 µm

Z-disc   Z   Z

sarcomere

sarcomere

0.5 µm

a-region   i-region

thick filament: myosin

0.025 µm

cross section of the
overlap volume within
the a-region
myosin filament

actin filament

thin filament: actin

Fig. 13.1   Scheme of muscle architecture. (Adapted from Di Prampero, 1985)

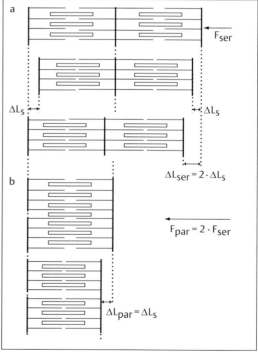

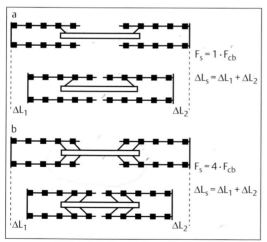

| 1 | | Myosin bridge attatched to actin-binding site |

Fig. 13.2 Sequence of events in cross-bridge construction and force generation. Starting from the initial state (1), the cycle begins with the detachment of the myosin head from the actin molecule (2). The head now moves to a new site (3), force is developed due to deformation of the molecule and the filaments shift relative to each other (4).

The force-length relationship

Sarcomeres arranged in series are called myofibrils. Muscle fibers are a collection of myofibrils arranged in parallel. Thus, muscle fibers are a collection of sarcomeres arranged in series as well as in parallel. The maximum force developed in a muscle fiber will increase in proportion to the quantity of myofibrils arranged in parallel, i.e. the force is proportional to the cross-sectional area of the muscle fiber (Fig. 13.**4**). Experiments have shown that the amount of force developed in a muscle fiber depends on the actual muscle fiber length and the shortening (contraction) velocity. These relationships are assumed to be determined by the filament system and by the parallel as well as the se-

Fig. 13.2 (figure, panels 1–4):
- 1: Myosin bridge attatched to actin-binding site
- 2: Myosin bridge detatched, ready to attatch to new actin site
- 3: Myosin bridge attatched to actin-binding site
- 4: Force development (Myosin head turns, actin filament tends to move in direction of arrow)

Fig. 13.3 Schematic illustration of the effects of parallel or series arrangement of bridges in a sarcomere. **a:** two bridges in series; **b:** four bridges in parallel. F_{cb} force in a bridge; F_s force of a sarcomere; ΔL_1, ΔL_2 changes in length of the halves of the sarcomere; ΔL_s change in length of the sarcomere. In case (**b**) the force is 4 times the force of case (**a**); the maximum change in length is the same in each case.

In the figure:
$$F_s = 1 \cdot F_{cb}$$
$$\Delta L_s = \Delta L_1 + \Delta L_2$$
$$F_s = 4 \cdot F_{cb}$$
$$\Delta L_s = \Delta L_1 + \Delta L_2$$

In Fig. 13.4:
$$F_{ser}$$
$$\Delta L_{ser} = 2 \cdot \Delta L_s$$
$$F_{par} = 2 \cdot F_{ser}$$
$$\Delta L_{par} = \Delta L_s$$

Fig. 13.4 Schematic illustration of the effect of a serial (**a**) or parallel (**b**) arrangement of sarcomeres. F_{ser} and F_{par} designate the maximum forces generated in the serial or parallel arrangement. ΔL_s is the change in length in a sarcomere; ΔL_{ser} and ΔL_{par} are the maximum attainable length changes in the serial or parallel arrangement. In case (**a**) the maximum force is half of the maximum force of case (**b**); in case (**a**) the maximum change in length is twice the maximum change in length in case (**b**).

ries arrangement of sarcomeres within a muscle fiber (Hill, 1938, 1964, 1970; Gordon *et al.*, 1966; Edman and Reggiani, 1987).

It has been known since the late nineteenth century that the force developed by a muscle of constant length, e.g. during isometric contraction, will vary with its starting length. In a very shortened or a very lengthened state, the muscle generates less force than in mid-ranges. The isometric force-length relationship can be measured directly when a muscle is maximally stimulated at a variety of discrete lengths and the resulting force is recorded. When maximum force at each length is plotted against length, a relationship like that shown in Fig. 13.**5** is obtained. The force-length curve represents the results of many experiments plotted on the same graph, i.e. an artificial connection of individual data points from isometric experiments. Therefore, the force-length relationship is strictly valid only for isometric contractions. The structural basis for the force-length relationship was elucidated in the early 1960s. Basically, the force-length relationship in skeletal muscle is assumed to be a direct function of the overlap between actin and myosin filaments (Huxley and Peachy, 1961; Gordon *et al.*, 1966).

Descending limb of the force-length curve. The region of the force-length curve in which the force decreases as the sarcomere length increases is known as the descending limb. Above a certain muscle fiber length, force development is no longer possible. The length of a myosin and of an actin filament is 1.65 μm and 2.0 μm respectively. At a sarcomere length of 3.65 μm, i.e. equal to the sum of the lengths of the filaments, there is no overlap between the actin and myosin filaments. Thus, in this situation, although biochemical processes might permit actin-myosin interaction by removing the inhibition on the actin filament, no myosin cross-bridges are located in the vicinity of the actin active sites and therefore no force generation can occur.

Plateau region of the force-length curve. Increasing force with decreasing muscle length occurs until the sarcomeres reach a length of 2.2 μm. When the sarcomere length ranges between 2.0 and 2.2 μm, muscle force remains constant. Thus, while sarcomere length shortening over the 2.2 to 2.0 μm range results in greater filament overlap, it does not result in increased force generation since no additional cross-bridge connections are made. This is due to the bare region (not containing cross-bridges) of the myosin molecule, which is 0.2 μm long. The region of the force-length curve over which change in length results in no change in force generation is called the plateau region. The maximum tetanic force of the muscle in this region is termed F_0. The length at which F_0 is attained is known as the optimal length, termed L_0.

Ascending region of the force-length curve. The region of the force-length curve where force increases as length increases is called the ascending limb. When sarcomeres shorten to below 2.0 μm, actin filaments from one side of the sarcomere double-overlap with the actin filaments on the opposite side. In other words, at these lengths, actin filaments overlap both with themselves and with the myosin filaments. Under these double-overlap conditions, the actin filament from one side of the

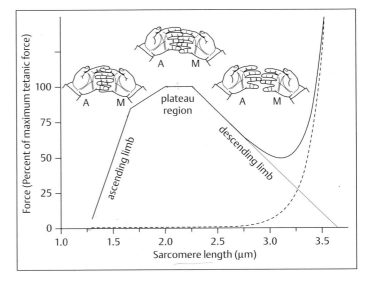

Fig. 13.**5** Maximum tetanic force in relation to sarcomere length. The dashed curve describes the elastic tensile force generated when a muscle is stretched beyond its optimal length. The solid curve describes the sum of active force and passive tensile force. At three sarcomere lengths the overlap of the myosin and actin filaments is visualized using the example of the fingers of the two hands sliding with respect to each other. In this example, the fingers of one hand represent the myosin (M) and the fingers of the other hand the actin (A) filaments.

sarcomere interferes with cross-bridge formation on the other side, resulting in decreased muscle force output. The region where shortening between 2.0 and 1.87 µm occurs is known as the shallow ascending limb of the force-length curve. This region is distinguished from the next portion of the force-length curve, which is known as the steep ascending limb. At these very short lengths, the myosin filament actually begins to interfere with shortening as it abuts the sarcomere Z-disk, leading to a rapid reduction of force.

Passive force-length curve. The dashed line in Fig. 13.**5** represents the force generated if a muscle is passively stretched to various lengths. Near the optimal length L_0, passive tension is almost zero. However, as the muscle is stretched to longer lengths, passive force increases dramatically. The increase in passive force, which occurs when the muscle is stretched, may play an important role in re-establishing myofilament overlap in the absence of muscle activation. These relatively long lengths can be attained physiologically. In such situations, large passive forces directed at re-establishing muscle length will be encountered.

The structures responsible for the increase in passive resistive force are located outside and inside the myofibrils. According to Cavagna (1977) and Heerkens *et al.* (1987) the parallel elastic elements of muscle (intramuscular connective tissue) are responsible for the force exerted by a passive muscle when it is stretched beyond its optimum length. As collagen is the major protein in muscle, tensile properties of passive muscles are primarily dependent on the amount and type of collagen (Kovanen *et al.*, 1984). Although intramuscular connective tissue enables forces (actively developed by the muscle or passively imposed on the muscle) to be transmitted safely and effectively by the entire tissue, information on the connective tissue component of skeletal muscle is relatively sparse.

Recent studies have shown the origin of passive muscle tension also to be located within the myofibrils themselves. A new structural protein, 'titin', sometimes referred to as 'connectin', may be the source of this passive tension (Wang *et al.*, 1993; Labeit and Kolmerer, 1995). This large protein molecule spans each half-sarcomere and is anchored to the Z-disk, connecting the thick myosin filaments end to end. Titin is thought to play a basic role in maintaining sarcomere structural integrity and to produce passive force when muscle sarcomeres are stretched. Furthermore, titin is assumed to produce a high percentage of the passive force that is developed in most muscles in the plateau region and the descending limb of the force-length curve. Once a sarcomere is stretched beyond thick and thin filament overlap, cross-bridge attachment becomes impossible, and the forces required to re-establish myofilament overlap are thought to come primarily from the passive elastic forces of the highly stretched titin. In addition to passively supporting the sarcomere, titin stabilizes the myosin lattice, so that high muscle forces do not disrupt the orderly hexagonal array. If titin is selectively destroyed, normal muscle contraction may cause significant myofibrillar disruption.

The force-velocity relationship

Skeletal muscle has an inherent capacity to adjust its active force to precisely match the load exerted on it during shortening, or to regulate the resistive force during muscle elongation. This property distinguishes muscles from a simple elastic structure and is based on the fact that active force generation is continuously adjusted to the speed of the contractile system. The maximum force development capacity of a muscle depends, not only on muscle length, but also on the velocity of contraction. It is observed that the active force development of a skeletal muscle is high when the velocity of contraction is low and that the force decreases with increasing velocity of contraction. Thus, when the load is high, the active muscle force is increased to the required level by reducing the speed of shortening. Conversely, when the load is low, the active force can be made correspondingly small by increasing the speed of shortening.

Fig. 13.**6** shows the relationship between force and velocity of an isolated whole sartorius muscle of the frog, published by Hill (1938). Experimentally, the force-velocity relationship, like the force-length relationship, is a curve that represents the results of a number of experiments plotted on the same graph. A muscle is stimulated maximally and allowed to shorten or to lengthen against a constant load. The muscle velocity during shortening or lengthening is measured and then plotted in relation to the load.

According to Hill, the relationship between force F and shortening velocity v during a concentric contraction may be described by the equation:

$$(F + a) \cdot v = b \cdot (F_{max} - F)$$

In this equation, a and b are experimentally derived constants. The values of a and b are estimated at approximately 0.25. F_{max} is the maximum tetanic force developed at a given muscle length. The maximum force development is achieved at a shortening velocity v equal to zero. The maximum shortening velocity v_{max} is observed at force F equal to zero (Fig. 13.**6**). The Hill equation can be used to predict the relative change in muscle force occurring as a muscle is allowed to shorten.

The force-velocity relationship is related to the cross-bridge cycling rate. The cross-bridges between actin and myosin have been found to attach and detach at certain rates (Hill, 1964; Pollack, 1983; Huxley, 1988). These are referred to as rate constants. At any point in time, the force generated by a muscle depends on the number of cross-bridges attached. When contraction velocity increases, the filaments slide past one another faster and faster; therefore, force decreases due to the lower number of cross-bridges attached. Conversely, as the relative filament velocity decreases, more cross-bridges have time to attach and generate force, so that force increases. This discussion is not aimed at giving a full description of the basis for the force-velocity relationship, but only at providing some insight into how cross-bridge rate constants can affect force generation as a function of velocity.

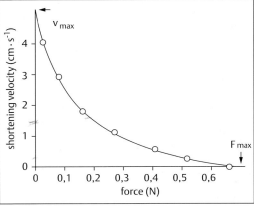

Fig. 13.**6** Empirical relation between force and contraction velocity of a muscle, documented for the sartorius muscle of the frog. The relation was described by Hill (1938) by means of a hyperbola.

Theoretical modeling of skeletal muscle behavior

The modeling of skeletal muscle serves the purpose of predicting static and dynamic behavior in different situations. The model of a muscle is constructed from single elements with known mechanical properties. Elements may be combined to represent properties of the whole muscle. Hill (1970) developed a muscle model consisting of two basic elements; a contractile element and an elastic element (Fig. 13.**7a**). The contractile element models the myofilaments responsible for active force development. The elastic element describes the passive elastic properties of the structure. The mechanical property of the elastic element equals the elastic property of a spring (see Chapter 7). Like a spring, the elastic elements store energy during elongation and release virtually all the energy as they return to their original length.

In its most simple form, the Hill model (Hill, 1958) is constructed from a contractile element connected in series with a passive elastic element. In this model, the contractile elements are considered to have force-length as well as force-velocity characteristics similar to those described for muscle fibers. As both elements are connected in series, both are subject to the identical tensile force. The change in length of the combined model is the sum of the length changes occurring in each element of the model. The velocity of shortening and lengthening of the model is the sum of the velocities of both elements of the model.

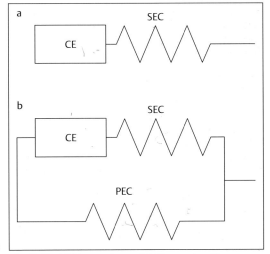

Fig. 13.**7** Hill's muscle model. The contractile properties are represented by the contractile element CE. The elastic properties are represented by the series elastic component SEC (in series to the contractile element) and the parallel elastic component PEC (parallel to the contractile element). (**a**) basic model for description of the active properties of a muscle. (**b**) basic model for description of the active and passive properties of a muscle.

The combined function of the elastic and contractile elements connected in series seems to be important for producing fine, coordinated movements (Joyce *et al.*, 1969; Rack and Westbury, 1984). It follows from the model that, during contraction of a muscle, force will increase slowly. This is assumed to be due to the simultaneous shortening of the contractile, and lengthening of the elastic, elements. The converse length changes of the contractile and elastic elements allow a smooth movement to occur without any 'rocking'. In other words, the elastic elements dampen rapid increases in muscle force (Bressler and Clinch, 1974).

If the length of a muscle fiber is below its optimum length, additional shortening of the muscle fiber leads to a decrease in force development accompanied by a simultaneous shortening of the series elastic elements. When the velocity of shortening of a muscle fiber increases, the force is reduced (because of the force velocity relationship) and the series elastic element is again allowed to shorten. As a consequence, the total length change in the combined model is greater than the isolated length change in the contractile element.

To explain the mechanical behavior of passive muscles, a third element is introduced: the parallel elastic element (Fig. 13.**7b**). The parallel elastic element is arranged in parallel to the contractile element. As the stiffness and the tensile strength of the contractile element are assumed to be negligibly small, the parallel elastic element is the source of the force preventing rupture of contractile elements during passive elongation of a muscle. On the other hand, the force of the parallel elastic element is negligibly small compared with the maximum force of the contractile element. In the case of maximum active force generation, the parallel elastic element will resist only a small fraction of the external force and will consequently shorten.

▨ **Mechanical properties of tendons**

Tendinous tissue behaves like a non-linear elastic structure. Fig. 13.**8** shows an example of a force-length characteristic of tendon, based on data published by Woo (1981). A specimen consisting of a tendon and its insertion into bone (tendon-bone complex) was investigated. Starting from its resting length, the bone-tendon complex was elongated up to rupture or failure at the site of insertion, and the opposing (resistive) force was measured. The stiffness of the complex at each point of the curve is defined as the ratio of force increase and length increase, i.e. $\Delta F/\Delta L$ [N/m]. The figure shows that the stiffness of the tendon is a function of elon-

gation. With minor elongation of the tendon, stiffness is low, e. g. small changes in force have relatively large effects on tendon length. As elongation increases, stiffness increases as well. In the linear portion of the curve, stiffness is virtually constant. The stress σ_{max} (force divided by cross-sectional area) of a tendon at the point of rupture amounts to approximately 100 MPa; the strain ε_{max} at rupture is in the region of 10 % of the starting length.

The series elastic elements located in tendinous tissue are important for an optimum function of active muscles. When a muscle develops force, the length of the tendon increases and the muscle is allowed to shorten. Because of the change in tendon length, a muscle-tendon unit will have an increased operating range relative to the range of muscle fibers alone. If the muscle-tendon unit is strained by small forces during a movement, the length change in the unit will occur at the tendon because of its lower stiffness. The result is that a fraction of the length change that would have to be accommodated by muscle fibers is actually taken up by tendons. Thus, by attaching muscles to bones via compliant (elastically elongating) tendons, the length changes of the muscle fibers are reduced. Length changes of muscles and their tendons may also have opposite signs. When the force of a muscle-tendon unit with constant length is reduced, the tendon is allowed to

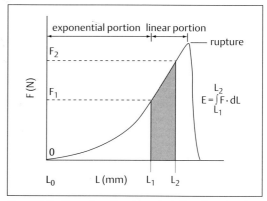

Fig. 13.**8** Force-length characteristic of a tendon, using the example of the flexor digitalis tendon of the pig (Woo, 1981). The graph shows the force of the tendon in relation to its length, starting from its length L_0 in the unloaded state. Force as function of length shows first an approximately exponential behavior pattern followed by an approximately linear portion. Upon further increase of the force, rupture occurs at the tendon-bone interface. The shaded area below the curve is a measure of the energy E stored when the force changes from F_1 to F_2 and the tendon length changes from L_1 to L_2.

shorten, while muscle length will increase. Length changes of tendons also dampen sharp increases in muscle force, i.e. the time elapsing until the muscle force reaches its maximum value is, in fact, increased (Rack and Westbury, 1984).

Plastic deformation of tendons is negligible, i.e. after release a stretched tendon will return to its original length. The energy expended on stretching the tendon is stored as potential energy and released almost completely as the force exerted on the tendon decreases to zero. The loss of energy is less than 10 %. The force-length characteristics of tendons are dependent only to a minor extent upon the velocity of stretching. Therefore, the deformation energy stored in a tendon during stretching is given by the area below the force-length curve (Butler *et al.*, 1978; Fung, 1981; Woo, 1981)

$$E = \int F \cdot dL \quad [Nm]$$

In this formula E denotes the energy, F the resistive force, and dL the change in length. The integral extends from the resting length of the tendon (with zero force F) up to the length reached under the force applied. The amount of stored energy increases as stretching increases (see Chapter 7). At higher forces the tendon is rather stiff and the change in length relative to the change in force will be small. Therefore, in this situation the increase in stored energy will be small as well. A greater amount of energy could be stored if the length change in the tendon were increased. In real life these increased ranges of elongation are obtained during stretch-shortening cycles occurring in a variety of movements. During a stretch-shortening cycle the initial stretching of the muscle-tendon unit is followed by active shortening of the complex. During the stretching phase energy is stored in the unit.

The potential energy stored in a muscle-tendon unit is released by decreasing the force exerted on the structure. If this is done slowly, the energy will become available slowly; if it is done at a rapid rate, the energy will be released rapidly as well. The amount of energy released per unit of time, the power P, is given by

$$P = F \cdot v$$

where F is the force and v the shortening velocity of the muscle-tendon unit.

It is of practical importance that tendons can store energy during a stretch-shortening cycle at a relatively low rate. Upon lengthening, the tendon then acts as an energy reservoir that can be emptied at a high rate to effect movements with high speed and power (Huijing, 1983). This situation may be compared to shooting an arrow with a bow.

The potential energy of the bow is increased when the active muscles pull on the string, thereby deforming the bow. When the string is suddenly released, the deformation energy is set free and the arrow will be launched with high power, resulting in a high velocity.

Force regulation in skeletal muscles

An excitatory impulse generated naturally in the central nervous system or artificially by an electrical signal generator creates a so-called action potential (specific electrical field) at the relevant muscle fibers. The tensile force developed by a single fiber in response to a single action potential invading the motor endplates is called a twitch. As the frequency of the stimulating impulses increases, twitches begin to overlap. At frequencies above a certain limit, single twitches can no longer be discriminated and tetanic contraction develops. The frequency limit, where tetanic contraction or tetanic force generation occurs, varies among different fibers and individual motor units. This limit is normally observed in the range between 10 and 100 Hz (Fig. 13.9). The higher the frequency of stimula-

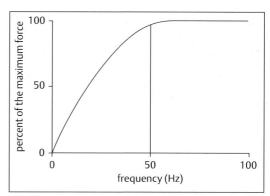

Fig. 13.**9**   Dependence of the force of a muscle fiber on the stimulation frequency, the force-frequency curve. At stimulation frequencies higher than about 10 Hz, single twitches merge to form a constant output force. In the lower region of the force-frequency curve, small changes in stimulation frequency effect large variations in force output. In contrast, at high frequencies a change in frequency effects only a small change in force, if any. Changing the frequency from 50 Hz to 100 Hz effects, for example, only a negligibly small change in force. Stimulation frequency of motor units is usually in the order of 10 to 60 Hz. In this region, force depends strongly on frequency.

Table 13.1 Relation between motor units and muscle fiber types

Designation of motor unit	Muscle fiber type
fast fatiguable unit (FF)	Type IIb, fast glycolytic fiber
fast fatigue resistant unit (FR)	Type IIa, fast oxidative glycolytic fibers
slow unit (S)	Type I, slow oxidative fiber

tion of the muscle fibers, the greater is the force produced in the muscle as a whole.

Skeletal muscle fibers possess a wide spectrum of morphologic, contractile, and metabolic properties. Muscle fibers are classified as fast or slow, oxidative or non-oxidative, and glycolytic or non-glycolytic (Brooke and Kaiser, 1970; Bruke, 1981). Often, only three different types are described; for details see Table 13.1. The three types differ characteristically with respect to speed of shortening, force generation, and endurance. Fast-contracting fiber types (Type IIb) shorten approximately two to three times faster than slow-contracting fibers (Type I). The specific tension (force divided by cross-sectional area) of fast muscle fiber types is higher than that of slow muscle fibers. In general, slow muscle fibers (Type I) have the greatest endurance, followed by Type IIa and Type IIb fibers.

The functional unit of force generation in a muscle is the sarcomere (in fact the half-sarcomere due to sarcomere symmetry). The functional unit of force generation of the muscle is the motor unit. A motor unit comprises an α-motoneuron and the muscle fibers innervated by it. This unit is the smallest part of the muscle that can be made to contract independently. Motoneurons have their cell bodies in the ventral root of the spinal cord. The axons of the neurons terminate at the motor endplate of the fibers. When stimulated, all the fibers of a motor unit respond simultaneously. The fibers of a motor unit are said to show an 'all-or-nothing response' to stimulation: they contract either maximally or not at all.

Motor units are usually classified according to the physiological properties of their muscle fibers (Bruke, 1981, Kernell 1996). These properties are the motor unit twitch tension, the tetanic tension recorded at an intermediate stimulation frequency, and the fatiguability of the unit in response to a specific stimulation protocol (Fig. 13.10). In general, motor units belong to three different groups. Those that have a fast contraction time and a low fatigue index are known as fast fatiguable (FF) units. Those that have a fast contraction time and a high fatigue index are designated fast fatigue resistant (FR) units. Those that have slow contraction times, and which are most resistant to fatigue, are classified as slow (S) units.

A whole muscle is subdivided into many motor units, each of which comprises a single motoneuron and its related muscle fibers. The muscle fibers belonging to one motoneuron have the same physiological, biochemical, and ultrastructural properties. The number of muscle fibers belonging to a motor unit, and the number of motor units within a whole muscle, vary widely. This is closely related to the degree of control required of the muscle. The muscle fibers within a motor unit are interspersed among fibers of other motor units. The functional consequence of this dispersion is that the forces generated by a unit will spread over a larger tissue area. This may minimize mechanical stress in focal regions within the muscle.

The nervous system can vary muscle force output by two mechanisms. By varying the stimulation frequency, the force will be changed, i.e. when the frequency of stimulation is increased, the force output will increase as well. Thus the force output is positively related to the discharge rate of a motor unit. This phenomenon is termed temporal summation. Alternatively, muscle force can be varied by changing the number of motor units that are active at a given time. For relatively low-force contractions, few motor units are activated, while for higher force generation, more units are activated (Bodine *et al.*, 1987). The process by which motor units are added as muscle force increases is termed recruitment.

In their classical study, Henneman *et al.* (1965) showed that, at very low forces, low amplitude voltage signals of short duration ('spikes') were observed at the nerve. As muscle force increased, the size of the spikes also increased in a very orderly fashion, i.e. as force continued to increase, the units recruited exhibited larger and larger spikes. The entire process was reversed as force decreased. From these observations it was concluded that, at low muscle force levels, motor units with the smallest axons and the lowest threshold and depolarization frequency were first recruited. As force increased, larger and larger axons with higher activation thresholds and higher excitation amplitudes were recruited. This is known as the 'size principle' and provides an anatomic basis for the orderly recruitment of motor units to produce a smooth contraction. In later studies, e.g. Binder and

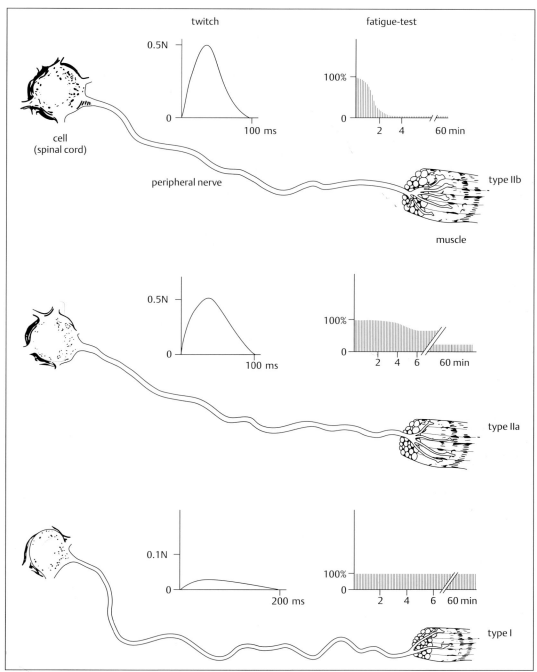

Fig. 13.**10** Schematic illustration of the anatomic and physiologic properties of three different types of motor units. Type IIb (upper diagram) has large axons innervating a large number of muscle fibers. Such units produce large forces but are subject to rapid fatigue. Type IIa (middle diagram) has medium size axons innervating a large number of muscle fibers. Such units produce lower forces than Type IIb but are less subject to fatigue. Type I (lower diagram) has small axons innervating only few fibers. Such a unit develops only a low force but is able to maintain this force over a longer period of time. (Adapted from Edington and Edgerton, 1976)

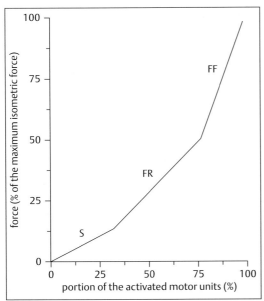

Fig. 13.11 Schematic illustration of the recruitment of motor units in relation to the active, isometric muscle force. At low force levels, units of type S (slow) are recruited first; with increasing force, units of type FR (fatigue resistant) and then of type FF (fast fatiguable) are recruited. (Adapted from Edgerton *et al.*, 1983)

Mendell (1990), it was determined that, in general, small motor axons innervate slow motor units (Type I) and larger motor axons innervate fast motor units (Types IIa and IIb). These findings were confirmed in studies on human motor units (Milner-Brown *et al.*, 1973, Edgerton *et al.*, 1983).

Based on the above findings, the following scheme was proposed for the voluntary recruitment of motor units (Fig. 13.**11**). At very low excitation levels, the smallest axons with the lowest threshold to activation are activated first. As voluntary effort increases, most of the next-larger axons are recruited, activating the Type IIa fibers. During maximal effort, the largest axons innervating Type IIb fibers are activated. This activation pattern seems reasonable, since the most frequently activated S-units are those with the greatest endurance. The FF units, which are rarely activated, have the lowest endurance. In addition, the S-units (Type I), which are activated first, develop the lowest tension, so that low tension is generated as contraction begins. This provides a mechanism for smoothly increasing tension as first S-units, then FR-units, and finally FF-units are recruited.

Relationship between force and electromyography (EMG)

Electromyography gives a method for recording and processing the electrical signals of an activated muscle. The twitch of a muscle fiber is initiated by electrochemical processes at the muscle fiber membrane. These electrical impulses propagate throughout the muscle fiber. The resulting electrical potentials are measured by fine intramuscular needle electrodes or electrodes attached to the skin. The electrical potential of a motor unit, representing the sum of the individual action potentials generated in the muscle fibers of the motor unit, has an amplitude in the range between 200 µV and 3 mV. The duration of the potentials is normally between 2 ms and 15 ms, depending on the muscle examined. When processing the EMG, it is usually the frequency and amplitude of the signals that are analyzed.

There is general agreement on the usefulness of the EMG as an indicator of the activation pattern of a motor pool. Electromyography is frequently used to study the activity of individual muscles in the maintenance of posture and during normal or abnormal patterns of movement (Basmajian, 1985). Such recordings can be combined with film or video recordings, helping to define the relationship between the position of a joint, or limb, and the EMG signal.

Some important, still unresolved problems in orthopedic biomechanics could be resolved if it were possible to predict the magnitude of the muscle force (in newtons) from the recorded electromyographic signal. In the past, several studies have been aimed at elucidating this relation. There is agreement that the EMG signal reflects the activity of a muscle. However, it is not possible at present to predict the resulting force from the recorded EMG signals. In most cases there is not even a proportionality between muscle force and signal amplitude. Only in special cases, i.e. under isometric contractions, a proportionality between integrated EMG (area below the curve) and force may be assumed. In such experiments it is important for the electrical activity from the total area of the muscle to be measured. If the moment arm of the muscle is known, the force can be calculated from the moment developed.

The derived factor of proportionality between EMG signal and force can be used to predict muscle force from the EMG signal only. However, this method has its limitations. The factor of proportionality between EMG signal and muscle force determined for one muscle may not be valid for another muscle. Other muscles may have different

S - FR - FF

moment arms, changing the relation between the EMG signal and force. Factors determined from one individual subject cannot be transferred to another subject, and placement of surface electrodes is poorly reproducible among subjects. In addition, the EMG signal seems to depend on the velocity of the change in muscle length. For example, EMG is being measured from a muscle that is shortening at 5 % v_{max}. The force generated by this muscle will be approximately 75 % of maximum isometric tension. If the EMG from the same muscle is measured under conditions where it is shortening at only 1 % of v_{max}, much more tension will be generated due to the slower contraction velocity. The EMG signal will, however, be identical in both situations. These findings are due to the fact that all motor units are already activated when generating 75 % of maximum force (Bigland-Ritchie et al., 1983a, 1983b; Loeb and Gans, 1986). Owing to the shortening of the muscle, not all cross-bridges are able to attach. When the velocity is reduced, the activity and the EMG signal remain virtually unchanged, but the force increases because more cross-bridges have sufficient time to attach. In an attempt to overcome these difficulties, efforts are made to obtain information on the velocity dependence of the EMG signal and to apply a theoretically derived or experimentally determined correction when predicting muscle force from the EMG signal of a contracting or elongating muscle.

In conclusion, EMG measurements provide valuable information on muscle activation patterns but an EMG record should be interpreted with caution in terms of force. In special circumstances, i.e. in purely isometric situations or when dealing with slow length changes, forces might be calibrated and estimated.

Muscle architecture

A typical muscle fiber in an adult man has a diameter in the range of 50 to 70 μm. The length varies from a few millimeters to more than ten centimeters. Muscle fibers are generally attached to tendon plates or aponeuroses, which have a continuous transition into the more rounded tendons that run outside the muscle. Skeletal muscles are distinguished from one another with respect to fiber length, ratio of fiber length to muscle length, and the orientation of the fibers relative to the long axis of the muscle (Woittiez *et al.*, 1983; Gans and De Vree, 1987; Otten, 1988, Huijing *et al.*, 1989; Lieber *et al.*, 1990). While muscle fibers have a relatively consistent fiber diameter between muscles of different sizes, the geometric arrangement (spatial ar-

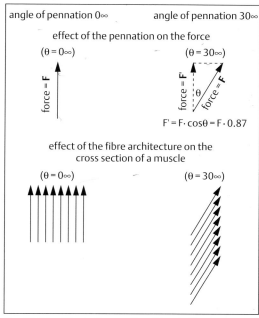

Fig. 13.**12**   Effect of pennation. Muscle fibers arranged in the longitudinal direction of the muscle transmit their entire force on the tendon. Muscle fibers directed at an angle with respect to the tendon transmit only part of their force in the longitudinal direction of the tendon. In the example shown, the longitudinal tendon force at an angle of pennation of 30° amounts to 87 % of the muscle fiber force.

chitecture) of these fibers can be quite different. The architecture of the muscle fibers at the microscopic level together with fiber type distribution is responsible for the contractile properties at the macroscopic level.

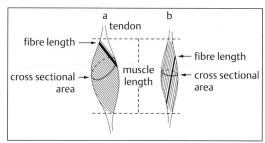

Fig. 13.**13**   Schematic illustration of muscles with differing architecture. **a**: muscle with short fibers and large physiologic cross section. **b**: muscle with long fibers and small physiologic cross section.

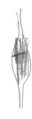

Most muscles may be seen as a collection of fibers arranged in parallel. In general, two types of fiber architecture are considered. Muscles with fibers extending parallel to the muscle force generating axis are termed parallel, or longitudinally arranged, muscles. Muscles with fibers oriented at an angle relative to the force-generating axis are termed pennate muscles (Fig. 13.**12**). For both parallel and pennate muscles, the ratio of muscle fiber length to muscle length ranges approximately between 0.2 and 0.6. In other words, even in the strictly longitudinally arranged muscles, the fibers extend at maximum over only 60 % of the muscle length.

The mechanical properties of muscles arranged in parallel are governed by the same principles of series and parallel arrangement as discussed above for sarcomeres. Based on this organization, it follows that the total change in length of a muscle equals the length change in the muscle fibers. The force-length and force-velocity relationship of a parallel muscle are similar to those of a single muscle fiber. The muscle force is equal to the sum of forces generated by the individual fibers. The mechanics of pennate muscle, however, are more complicated. The geometric arrangement of the individual muscle fibers in relation to the longitudinal axis of the muscle affects the relationship between muscle fiber and muscle length change. A number of architectural studies performed in human upper and lower limb muscles have demonstrated that pennation angles range from 0° to 30° (Lieber *et al.*, 1990, Kawakami *et al.*, 1998). If muscle fibers are arranged at an angle φ in relation to the longitudinal axis of the tendon, the magnitude of the force component **F'** of the force **F** developed in the muscle fibers and transmitted to the tendon (Fig. 13.**12**) will be

$$|\mathbf{F'}| = |\mathbf{F}| \cdot \cos \phi$$

At an angle of pennation greater than zero, cos φ will always be less than 1 and only a fraction of the muscle fiber force will be transmitted in the direction of the axis of the tendon. Therefore, in pennate muscles, the force actually transmitted to the tendon will be less than the sum of forces developed in the individual muscle fibers. When a pennate muscle contracts, the angle of pennation increases.

What is the rationale behind a design inducing part of the force generated not to be transmitted to the tendon? In a number of locations in the body it would be difficult to accommodate muscles with pennation angles equal to zero because large numbers of longitudinally arranged fibers lead to large cross sections of the muscles. Thus it may be hypothesized that pennation is a space-saving strategy, as it reduces the anatomical cross-sectional area at the expense of reducing the longitudinal

force transmission to the tendon. On the other hand, pennation permits more muscle fibers to be attached along a tendon, thus compensating for the reduced force.

Different models are proposed to explain the effect of pennation on the force-producing capacities of skeletal muscle (Huijing, 1983; Gans and de Vree, 1987; Otten, 1988, Epstein and Herzog, 1998). These models, in general, are based on muscle geometry, volume constraints, pennation angles between muscle fibers and tendon, homogeneity of sarcomere length, and numbers of sarcomeres in series, as well as on the relationship between the force-length characteristics of muscle fibers and tendon elasticity. The issue is, however, still under discussion.

The anatomical cross-sectional area of a muscle is, in general, not proportional to its maximum force because of differences in fiber architecture. To correlate the maximum force capacity with the cross-sectional area of a muscle, the physiological cross-sectional area (PCSA) has to be calculated. The PCSA represents the sum of cross-sectional areas of the muscle fibers, measured perpendicular to their longitudinal direction (Fig. 13.**13**). The physiological cross-sectional area is proportional to the maximum force capacity of a muscle. This area is hardly ever identical to the cross-sectional area of a muscle in the traditional anatomic planes, as seen, for example, in magnetic resonance imaging (MRI). The physiological cross-sectional area is calculated as follows

$$PCSA = m / (\rho \cdot l)$$

In this equation m represents muscle mass (g), ρ muscle density (1.056 g/cm³ for mammalian muscle), and l the mean length of the muscle fibers within the muscle.

The content of this formula may be visualized as follows. Muscle mass divided by density equals muscle volume. If the muscle were cylindrical in shape, dividing volume by length (fiber length) would represent the cylinder cross-sectional area. Since fiber length is not equal to cylinder length, the area calculated according to the above formula is only a theoretical parameter characterizing a cylinder with a length equal to that of the fibers. In general, PCSA and maximum force development are not strictly proportional to muscle mass. Knowledge of the muscle mass or its changes thus permits no prediction with respect to the magnitude of the muscle force or its change.

Each muscle is unique in terms of its architecture. However, taken as functional groups, some generalizations can be made (Table 13.**2**). Muscles with greater angles of pennation generally contain

Table 13.**2**   Effect of fiber architecture on mechanical properties of skeletal muscle

Orientation to tendon	Functional advantage	Types of muscles
parallel arrangement (angle of pennation < 10°)	1. more effective transmission of force on tendon. 2. greater extent and speed of shortening. 3. greater economy of maintaining tension	predominantly Type I fibers
pennate arrangement (angle of pennation >10°	greater physiological cross-sectional area to enhance force and power generation	predominantly Type II fibers

more fibers and thus can exert greater total force. In contrast, a muscle containing fibers with a small angle of pennation generally benefits from a more effective transmission of force to the tendon. In addition, muscles with long fibers appear to be designed for a large working range because excursion range is proportional to the length of the muscle fibers. This occurs primarily because there are more functional units (sarcomeres) arranged in series in the direction of movement. The gross archi-

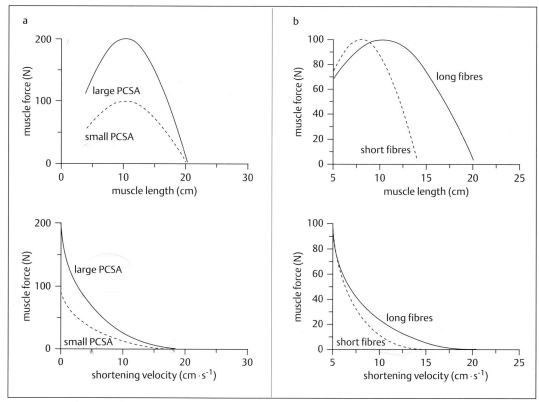

Fig. 13.**14**   Schematic illustration of the force-length and force-velocity relation of muscles with differing architecture. **a**: force-length and force-velocity relation of two muscles with equal fiber length but different physi-ological cross-sectional areas PCSA. **b**: force-length and force-velocity relation of two muscles with different fiber length but equal physiological cross-sectional areas (PCSA).

tecture of a muscle may also influence its shortening properties. In general, the longer a given muscle and the more parallel the alignment of its fibers, the greater its capacity for length changes and shortening velocity. Consequently, a muscle's architectural features need to be considered when evaluating its functional role in various activities.

Fig. 13.**14a** compares the force-length and force-velocity curves of two muscles with equal muscle fiber lengths and pennation angles. The muscle mass of the second muscle is assumed to be twice the mass of the first. Both muscles have the same basic shape of the force-length curve; however, the force curve from the muscle with the greater mass is shifted to larger force values. The same holds for the force-velocity curves. If the force equals zero, however, both muscles have the same maximum shortening velocity v_{max}. The muscle with the greater mass exhibits a larger maximum force F_{max},

but both curves exhibit the same basic shape. If both curves were plotted on relative scales, the two muscles would appear to have identical properties. Stress, i.e. force divided by cross-sectional area, is equal between the two muscles.

Fig. 13.**14b** shows two muscles with identical physiological cross section and pennation angles but with different fiber lengths. As shown in the figure, the peak force of the force-length curve is identical but the muscle with the longer fibers exhibits a greater range of length changes and an increased maximum shortening velocity v_{max} compared with the muscle with the shorter fibers. These two examples show that muscle architecture has a profound influence on functional properties. The contractile units, i.e. the sarcomeres, are identical in both examples.

As a joint rotates, the change in length of a muscle is dependent on the distance between the insertion of the muscle and the center of rotation. Fig. 13.**15** compares two muscles with different distances between their insertion and the center of rotation. When movement occurs with a given interval of rotation, the change in length of the muscle with the shorter distance will, for purely geometric reasons, be less than that of the muscle with the longer distance. In general, a muscle with a long distance between insertion and center of rotation will have longer muscle fibers. This is interpreted as adaptation to the mechanical requirements. However, the range of length changes made possible by the architectural design is not always fully exploited in real life. The architectural design of a muscle is also assumed to be adapted to parameters like velocity and acceleration of joint movements (Lieber and Boakes, 1988). However, knowledge in this field is still fragmentary.

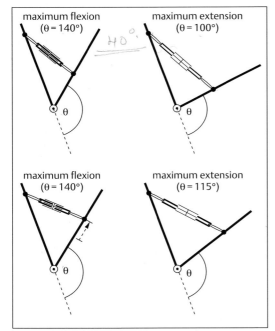

Fig. 13.**15** Change in the range of motion of a joint due to a change in the distance between the insertion of a muscle and the center of rotation. The joint in the upper part of the figure may have a range of movement (difference between maximum extension and flexion) of 40°. When the distance between the insertion and the center of rotation is increased (lower part of the figure), the range of motion decreases to 25°. This decrease is due to the fact that, because of the increase in the distance between insertion and center of rotation, the length change in the sarcomeres per degree of rotation increases.

Skeletal muscle mechanics

Skeletal muscles are designed to initiate movements, to decelerate movements, to resist external loads so that movement does not occur, and to provide the body with a substantial part of its necessary heat. Muscle activity may be static or dynamic. Static muscle work is defined as contraction with constant muscle length. Dynamic muscle activity is defined as contraction during which muscle length changes. Contractions may be classified into three types:

Isometric contraction. When a muscle develops force but no movement occurs, as muscle length remains constant, static equilibrium exists. This contraction is called isometric. Often, a situation in which force increases with no observable change in length of the muscle-tendon unit, is also called isometric contraction. In reality, there is shortening of the muscle fibers and simultaneous elongation of the tendon in this case.

Concentric contraction. When a muscle is able to shorten against a given load, movement occurs. This type of contraction is termed concentric. The force developed under concentric muscular action is always less than the maximum isometric force F_{max} developed at optimum muscle length. The shortening velocity of contraction is increased when muscles work against small loads. When the load against which the muscle contracts is reduced almost to zero, the maximum velocity of contraction v_{max} is achieved. The velocity of contraction v_{max} is characteristic of each muscle and depends on muscle fiber distribution and architectural characteristics. During concentric muscular activity, mechanical work E is performed

$$E = F \cdot (-\Delta L)$$

In this equation F and ΔL designate the force and the length change in the muscle. When muscles shorten, the change in length is counted negative and thus mechanical work is positive. The mechanical power P of a muscle is defined as the work performed per unit of time

$$P = F \cdot (-v)$$

In this equation v is the contraction velocity of the muscle. The velocity is counted negative when a muscle shortens and the power is thus positive. Because of the relationship between force and contraction velocity (see section above on the force-velocity relationship), maximum power occurs at a shortening velocity of approximately 1/3 of v_{max}.

Eccentric contraction. If a muscle is activated in such a fashion that its length under a given external load is observed to increase, the contraction is designated eccentric. According to the above equations, the work and power delivered during eccentric contractions are negative. This means that the muscle absorbs energy. During eccentric contractions, the muscle force may exceed by far the maximum isometric force F_{max}. The increase in force is due to summing of active and passive resistive force. This passive force is directed at restoring muscle length when muscles are stretched during an activity (see Fig. 13.**5**). This property is fundamental to many everyday movement patterns. There is currently considerable scientific interest in studying the behavior of muscles during eccentric contractions. Eccentric contractions are physiologically common. In addition, muscle pain and some muscle injuries seem to be associated with eccentric muscular activity.

Note: Muscle contractions are sometimes classified as isometric, concentric, or eccentric depending on whether 'the external force equals the muscle force, or is smaller or larger than the muscle force'. Mechanically, this statement is incorrect as, according to Newton's third law, the muscle force is invariably opposite and equal to the external force exerted on the muscle. This holds for all three types of muscle contraction. The difference between the different contractions is defined by the length change in the muscle and the resulting movement under application of the force.

Muscle activity during movements of the body seldom involves pure forms of isometric, concentric, or eccentric contractions. This is due to body segments being periodically subjected to impact forces, as in walking or running, or to gravity lengthening the muscles. A sequence of eccentric and concentric actions defines a stretch-shortening cycle. The purpose of stretching is to make the final concentric contraction more powerful than that resulting from a pure concentric contraction alone. The observed increase in force is due to summing the active force and the passive force originating from the initial lengthening beyond optimum length.

If the force output of the muscle is enhanced during a stretch-shortening cycle, it is to be expected that the work efficiency will be increased as well. Mechanical efficiency is defined as the ratio of external work performed to the extra energy production:

$$\text{mechanical efficiency } (\%) = E_{ext} \cdot 100/(E_{tot} - e)$$

In this equation E_{ext} is the external work, E_{tot} the energy expended, and e the resting metabolic rate (Aura and Komi, 1986a, 1986b). The increase in mechanical efficiency is assumed to be related to the enhancement of resistive forces when elastic structures in the muscle or at the muscle-tendon unit are lengthened (Cavagna, 1977; Cavagna *et al.*, 1968, 1981; Bressler and Clinch, 1974; Bobbert *et al.*, 1986; Alexander 1988a, 1988b).

Muscles generate force and transmit this force via tendons to the bones. With respect to the axis of rotation of a joint, a muscle force **F** produces a moment (or torque) **M**. The moment is defined as the cross product of the vectors **L** and the muscle force **F**

$$M = L \times F$$

Vector **L** points from the axis of rotation to the point of force application at the bone. The moment

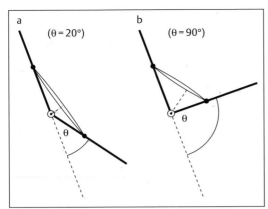

Fig. 13.16 Change in the moment arm of a muscle in relation to the state of flexion of a joint. The dashed line designates the moment arm, i.e. the perpendicular distance of the line of action of the muscle force from the center of rotation. At a small flexion angle ($\theta = 20°$) the moment arm is relatively small. With increasing flexion of the joint (for example $\theta = 90°$) the moment arm increases. The moment arm reaches its maximum value at $\theta = 180°$. The moment arm is only one of the two factors determining the moment. In addition, the moment depends on the muscle force.

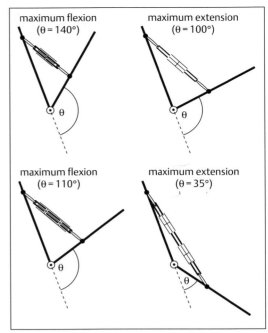

Fig. 13.17 Change in the range of motion of a joint due to a change in muscle length. With short muscle fibers (upper diagrams) the joint may be mobile between 140° and 100°. Longer muscle fibers (lower diagrams) influence the minimum and maximum length of the muscle. Thus the limits of flexion and extension change to 110° and 35°, so that the range of motion changes to 75°.

developed thus depends on the amount of force developed, the magnitude of **L**, and the angle between the line of force and the direction of **L**. Therefore, the moment may be changed by changing the force, or the point of force application, and thus the angle.

The moment arm of a muscle is defined as the perpendicular distance between the line of application of the muscle force and the center of rotation of a joint. For purely geometric reasons the moment arm of a muscle will change as a function of joint position, i.e. in the range between maximum extension and maximum flexion. Fig. 13.16 illustrates this with the case of a simple hinge joint crossed by a muscle. It is observed that, close to maximum extension of the joint, the moment arm is small. As flexion of the joint increases, the moment arm of the muscle also increases. The moment arm would assume its maximum value at a flexion angle of 180° (not attainable *in vivo*). If the distances of the points of insertion of a muscle from the axis of rotation are equal to both sides of the axis, the moment arm will change in proportion to the sine of half the flexion angle. Thus, close to maximum extension, a given force will effect a low moment; as the flexion angle increases the moment will increase as well.

As described above (see Chapter 3), the moment depends on the product of moment arm and force. During actual activities the moment varies within broad limits. This variation is due to the fact that muscle force varies in relation to muscle length, shortening velocity, and the number of motor units recruited. The relationship between muscle length, state of rotation of a joint and moment is illustrated in Fig. 13.17. Supposing a muscle-joint system is configured in such a way that, when extending from 140° to 100°, the muscle changes from its minimum to its maximum length. What would happen if the muscle length were significantly increased? Since more sarcomeres are added in series to take up the length change, the range of length change will increase. As shown in the illustration, the muscle could now extend to 35° (instead of 100°). The minimum length at which the longer muscle is not able to develop force will also increase. Therefore, the lower limit of range of motion will be changed as well, i.e. from 140° to 110°.

When the joint angle changes, the relative change in sarcomere length will depend on muscle fiber length. In muscles with long fiber lengths, the relative change in sarcomere length per degree of rotation will be small. Therefore, according to the force-length relationship, the change in force as the joint rotates will be minor. If, however, muscle fiber length is short, the change in length of the sarcomeres will be increased and the force developed will change during movement of the joint.

For skeletal muscle, a close relationship can be assumed to exist between muscle architecture, geometric relation to bones and joints, and mechanical muscle properties like force generation, length change, and velocity. This indicates that the architectural specialization observed in numerous muscles has profound functional consequences. Muscles might be able to perform a large range of tasks, mainly as a result of their intrinsic design rather than by being triggered by a specific set of command signals from the central nervous system (CNS). This design probably allows the central nervous system to act as a coordinator of different actions rather than as a definer of a particular activity.

Further reading

Textbooks and review papers

Fitts RH, Widrick JJ. Muscle mechanics: adaptation with exercise training. *Excerc Sport Sci Rev.* 1996; **24**: 427–473 [review paper, 139 references]

Herzog W (ed) *Skeletal muscle mechanics.* 'From Mechanism to Function'. Chichester: John Wiley & Sons; 2000

Tillmann B. Binde- und Stützgewebe des Bewegungsapparates. In: Tillmann B, Töndury G (eds). Rauber Kopsch. *Anatomie des Menschen.* Band 1, 2nd ed. Stuttgart: Thieme; 1998

Zajac FE. Muscle and tendon: properties, models, scaling and application to biomechanics and motor control. *Crit Rev Biomed Eng.* 1989; **17**: 359–411 [review paper, 177 references]

Scientific papers, cited in the text or in the figures

Alexander R. *Elastic Mechanisms in Animal Movement.* Cambridge: Cambridge University Press; 1988a

Alexander R. The spring of your step: The role of elastic mechanisms in human running. In: de Groot G, Hollander AP, Huijing PA, van Ingen Schenau GJ (eds). *Biomechanics XI-A.* Amsterdam: Free University Press; 1988b, 17–25

Aura O, Komi PV. Mechanical efficiency of pure positive and negative work with specific reference to the work intensity. *Int J Sports Med.* 1986a; **7**: 44

Aura O, Komi PV. Effects of prestretch intensity on mechanical efficiency of positive work and on elastic behavior of skeletal muscle in stretch-shortening cycle exercise. *Int J Sports Med.* 1986b; **7**: 137

Basmajian JV, DeLuca CJ. *Muscles alive. Their Functions Revealed by Electromyography.* 5th ed. Baltimore: Williams & Wilkins; 1985

Bigland-Ritchie B, Johansson R, Lippold OCJ, Smith S, Woods J. Changes in motorneurone firing rates during sustained maximal voluntary contractions. *J Physiol.* 1983a; **340**: 335–346

Bigland-Ritchie B, Johansson R, Lippold OCJ, Smith S, Woods J. Contractile speed and EMG changes during fatigue of sustained maximal voluntary contraction. *J Neurophysiol.* 1983b; **50**: 313–324

Binder MD, Mendell LM (eds). *The Segmental Motor System.* New York: Oxford University Press; 1990

Bobbert MF, Huijing PA, Ingen Schenau GJ van. An estimation of power output and work done by the human triceps surae muscle-tendon complex in jumping. *J Biomech.* 1986; **19**: 899–906

Bodine SC, Roy RR, Eldered E, Edgerton VR. Maximal force as a function of anatomical features of motor units in the cat tibialis anterior. *J Neurophysiol.* 1987; **6**: 1730–1745

Bressler BH, Clinch NF. The compliance of contracting skeletal muscle. *J Physiol.* 1974; **237**: 477–493

Brooke MH, Kaiser KK. Muscle fibre types: how many and what kind? *Arch Neurol.* 1970; **23**: 369–379

Bruke RE. Motor units anatomy, physiology, and functional organization. In: Brookhart JM, Mountcastle VB, Brooks VB, Geiger SR (eds). *Handbook of physiology.* Bethesda MD: American Physiological Society; 1981, 345–422

Butler DL, Grood ES, Noyes FR, Zernike RF. Biomechanics of ligaments and tendons. *Exerc Sports Sci Rev.* 1978; **6**: 125–182

Cavagna GA. Storage and utilization of elastic energy in skeletal muscle. *Exerx Sport Sci Rev.* 1977; **5**: 89–129

Cavagna GA, Citterio G, Jacini P. Effects of speed and extent of stretching on the elastic properties of active frog muscle. *J Exp Biol.* 1981; **91**: 131–143

Cavagna GA, Dusman B, Margaria R. Positive work done by a previously stretched muscle. *J Appl Physiol.* 1968; **24**: 21–32

Di Prampero PE. Metabolic and circulatory limitations to VO2max at the whole animal level. *J Exp Biol.* 1985; **115**: 319–332

Edgerton VR, Roy RR, Bodine SC, Sacks RD. The matching of neuronal and muscular physiology. In: Borer KT, Edington DW, White TP (eds). *Frontiers of Exercise Biology.* Illinois: Human Kinetic Publishers; 1983

Edington DW, Edgerton VR. *Biology of physical activity.* Boston: Houghton Mifflin; 1976

Edman KAP, Reggiani C. The sarcomere length-tension relation determined in short segments of intact muscle fibres of the frog. *J Physiol.* 1987; **385**: 709–32

Epstein M, Herzog W. *Theoretical Models of Skeletal Muscle: Biological and Mathematical Considerations.* Chichester: John Wiley & Sons Ltd; 1998

Fung YC. *Biomechanics. Mechanical Properties of Living Tissues.* New York: Springer; 1981

Gans C, De Vree F. Functional bases of fibre length and angulation in muscle. *J Morphol.* 1987; **192**: 63–85

Gordon AM, Huxley AF, Julian FJ. The variation in isometric tension with sarcomere length in vertebrate muscle fibres. *J Physiol.* 1966; **184**: 170–192

Henneman E, Somjen G, Carpenter DO. Functional significance of cell size in spinal motorneurons. *J Neurophysiol.* 1965; **28**: 560–580

Heerkens YF, Woittiez RD, Kiela J. Mechanical properties of passive rat muscle during sinusoidal stretching. *Pflueg Arch.* 1987; **409**: 438–447

Hill AV. The heat of shortening and the dynamic constants of muscle. *Proc R Soc Lond (Biol).* 1938; **126**: 136–195

Hill AV. The series elastic component of muscle. *Proc R Soc Lond.* 1958; **B137**: 273–280

Hill AV. The effect of load on the heat of shortening of muscle. *Proc R Soc Lond (Biol).* 1964; **159**: 297–318

Hill AV. *First and Last Experiments in Muscle Mechanics.* Cambridge: Cambridge University Press; 1970

Huijing PA, van Lockeren Campagne AHH, Koper JF. Muscle architecture and fibre characteristics of rat gastrocnemius and semimembranosus muscles during isometric contraction. *Acta Anat.* 1989; **135**, 46–52

Huijing PA. Elastic Potential of Muscle. In: *Strength and Power in Sport.* Komi V (ed.). Oxford: Blackwell Scientific Publications; 1983, 151–168

Huxley AF. Muscle structure and theories of contraction. *Progress in Biophysics and Biophysical Chemistry.* 1957; **7**: 255–318

Huxley AF. Muscular contraction. *Ann Rev Physiol.* 1988; **50**, 1–16

Huxley AF, Peachy LD. The maximal length for contraction in vertebrate striated muscle. *J Physiol.* 1961; **156**: 150–165

Huxley HE. Molecular basis of contraction in cross-striated muscle. In G Bourne (ed.) *The structure and function of muscle,* Vol. 1, 2nd ed., New York: Academic Press; 1973, 301–387

Joyce GC, Rack PMH, Westbury DR. The mechanical properties of cat soleus muscle during controlled lengthening and shortening movements. *J Physiol.* 1969; **204**: 461–474

Kawakami Y, Ichinose Y, Fukunaga T. Architectural and functional features of human triceps surae muscles during contraction. *J Appl Physiol.* 1998; **85**: 398–404

Kernell D. Organization and properties of spinal motoneurons and motor units. *Prog Brain Res.* 1996; **54**(1): 41–51

Kovanen V, Suominen H, Hekkinen E. Mechanical properties of fast and slow skeletal muscles with special references to collagen and endurance training. *J Biomech.* 1984; **17**: 725–735

Labeit S, Kolmerer B. Titins: giant proteins in charge of muscle ultrastructure and elasticity. *Science.* 1995; **270**: 293–296

Lieber RL, Boakes JL. Sarcomere length and joint kinematics during torque productions in the frog hindlimb. *Am J Physiol.* 1988; **254**:C759–C768

Lieber RL, Fazeli BM, Botte MJ. Architecture of selected wrist flexors and extensor muscles. *J Hand Surg.* 1990; **15**: 244–250

Loeb GE, Gans C. *Electromyography for Experimentalists.* Chicago: University of Chicago Press; 1986

Milner-Brown HS, Stein RB, Yemm R. The contractile properties of human motor units during voluntary isometric contractions. *J Physiol.* 1973; **228**: 285–306

Otten E. Concepts and models of functional architecture in skeletal muscle. *Exe Sport Sci Rev.* 1988; **16**: 89–137

Pollack GH. The cross-bridge theory. *Physiol Rev.* 1983; **63**: 1049–1113.

Rack PMH, Westbury DR. Elastic properties of the cat soleus tendon and their functional importance. *J Physiol.* 1984; **347**: 479–495

Wang K, McCarter R, Wright J, Beverly J, Ramirez-Mitchell R. Viscoelasticity of the sarcomere matrix of skeletal muscles: The titin-myosin composite filament is a dual-stage molecular spring. *J Biophys.* 1993; **64**:1161–1177

Woittiez RD, Huijing PA, Rozendahl RH. Influence of muscle architecture on the force-length diagram of mammalian muscle. *Pflueg Arch.* 1983; **399**: 275–279

Woo SLY. The effects of exercise on the biomechanical and biochemical properties of swine digital flexor tendons. *J Biomech Eng.* 1981; **103**: 51–56

14 Mechanical Properties of Bones

An organism composed only of soft tissues could survive without great problems in the ocean. When living on land or in the air, rigid and fracture-resistant structural elements are indispensable for maintenance of the body shape and for locomotion. Fig. 14.**1** illustrates the mechanical demands on our skeleton. The ultimate strength of bones must be high enough to ensure that fractures are not encountered under everyday, physiological loading. In addition, bones must be rigid, i. e. their deformation under applied loads must be small. Muscles would otherwise be unable to stabilize postures or to produce movement.

In addition, bones protect vital organs such as the brain, spinal cord, heart, and lungs. Structural properties such as strength and rigidity are of importance here, too. Apart from their duties in the mechanical field, bones play an important role in the calcium metabolism and provide space for the blood-generating cells. For this reason the mechanical properties and architecture of the bones are inextricably linked with metabolic processes. One example of this interrelation is the decrease in bone density observed with increasing age or in the course of certain diseases.

▨ Architecture of the bone tissue

The material properties and architecture of bones can be discussed at different levels, under ultramicroscopic, or microscopic magnification, as well as macroscopically (as seen with the naked eye). This section does not aim to give a comprehensive description of the composition and properties of bones but is confined to those items that explain the unique mechanical properties of bones and which highlight the difficulties encountered in an exact description of these properties. For comprehensive information the reader is referred to the writings of Currey (1984, 1999), Martin and Burr (1989), Martin *et al.* (1998), and Tillmann (1998a, b).

Ultramicroscopic findings. Bone is composed of cells embedded in a fibrous, organic ground substance (extracellular matrix). The extracellular matrix of mature bone consists of about 20% water. The dry material consists of 30–40% organic and 60–70% inorganic components. The organic component consists of 90% collagen, with the remaining 10% being composed essentially of glycosaminoglycans and glycoproteins.

The collagen of the bones is identical with the material employed in other tissues of the body subjected to tensile stress, such as ligaments or connective tissue. In primary woven bone, the collagen fibrils are not aligned in any preferred direction. In mature lamellar bone, in contrast, the collagen fibrils can form a meshed or spiral arrangement,

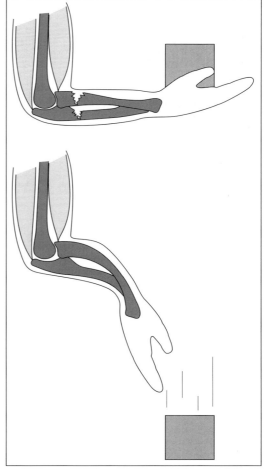

Fig. 14.**1** Mechanical demands on bones. Excessively fragile or flexible bones are unable to stabilize postures or to control movements. (adapted from Currey, 1984)

aligned preferentially in the longitudinal direction of the long bones.

The rigidity and strength characteristic of bone material are effected by the deposition of mineral substances in the organic ground substance (matrix). These inorganic salts comprise about 85 % calcium phosphate, 6–10 % calcium carbonate, and small admixtures of other alkaline salts. After generation of the organic matrix these salts are first deposited in an amorphous phase; subsequently crystals bearing a close resemblance to hydroxyapatite $Ca_{10}(PO_4)_6(OH)_2$ are formed. These crystals are between 20 and 100 nm long and between 1.5 and 3.0 nm in diameter (1 nm = 10^{-9} m). They are aligned in their long axis to the collagen fibrils and are attached to the fibrils in several layers.

Microscopic findings. The bone cells comprise the bone building cells (osteoblasts), the bone resorbing cells (osteoclasts), and the mature cells enclosed in the extracellular matrix (osteocytes). Osteoblasts produce an early stage of bone tissue, the osteoid. In the course of this phase the osteoblasts remain enclosed in the matrix and become osteocytes. Within a few days the osteoid is mineralized to about 70 %; mineralization is completed within a few months. Osteoclasts resorb the collagen component of the bone tissue by an enzymatic process. The mineral component is dissolved by creation of an acid environment.

During the growth phase, as well as during the entire lifetime, bone tissue is continuously remodeled, as osteoclasts remove bone and osteoblasts rebuild new bone, often in a different architecture. For this reason, a distinction is made between primary bone (created initially) and secondary bone (created by reconstruction). Almost all bone present at birth, and the callus produced for the purpose of stabilization around fractures, consists of so-called 'woven bone'. The collagen fibers of woven bone have diameters in the region of 0.1 μm (1 μm = 10^{-6} m) and exhibit no preferred direction. Unordered trabeculae, the so-called 'primary spongy bone', develop from woven bone. Under the influence of mechanical loading, the primary spongy bone is transformed into spatially ordered, secondary trabecular (or spongy) bone. The lamellar bone material of cortical bone also originates from woven bone. In lamellar bone, mineral and collagen are deposited in layers of about 5 μm thickness. The collagen fibers of lamellar bone have diameters in the region of 2–3 μm and definitely preferred orientations. The architecture of lamellar bone bears some similarity to that of technical fiber composite materials (Currey, 1964; Tillmann, 1998a). The lamellar, cortical bone is interspersed with osteons. Osteons are created, when bone is resorbed by osteoclasts, in the form of a thin channel,

which is subsequently filled with new bone deposited in layers by osteoblasts.

Macroscopic findings. The small difference in density of woven bone and lamellar bone material is due to minor differences in their organic and inorganic composition. Major differences in the density of bone tissue samples are due to the porosity of the tissue. In the cross section of long bones, an outer layer of compact bone, known as cortical bone, is visible. The internal volume of long bones is usually filled with a structure composed of thin rods (trabeculae) and plates. Bone displaying this architecture is termed trabecular (or: spongy) bone. The architecture of trabecular bone is not unlike that of technical foams with open pores. There is no abrupt transition from cortical to trabecular bone. The outermost bony layer of the long bones beneath the articular cartilage, for example, is called cortical bone, despite the fact that its thickness at this location is virtually the same as that typical of trabeculae.

As a rough categorization, the apparent density of cortical bone is above 1.5 g/cm^3, and the apparent density of trabecular bone between 0.1 and 1.0 g/cm^3. The qualifier 'apparent' points to the fact that this density measurement allows for porosity; it does not describe the true density of the compact material (i.e. measured without voids). The apparent density is obtained by dividing the mass of a bone sample, cleaned of marrow and body fluids, by its volume. The apparent density should be distinguished from the density measured in the material in its compressed state, i.e. without pores. With regard to this latter density, cortical and trabecular bone would exhibit only minor differences because both bone types are constructed essentially from lamellar bone. Deformation and strength of bones depend strongly on the apparent density. This justifies the measurement in vivo of apparent bone density, because such data allow conclusions to be drawn on the mechanical properties of the bones under investigation.

Stress and strain of inhomogeneous, anisotropic materials

Bone material is inhomogeneous because it is composed of a crystallized mineral and a fibrous organic component. Due to the spatial alignment of the organic fibers in lamellar bone, to the architecture of the layered lamellae in cortical bone, and to the spatial configuration of the trabeculae in trabecular bone, the mechanical properties of bone (moduli of elasticity and shear etc.) depend on the orientation in which they have been measured. Materials whose mechanical properties depend on the orientation of measurement are described as 'anisotropic'.

Unlike isotropic materials, the strain occurring in anisotropic materials is not necessarily in the same direction as the applied stress. Under tensile stress a beam made of an anisotropic material may, for example, not only lengthen but also exhibit an angular deformation (Fig. 14.**2**). The deformation of inhomogeneous, anisotropic materials under the influence of external forces cannot be characterized by the three material constants (modulus of elasticity E, shear modulus G and Poisson's ratio μ) as is the case with homogeneous, isotropic materials. To describe the relation between stress and strain, Hooke's law and the law describing shear deformation (see Chapter 6)

$$\sigma = E \cdot \varepsilon$$
$$\tau = G \cdot \alpha$$

have to be generalized. In this generalized law the modulus of elasticity E and the shear modulus G are replaced by a term c, known as the 'stiffness matrix'. In the general case, this term depends on 21 material constants. (We are dealing here with a symmetric 6 x 6 tensor with 21 independent elements.) The stress σ is replaced by a mathematical expression (a vector with six components) which depends on the three normal and the three shear stresses. The strain ε is replaced by a mathematical expression (vector with 6 components) which depends on the linear strains in the three spatial directions and on three angular deformations. In this formulation, the generalized Hooke's law (Currey, 1984; Katz and Meunier, 1987; Sommerfeld, 1992) is written as

$$\sigma_i = \sum c_{ij} \cdot \varepsilon_j$$

The index i assumes values from 1 to 6. The mathematical sum sign Σ indicates that, to calculate the i-th component σ_i of the stress vector, all products $c_{ij} \cdot \varepsilon_j$ have to be added together. The index j runs from j = 1 to j = 6. Thus, in contrast to the case of isotropic materials, the stress in a certain spatial direction will depend on the strain and the angular deformation in all three spatial directions. Conversely, a normal stress effects not only a deformation in the direction of the stress but also an angular deformation. This was the very case in the example shown in Fig. 14.**2**.

In the technical domain the generalized Hooke's law forms the basis for a description of the mechanical properties of fiber-reinforced materials. But even in such applications, it proves difficult to determine the complete set of 21 material con-

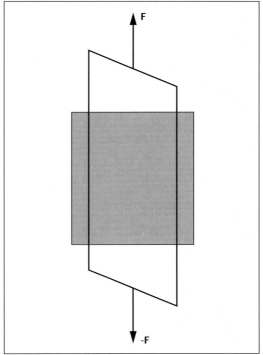

Fig. 14.2   An anisotropic material loaded by a force (in this case illustrated by a tensile force) exhibits not only a change in length in the direction of the force but also an angular deformation.

stants experimentally. When dealing with bone material, additional difficulties arise. Due to changes in bone density and architecture, the mechanical properties of bone change from one volume element to the next. In addition, bone is non-linearly elastic, i.e. the material properties depend on the magnitude of the applied strain and on the deformation velocity. In technical materials there is no equivalent to the repair and adaptation processes *in vivo*, as encountered in bone.

These comments are aimed at making it clear that, other than for those situations where a crude, approximate description of the mechanical behavior of bone will suffice, a detailed description has to be based on intricate theory and on experimental determination of a large set of material constants. For this reason, lines of reasoning are often complex and may fail to come across vividly. However, a detailed description is indispensable if, for example, the relation between mechanical stimuli and bone adaptation is to be investigated. To this end, the state of stress and deformation under the application of external forces and moments must be known as accurately as possible. Estimates based on the properties of a homogeneous, isotropic material are insufficient.

Material properties of cortical bone

When, in the following, the mechanical properties of bone are characterized by only few material constants, it must be kept in mind that this constitutes a crude approximation to reality. Table 14.1 gives an overview of the properties of human cortical bone. The numbers quoted are only approximate. The ranges of variation are due, in part, to the biological variation of the individual bones investigated and, in some cases, to varying examination methods. The stress σ_u, which effects the destruction of a sample, is called the 'ultimate' (or 'maximal') stress.

The anisotropy of bone material becomes apparent when samples cut in different directions from the cortical layer of a long bone are compared. As an illustration, Table 14.2 quotes measured results for the modulus of elasticity and the ultimate stress for samples cut in longitudinal and transverse direction with respect to the long axis of a bone.

Bone material is viscoelastic; the values of the material constants depend on the deformation velocity (i.e. whether deformation occurs over a short or long time interval). As an example, Fig. 14.3 shows the relation between the modulus of elasticity E and of the ultimate stress σ_u on the deformation velocity. The observed increase of E and σ_u with increasing deformation velocity indicates that the material is becoming 'harder' and 'stronger'.

Table 14.1 Material properties of human cortical bone (from Reilly and Burstein, 1974)

Modulus of elasticity E	$6 \dots 25 \cdot 10^9$ N/m^2
Poisson's ratio μ	$0.08 \dots 0.45$
Shear modulus G	$0.31 \cdot 10^9$ N/m^2
Ultimate stress in tension	$87 \dots 151 \cdot 10^6$ N/m^2
Ultimate stress in compression	$106 \dots 193 \cdot 10^6$ N/m^2
Ultimate stress in shear	$53 \dots 82 \cdot 10^6$ N/m^2

Table 14.2 Orientation-dependence of the material properties of human cortical bone (from Reilly and Burstein, 1975)

Modulus of elasticity, sample oriented in longitudinal direction	$17.0 \cdot 10^9$ N/m^2
Modulus of elasticity, sample oriented in transverse direction	$11.5 \cdot 10^9$ N/m^2
Ultimate tensile stress, sample oriented in longitudinal direction	$133 \cdot 10^6$ N/m^2
Ultimate tensile stress, sample oriented in transverse direction	$51 \cdot 10^6$ N/m^2
Ultimate compressive stress, sample oriented in longitudinal direction	$193 \cdot 10^6$ N/m^2
Ultimate compressive stress, sample oriented in transverse direction	$133 \cdot 10^6$ N/m^2

Like many other materials, cortical bone exhibits mechanical fatigue under repeated loading. The stress at which fracture of a sample is observed decreases with increasing numbers of load cycles.

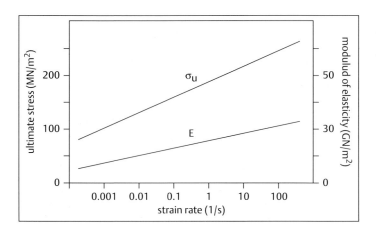

Fig. 14.3 Modulus of elasticity E and ultimate stress σ_u of cortical bone related to strain rate (adapted from Wright and Hayes, 1976)

Fig. 14.**4** Fatigue properties of human cortical bone in relation to the magnitude of the strain. In addition, regions of strain of the bones of the lower extremity expected to occur during strenuous exercises, running, or walking are shown (adapted from Carter *et al.*, 1981b)

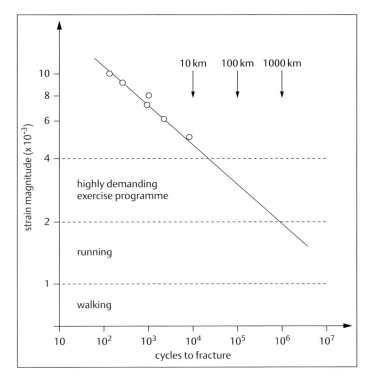

Carter *et al.* (1981a, 1981b) and Carter and Caler (1983) reported that material fatigue depended predominantly on the magnitude of the strain, with bone density or ash content having only little influence on fatigue strength. According to these authors, the ultimate stress after 10^7 load cycles is in the region of $7 \cdot 10^6$ N/m^2. This is considerably lower than the ultimate stress under a single load cycle as quoted in Table 14.**1**.

Fig. 14.**4** shows the number of cycles to fracture in dependence on the magnitude of the strain as measured by Carter *et al.* (1981). To check how high the risk of a fatigue fracture is when walking, running, or performing strenuous athletic exercises, estimated regions of the strain in the lower extremity are also shown in this diagram. It is concluded that fatigue fractures are not to be expected when walking. When running over long distances, occurrence of fatigue fractures is possible, especially if an individual running style with high repetitive loading coincides with low individual bone strength. Indeed, fractures of the lower extremity, occasionally observed in young soldiers after running long distances or marching with heavy field packs, are interpreted as fatigue fractures.

The mechanical properties of cortical bone change with age (Kiebzak, 1991). These changes are assumed to be caused by structural changes in the organic and inorganic bone components. According to Burstein *et al.* (1976), the modulus of elasticity, the ultimate stress, and the ultimate strain decrease with age. In other words, bone becomes softer and more brittle with increasing age. In the material investigated by Burstein and colleagues no gender-related difference in the mechanical properties was noted. For unknown reasons, age-related changes in cortical bone samples from the femur were more pronounced than in samples from the tibia.

Architecture and material properties of trabecular bone

Trabecular bone is composed of a three-dimensional mesh of interconnected bone beams and plates, arranged similarly to that of open-pore technical foam materials. With the exception of woven bone, the beams and plates are oriented in

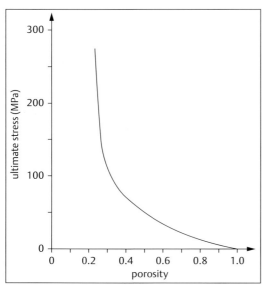

Fig. 14.5 Ultimate compressive stress of human bone in relation to porosity (adapted from Martin and Burr, 1989)

$$E = 15 \cdot (1 - p)^3 \ [\text{GPa}]$$

This formula tells us that, with increasing porosity p (with increasing void space in the sample), the modulus of elasticity E exhibits a marked decrease. Quantitatively, the modulus of elasticity of trabecular bone ranges between 1.4 and 9800 MPa (Goldstein, 1987).

Fig. 14.5 shows the ultimate stress of samples of trabecular bone in dependence on porosity. The ultimate stress is seen to decrease substantially with increasing porosity. With increasing porosity (or decreasing apparent density) trabecular bone becomes 'softer' and 'weaker'. The ultimate stress observed in samples of trabecular bone covers the entire stress range depicted in Fig. 14.5. Depending on the type of bone and the source of the samples, published data range between 0.2 MPa and 378 MPa (Goldstein, 1987). The maximum strain of trabecular bone is about 4 % (Ford and Keaveny, 1996). The ultimate strain is independent of the porosity and the apparent density. Samples of trabecular bone are usually not irreparably damaged by one single overload episode, but subsequently still exhibit some strength, though at a reduced level (see, for example, Keaveny et al., 1999). The residual strength of mechanically damaged bones, e.g. of fractured osteoporotic vertebrae, constitutes a vital safety factor for the functioning of the locomotor system.

When a sample of trabecular bone is viewed with the naked eye, the alignment of the trabeculae in preferred directions is obvious beyond any doubt. In the past, to describe the intuitively observed anisotropy in quantitative, mathematical terms posed considerable difficulties. The remarkable progress made in recent years, however, allows the spatial anisotropy of the mesh to be described in numerical terms and these data to be linked with the anisotropy of the mechanical properties. Parameters describing the local anisotropy ('fabric') of the spatial mesh can be defined. In parallel, the deformation of such meshes under the influence of external forces can be computed using the finite elements method (FEM) or, alternatively, can be measured directly. The comparison of calculated and measured results reveals how well a specific anisotropy parameter actually describes the mechanical properties of a sample of trabecular bone (Odgaard, 1997; Odgaard et al., 1997, Cowin, 1997).

Fig. 14.6 illustrates three proposals for a quantitative description of the local anisotropy of trabecular bone (Odgaard et al., 1997). Fig. 14.6 illustrates these proposals using a two-dimensional model; the concepts are, however, applied in three dimensions. The sample of trabecular bone shown appears intuitively to be preferentially oriented in a

preferred directions that are readily discernible to the naked eye on bone sections. Below the cartilaginous layer of joints, for example, the trabeculae are preferentially oriented perpendicular to the joint surface. There appears to be a second preferred direction, oriented at approximately 90° to the first, where the beams and plates are interconnected, thus reinforcing the mesh. It is understandable from these observations that the elastic properties and the strength of trabecular bone are determined by the density, the distance, and the relative orientation and interconnection of the beams and plates. It follows furthermore that measured material properties of trabecular bone depend on the direction of testing. Trabecular bone is an anisotropic material (Keaveny and Hayes, 1993).

If the material properties of cortical bone, and those of the beams and plates of trabecular bone, are assumed to be approximately equal, the material properties of samples of cortical and trabecular bone (save for anisotropic effects) can be expected to vary in relation to the degree of porosity. The term 'porosity' designates that fraction of the volume of a sample that is not filled by bone material. The porosity of a sample of cortical bone with no voids would be zero; the porosity of trabecular bone can approach (though not reach) the value 1.

The modulus of elasticity of trabecular bone with porosity p can be approximated (Martin, 1991) by

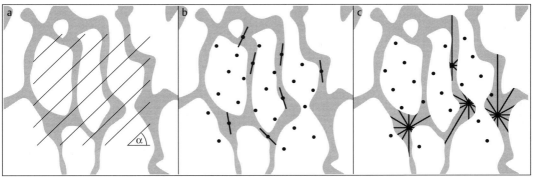

Fig. 14.**6a**   Illustration of the parameter 'mean intercept length' used to describe the spatial anisotropy of trabecular bone (adapted from Odgaard *et al.*, 1997)

Fig. 14.**6b**   Illustration of the parameter 'volume orientation' used to describe the spatial anisotropy of trabecular bone (adapted from Odgaard *et al.*, 1997)

Fig. 14.**6c**   Illustration of the parameter 'star volume distribution' used to describe the spatial anisotropy of trabecular bone (adapted from Odgaard *et al.*, 1997)

vertical direction. An attempt can be made to describe the preferred direction by superimposing a line grid in different orientations (Fig. 14.**6a**) and observing the lengths of the grid lines ('intercept length') intersecting the trabeculae. In the example shown, we expect long intercept lengths when the grid is oriented vertically and short lengths when the grid is oriented horizontally.

Alternatively (Fig. 14.**6b**), points can be selected at random within the bone volume and the direction in which straight lines through these points exhibit the longest intercept with the bone volume ('volume orientation') is observed. In the example shown, these directions would preferentially point to the vertical; a second preferred direction would point approximately to the horizontal. As a further alternative (Fig. 14.**6c**), the orientation of local bone volume elements can be quantified if points are again selected at random within the bone volume and the distance of the bone surface as seen from these points in different directions is recorded (described as 'star length' and 'star volume'). In addition to orientation, these parameters also quantify the interconnection of the beams and plates in the trabecular bone.

The spatial resolution of computed tomography (CT) performed *in vivo* on humans is at present not fine enough to image single beams and plates of trabecular bone. For this reason, the procedures for quantifying anisotropy are, as yet, confined to investigations *in vitro*. If the manufacturers of CT apparatus succeed in the future in increasing the spatial resolution, so that the architecture of trabecular bone can be imaged *in vivo*, interesting and important new insights into the adaptation

and remodeling processes of bone can be expected.

Measurement of bone density and bone mineral content *in vivo*

The strength of bones under compression, bending, or torsion is determined by the shape and thickness of the cortical bone, and by the density and architecture of the trabecular bone. Up to now, parameters describing the trabecular architecture in quantitative terms could not be determined in vivo. Estimation of the fracture risk in individual cases, and monitoring of the success of therapeutic interventions aimed at improving the strength of bones, must, therefore, rely on measurements of the bone geometry, the bone density, or the bone mineral content. To this end, measurement of the bone mineral density from the absorption of γ or roentgen radiation, and density measurement by computed tomography, can be employed.

Absorption of γ or roentgen radiation (SPA, DPA, DEXA). When passing through matter, the intensity of γ or roentgen (X-) radiation is attenuated. For radiation of a given energy it holds that

$$I = I_0 \cdot e^{-\mu \cdot x}$$

In this formula I_0 and I denote the intensity of the incoming and outgoing beam; e = 2.718... is the Euler number; x is the thickness of the layer of matter; μ is the coefficient of absorption of the material. μ depends on the atomic number (ordinal number in the periodic system of elements) of the irradiated element (or the atomic numbers of all elements contained in a mixed sample), on the density of the matter, and on the energy of the radiation.

If the coefficient of absorption μ of the mineral component of bone is known, and if the intensities of the incoming and outgoing beams are measured, the thickness x of the mineral layer can be determined. This is the basis of single photon absorptiometry (SPA). If, in addition to bone mineral, soft tissue is located in the path of the radiation, an error occurs when using the above formula, because the soft tissue also contributes to the absorption of the radiation (though to a much lesser extent than the mineral component). This systematic error can be corrected by measuring the absorption in a layer of water of equal thickness, in addition to the object of interest, composed of bone and soft tissue. The water is used here as substitute for soft tissue and the thickness of the mineral layer is determined from the difference between the two measurements.

Alternatively, the object can be irradiated with radiation of two different energies. With a mixture of two materials in the path of the radiation, the attenuation of the rays is given by

$$I = I_0 \cdot e^{-\mu_1 \cdot x_1 - \mu_2 \cdot x_2}$$

with μ_1 and μ_2 as coefficients of absorption and x_1 and x_2 as thicknesses of the layers of both materials. The fact that the coefficients of absorption are energy-dependent is utilized to determine the thickness of both layers if the absorption is measured at two different energies of radiation. Performing measurements at the energies A and B of the radiation provides two equations

$$I_A = I_{0A} \cdot e^{-\mu_{1A} \cdot x_1 - \mu_{2A} \cdot x_2}$$
$$I_B = I_{0B} \cdot e^{-\mu_{1B} \cdot x_1 - \mu_{2B} \cdot x_2}$$

from which, with knowledge of the energy-dependent absorption coefficients μ_{1A}, μ_{2A}, μ_{1B}, and μ_{2B}, the thickness x_1 and x_2 of the layers can be determined. The source of radiation utilized comprises either two radioactive elements (dual photon absorptiometry, DPA) or X-ray tubes driven by two different voltages (dual energy X-ray absorptiometry, DEXA). If X-ray tubes are employed, it has to be noted that they do not emit radiation of a fixed energy but an energy spectrum with a fixed maximum energy, determined by the input voltage. The determination of the thickness of the two layers then relies on formulae similar to those quoted above.

As an irradiating beam (irrespective of whether it originates from radioactive sources or X-ray tubes) is never concentrated on one point, but is always extended over a certain area, an absorption measurement does not record the thickness of a layer but rather the area density of materials. The area density of bone mineral is designated as 'bone mineral density' (BMD) and is given in units of g/cm². It designates the amount of mineral (in grams) per square centimeter as seen from the direction of the radiation source. When measuring the mineral density of the lumbar spine, the BMD is occasionally also quoted in units of g/cm. Such data designate the amount of bone mineral (in grams) per centimeter, for example of the lumbar spine measured in a craniocaudal direction. The bone mineral content (BMC) designates the mineral content of a whole organ, for example, a vertebra. The mineral content is given in units of grams (g). Some authors determine the mineral content of an organ by an absorption method and the volume of the organ by an additional measurement. As a result, a bone mineral density (volumetric density) in units of g/cm³ is obtained. If the bone mineral is measured by SPA, DPA, or DEXA, all bone mineral in the path of the beam is registered. These methods cannot discriminate which fraction of the bone mineral is located in the cortical and the trabecular bone of an organ under investigation. (N.B.: The designations BMD for line, area, or volumetric density, and BMC for total content are, unfortunately, not used in a standardized fashion in the scientific literature.)

Quantitative computed tomography (QCT). Based on the absorption data of an object irradiated by X-rays in a number of different directions, computed tomography calculates a three-dimensional model of the density distribution of the object under investigation. When applied to the human body, volume elements exhibiting large differences with respect to absorption of X-rays, i. e. bone, soft tissue, void spaces, and surrounding air, are dealt with. For this reason the density calculated in each volume element is not quoted in absolute units but in Hounsfield units, H

$$H = 1000 \cdot ((\rho / \rho_w) - 1.0)$$

In this formula ρ designates the computed density of the material and ρ_w the density of water. According to this formula a volume filled with water has zero density in Hounsfield units. A volume filled with fat has negative values in Hounsfield units, because the density ρ of fat is lower than that of water. A volume filled with bone has positive values in Hounsfield units, because the density ρ of bone is higher than that of water.

To convert density values given in Hounsfield units into density values of bone mineral, calibration objects are measured together with the bones or body segments under investigation. Following a proposal by Genant *et al.* (1985), differently concentrated solutions of K_2HPO_4 in water are used for this purpose. The absorption of X-rays by K_2HPO_4 is very similar to the absorption by the mineral component of bone. The measured Hounsfield units of a calibration object are employed to convert the density of the object into an equivalent density of K_2HPO_4 in units of mg/cm^3. This protocol is designated as 'quantitative computed tomography' (QCT). Whereas density values in Hounsfield units measured on different X-ray units are not directly comparable due to inadvertent or uncontrolled shifts in machine calibration or changes in tube voltage, density data given in units of mg/cm^3 K_2HPO_4 are independent of the apparatus and thus permit direct comparisons. As QCT determines real density data and not only area or line densities, it is possible – unlike with SPA, DPA or DEXA – to obtain data separately for partial volumes filled with cortical or trabecular bone.

If the tomograph employs one fixed tube voltage, the density of only one material can be determined in each volume element. If more than one material is present, for example bone and fat, a systematic error occurs. Repetition of the measurement with a different X-ray energy (double energy quantitative computed tomography, DQCT) would allow two materials to be discriminated, as with DPA and DEXA. This procedure, however, has not been adopted for routine clinical application, due to the increased radiation exposure and the comparatively small diagnostic benefit. For a comparison of the precision and reproducibility of QCT, DPA, and DEXA when determining bone density and bone mineral density, the reader is referred to Mazess (1990).

Determination of the fracture risk of proximal femur and lumbar vertebrae *in vivo*

Before attempting to determine *in vivo* the risk of fracture of a bone, the extent to which the strength depends on the geometrical dimensions (e. g. diameter, cross-sectional area, wall thickness) and the densities of the cortical and trabecular bone must be investigated *in vitro*. When these parameters are subsequently determined *in vivo*, high-risk subjects, in whom the strength of certain bones is unduly decreased, can be identified.

One issue, independent of the determination of a fracture risk, is to find out which of the aforementioned parameters can be influenced by therapeu-

tic measures, with the aim of improving bone strength. As the outer dimensions of bones seem to undergo virtually no change after maturation of the skeleton (i. e. after the age of 16–18 years), an attempt can only be made to exert a positive influence on the bone density or on the bone mineral content according to the state of the art. In other words, monitoring the bone or mineral density offers an adequate control of therapeutic outcome. For determination of the fracture risk, density measurements alone do not suffice because the outer dimensions of the bones have to be taken into account as well.

Due to the serious clinical problems associated with fractures of the proximal femur and lumbar vertebrae, past attempts to predict fracture risk concentrated on these two bones. Lotz and Hayes (1990) investigated the relation between the density of the trabecular bone in the region of the junction of femoral neck and femur by QCT and the strength of the bone. The experimental setup was designed to simulate a fall on to the side. The authors considered this type of fall to be the primary cause of fractures of the proximal femur occurring in the elderly. Fig. 14.**7** shows the relation between the bone density and the strength of the specimens investigated, together with the regression line describing the mean, statistical relation between these parameters. The graph shown in Fig. 14.**7** permits the individual fracture risk to be estimat-

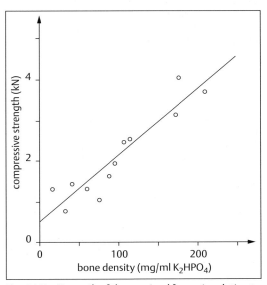

Fig. 14.**7**   Strength of the proximal femur in relation to bone density (adapted from Hayes *et al.*, 1991)

ed (Hayes *et al.*, 1991). A close relationship between fracture load of the proximal femur *in vitro* and its ash content or bone mineral content has also been demonstrated (Lochmüller *et al.*, 2000) in a loading mode simulating loading in erect stance.

In order not to misjudge the experimental results quoted above, it has to be pointed out that the time sequence and the type of fall causing fracture of the proximal femur are currently subjects of controversial discussion. Some authors (see above) postulate that the bone is fractured through the force exerted when falling sideways and hitting the floor. Others propose that a fall occurs because the bone was fractured. Depending on which mechanism is relevant, i. e. spontaneous fracture due to loading of the femur approximately in the direction of its long axis, or traumatic fracture with the force essentially directed laterally, the strength is definitely determined by different architectural parameters (Keyak, 2000). An experimental setup aimed at simulating fractures of the proximal femur must be designed to comply with the investigator's hypothesis on the fracture mechanism. (Things would be much easier, and suggestions for prevention could be given, if detailed observations of subjects at the very moment of fracture were available. For obvious reasons, such data do not exist.)

Prompted by the high incidence of vertebral fractures in subjects with osteoporosis, attempts were made in a number of laboratories to predict the strength of vertebral bodies in vivo from measurements of the bone mineral density, or the density of vertebral, trabecular bone. Two examples of such work, that of Hansson *et al.* (1980) and that of Brinckmann *et al.* (1989) are given below. Hansson *et al.* (1980) measured the compressive strength of lumbar vertebrae in relation to the bone mineral density, determined by DPA in units of g/cm. The results of the experiments showed that strength and bone mineral density were positively, linearly correlated. With a known mineral density, the data permit compressive strength to be predicted with an error (standard error of estimate, SE) of 0.89 kN.

Brinckmann *et al.* (1989) measured the compressive strength of lumbar vertebrae in relation to the density of the trabecular bone in the central volume of the vertebral bodies, measured by QCT in units of mg/cm^3 K$_2$HPO$_4$, and the endplate area, measured by CT in units of cm^2. The results of this investigation show (see also Chapter 11) that the compressive strength is proportional to the product of bone density and endplate area. In other words, the compressive strength increases with increasing bone density, as well as with increasing dimensions of the vertebral body. Based on measured data of the density and the endplate area, the compressive strength can be predicted with an error of 1 kN.

It may be surprising on first sight that the compressive strength seems to depend, with virtually equal accuracy, on the bone mineral density on the one hand, and on the product of trabecular bone density and endplate area on the other. This apparent discrepancy can be resolved by considering the units (dimensions) of the input data. Bone mineral density was measured by Hansson *et al.* in units of g/cm; thus the width of the vertebral body is taken into account. Using DPA (or any other method relying on the attenuation of a γ- or X-ray beams), the depth of the bone investigated, *per se*, enters into the result. The product of bone density and area measured by QCT has a dimension identical to the bone mineral density measured by Hansson and colleagues, i. e. g/cm$^3 \cdot$ cm^2 = g/cm. The real difference between the two procedures is that DPA includes contributions from the cortical bone while QCT considers only the density of the trabecular bone. The finding that both procedures allow compressive strength to be predicted with approximately equal accuracy supports the assumption that, in vertebral bodies, the density of the trabecular bone and the amount of cortical bone in the outer shell are proportionally related to each other. For a comparison of strength prediction based on QCT with that based on DEXA or ash content data, see, for example, Ebbesen *et al.* (1999).

Both in fractures of the femoral neck and in compression fractures of lumbar vertebrae, the scatter of the measured data with respect to the regression lines indicates that strength depends on parameters in addition to bone density and size, though to a lesser extent. A number of different factors may be responsible for the unexplained portion of the variation of the measured data. It is possible that experimental methods *in vitro* producing femoral or vertebral fracture provide inadequate simulation of the fracture event *in vivo*. The material properties of bones might have inter-individual differences not detected by a density measurement. Differences in the individual architecture of trabecular and cortical bone certainly influence compressive strength. However, attempts to improve the accuracy of strength prediction by taking account of architectural parameters determined *in vivo* have been unsuccessful. It is quite possible that the relevant parameter has not been identified or that, up to now, such a parameter could not be measured with sufficient accuracy. Alternatively, it is possible that architectural parameters are closely correlated with bone density. In this case, a prediction based on density as well as on parameter data would be expected to improve the accuracy of the compressive strength only marginally (see, for example, McCalden *et al.*, 1997).

Adaptation of bones to mechanical demands

Long before the cellular basis for bone adaptation and remodeling had been discovered, it was conjectured that bones are not unchangeable structures, but can adapt to their mechanical demands in the human locomotor system. Meyer (1867) demonstrated surprising similarities between the alignment of trabeculae in the vicinity of joints and the latticework of iron bridges. Wolff (1892) hypothesized that trabecular bone represented a latticework reaching maximum strength while employing a minimum of bone material. In the interim, the work of Meyer and of Wolff has proved to be extremely stimulating and inspiring to researchers. For a historical overview the reader is referred to Roesler (1987).

When discussing the adaptation of bones to their mechanical demands, 'Wolff's law of the transformation of bones' is frequently cited. It has to be pointed out that we are not dealing here with a law in terms of physics, e. g. Kepler's law governing the motion of the planets. No specific conclusions can be drawn from Wolff's law. The frequent reference to 'Wolff's law' in the scientific literature is a somewhat meaningless phrase. What is really meant is the hypothesis that a change in mechanical demands induces changes in bone structure or, conversely, that an observed change in bone structure permits conclusions to be drawn on changed mechanical demands. Incidentally, with respect to adaptation to mechanical demands, bones are not an exception. Muscles, tendons, skin, and all other tissues of the body exhibit such adaptation as well.

Specific conclusions derived from Wolff's law by some authors, e. g. 'the architecture of bones can be deduced exclusively from basic mechanical principles', or 'the trabeculae of trabecular bone are aligned in the direction of the principal stresses (directions where only compressive or tensile stresses exist)', have proved to be incorrect. In addition, our present knowledge suggests that adaptation and remodeling processes of bone are often masked by other processes. If, for example, the adaptation of proximal femur and vertebral body to their mechanical demands at increasing age were the number one priority, it might be concluded from Wolff's law (naively viewed) that more new bone is deposited than old bone removed. This is, unfortunately, not the case in reality. However, the fact that some aspects of bone mechanics are nowa-

days, more than one hundred years after the pioneering conjectures of Meyer and Wolff, viewed differently should not diminish our admiration for the remarkable powers of observation displayed by these ingenious researchers.

From the great number of observations relating to the response of bone to mechanical demands, two representative examples are discussed below. Further examples are described in Appendix A3. Fig. 14.**8** shows the result of an experiment designed to observe the change in cross-sectional area of the cortical bone of the turkey ulna in relation to the strain applied. At a strain of approximately 0.001 mm/mm no change was observed. At lower strains, the cross-sectional area decreased, at higher strains it increased through apposition of new bone. Experiments of this type are aimed at determining which mechanical stimuli are adequate to trigger the adaptation of bone.

Fig. 14.**9** shows the change in alignment of trabeculae in the human femoral neck before and 10 years after execution of a varization osteotomy as documented by Pauwels (1973). In a varization osteotomy a medially opened wedge of bone is removed from the intertrochanteric region. This decreases the angle between the neck and the femoral shaft. In addition to decreasing the load on the

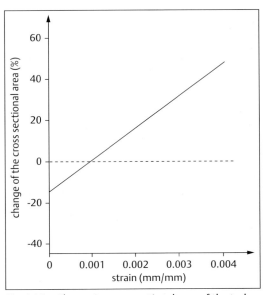

Fig. 14.**8** Change in cross-sectional area of the turkey ulna in relation to the peak value of the strain exerted experimentally *in vivo* (adapted from Rubin and Lanyon, 1985)

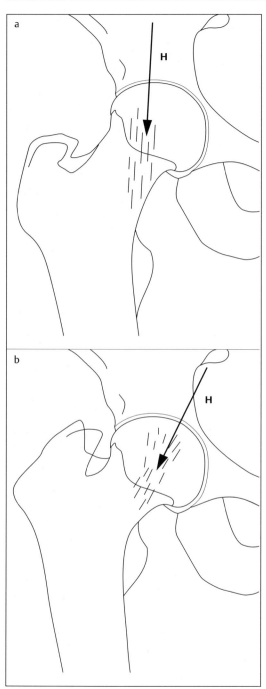

Fig. 14.9 Orientation of the trabeculae in the femoral neck (**a**) before and (**b**) 10 years after execution of a varization osteotomy (adapted from Pauwels, 1973)

hip joint, this surgical intervention also changes the direction of the load vector **H**. Postoperatively this vector is more inclined to the vertical than it was preoperatively. Pauwels documented that a change in the direction of loading effected a change in the alignment of the trabeculae in the long term.

While it is agreed that the functional adaptation of bones is triggered and controlled by mechanical stimuli, there is disagreement on which specific mechanical signal, or combination of signals, actually induces the cell system of osteoclasts, osteoblasts, and osteocytes to either resorb or produce bone at specific sites in cortical or trabecular bone. This is an intricate problem, because the complex mechanical properties of bone material make it very difficult to determine the local stress and strain even under simple loading conditions. Mechanical stimuli currently under discussion that might control the adaptation of bones are magnitude of the deformation, frequency of the deformation, difference in deformation in adjacent volumina (deformation gradients), deformation rate, sum of the deformations encountered in the past (deformation history) and density of the deformation energy (Cowin, 1993; Rubin *et al.*, 1996). Processes accompanying deformation of bones are pressure changes and flux of the water contained in the bone material or piezoelectric voltages originating from the deformation of the crystalline component of bone. The problem is in deciding whether certain signals (e.g. piezoelectric signals) are merely a by-product of the mechanical influences on bone, or whether such signals have an important role in transmitting the mechanical information to the cell system.

Furthermore, the role of microfractures of the trabecular bone in the adaptation process is debated controversially. Such microfractures are frequently seen in the trabecular bone in the region of the hip joint and in vertebral bodies (Vernon-Roberts and Pirie, 1973; Kitahara, 1980; Ohtani and Azuma, 1984; Burr *et al.*, 1997). Such fractures can be regarded as pathologic because they indicate insufficient strength in relation to the mechanical loading. On the other hand it is quite feasible that these fractures occur in the course of a physiologic process in which old, brittle bone is removed and replaced with newly formed, better adapted bone. It is hypothesized that the fracture callus in the trabecular mesh might also enable growth of new trabeculae, bridging between formerly separated trabeculae (Delling *et al.*, 1997). A better understanding in the future of how signals are transmitted to osteoclasts and osteoblasts, and of how remodeling and adaptation depend on factors like local circulation and hormonal influences, would certainly pave the way for substantial therapeutic progress.

Further reading

Textbooks and review papers

Currey JD. *The mechanical adaptations of bones.* Princeton: Princeton University Press; 1984

Currey JD. The design of mineralised hard tissues for their mechanical functions. *J Exp Biology.* 1999; **202**: 3285–3294

Huiskes R. If bone is the answer, then what was the question? *J Anat.* 2000; **197**: 145–156

Keaveny TM, Hayes WC. A 20-year perspective on the mechanical properties of trabecular bone. *J Biomechanical Engng.* 1993; **115**: 534–542 [review paper, 108 references]

Kiebzak GM. Age-related bone changes. *Experimental Gerontology.* 1991; **26**: 171–187 [review paper, 100 references]

Kummer BKF. Biomechanics of bone: mechanical properties, functional structure, functional adaptation. In: Fung *et al.* (eds). *Biomechanics: Its foundations and objectives.* Englewood Cliffs: Prentice Hall; 1972, 237–271

Martin RB, Burr DB. *Structure, function and adaptation of compact bone.* New York: Raven Press; 1989

Martin RB. Determinants of the mechanical properties of bones. *J Biomechanics.* 1991; **24** Suppl 1: 79–88 [review paper, 67 references]

Martin RB, Burr DB, Sharkey NA. *Skeletal tissue mechanics.* New York: Springer; 1998

Odgaard A, Three-dimensional methods for quantification of cancellous bone architecture. *Bone.* 1997; **20**: 315–328 [review paper, 189 references]

Sommerfeld A. *Mechanik der deformierbaren Medien.* Fues E, Kröner E (eds). Reprint of the 6th ed. Thun: Deutsch; 1992

Tillmann B. Binde- und Stützgewebe des Bewegungsapparates. In: Tillmann B, Töndury G (eds). *Rauber Kopsch. Anatomie des Menschen.* Band 1. 2nd ed. Stuttgart: Thieme; 1998a

Tillmann B. Skelettsystem. In: Tillmann B, Töndury G (eds). *Rauber Kopsch. Anatomie des Menschen.* Band 1. 2nd ed. Stuttgart: Thieme; 1998b

Scientific papers, cited in the text or legends

Brinckmann P, Biggemann M, Hilweg D. Prediction of the compressive strength of human lumbar vertebrae. *Clin Biomechanics.* 1989; **4** Suppl 2: S1–S27

Burr DB, Forwood MR, Fyhrie DP, Martin RB, Schaffler MB, Turner CH. Bone microdamage and skeletal fragility in osteoporotic and stress fractures. *J Bone Min Res.* 1997; **12**: 6–15

Burstein AH, Reilly DT, Martens M. Aging of bone tissue: mechanical properties. *J Bone Jt Surg.* 1976; **58 A**: 82–86

Carter DR, Caler WE, Spengler DM, Frankel VH. Uniaxial fatigue of human cortical bone. The influence of tissue physical characteristics. *J Biomechanics.* 1981a; **14**: 461–470

Carter DR, Caler WE, Spengler DM, Frankel VH. Fatigue behavior of adult cortical bone: The influence of mean strain and strain range. *Acta Orthop Scand.* 1981b; **52**: 481–490

Carter DR, Caler WE. Cycle-dependent and time-dependent bone fracture with repeated loading. *J Biomech Engng.* 1983; **105**: 166–170

Cowin SC. Bone stress adaptation models. *J Biomech Engng.* 1993; **115**: 528–533

Cowin SC. Remarks on the paper entitled 'fabric and elastic principal directions of cancellous bone are closely related'. *J Biomechanics.* 1997; **30**: 1191–1192

Currey JD. Three analogies to explain the mechanical properties of bone. *Biorheology.* 1964; **2**: 1–10

Delling G, Vogel M, Hahn M. Neue Vorstellungen zu Bau und Funktion der menschlichen Spongiosa – Ist die Theorie von der Imbalance zwischen Osteoklasten und Osteoblasten noch haltbar? In: Schneider E (ed). *Hefte zu Der Unfallchirurg.* Berlin: Springer; 1997, 173–184

Ebbesen EN, Thomsen JS, Beck-Nielsen H, Nepper-Rasmussen HJ, Mosekilde L. Lumbar vertebral body compressive strength evaluated by dual energy x-ray absorptiometry, quantitative computed tomography and ashing. *Bone.* 1999; **25**: 713–724

Ford CM, Keaveny TM. The dependence of shear failure properties of trabecular bone on apparent density and trabecular orientation. *J Biomechanics.* 1996; **29**: 1309–1317

Genant HK, Ettinger B, Cann CE, Reiser U, Gordan GS, Kolb FO. Osteoporosis: assessment by quantitative computed tomography. *Orthop Clin North Am* 1985; 16: 557–568

Goldstein SA. The mechanical properties of trabecular bone: dependence on anatomic location and function. *J Biomechanics.* 1987; **20**: 1055–1061

Hansson T, Roos B, Nachemson A. The bone mineral content and ultimate compressive strength of lumbar vertebrae. *Spine.* 1980; **5**: 46–55

Hayes WC, Piazza SJ, Zysset PK. Biomechanics of fracture risk prediction of the hip and spine by quantitative computed tomography. *Radiol Clin North Am.* 1991; **29**: 1–18

Katz JL, Meunier A. The elastic anisotropy of bone. *J Biomechanics.* 1987; **20**: 1063–1070

Keaveny TM, Wachtel EF, Kopperdahl DL. Mechanical behavior of human trabecular bone after overloading. *J Orthop Res.* 1999; **17**: 346–353

Keyak JH. Relationships between femoral fracture loads for two load configurations. *J Biomechanics.* 2000; **33**: 499–502

Kitahara H. Morphological observations on trabecular microfractures in the lumbar vertebrae. *J Jpn Orthop Ass.* 1980; **54**: 449–460

Lochmüller EM, Miller P, Bürklein D, Wehr U, Rambeck W, Eckstein F. In situ femoral dual energy x-ray absorptiometry related to ash weight, bone size and density, and its relationship with mechanical failure loads of the proximal femur. *Osteoporosis Int.* 2000; **11**: 361–367

Lotz JC, Hayes WC. The use of quantitative computed tomography to estimate risk of fracture of the hip from falls. *J Bone Surg Am.* 1990; **72A**: 689–700

Mazess RB. Bone densitometry of the axial skeleton. *Orthop Clin North Am.* 1990; **21**: 51–63

McCalden RW, McGeough JA, Court-Brown CM. Age-related changes in the compressive strength of cancellous bone. *J Bone Jt Surg.* 1997; **79 A**: 421–427

Meyer H. Die Architektur der Spongiosa. *Arch Anat Physiol wiss Med.* 1867; **34**: 615–628

Odgaard A, Kabel J, van Rietbergen B, Dalstra M, Huiskes R. Fabric and elastic principal directions of cancellous bone are closely related. *J Biomechanics.* 1997; **30**: 487–495

Ohtani T, Azuma H. Trabecular microfractures in the acetabulum. *Acta Orthop Scand.* 1984; **55**: 419–422

Pauwels F. *Atlas zur Biomechanik der gesunden und kranken Hüfte.* Berlin: Springer; 1973, Fig. 219, p. 181

Reilly DT, Burstein AH. The mechanical properties of cortical bone. *J Bone Jt Surg.* 1974; **56A**: 1001–1022

Reilly DT, Burstein AH. The elastic and ultimate properties of compact bone tissue. *J Biomechanics.* 1975; **8**: 393–405

Roesler H. The history of some fundamental concepts in bone biomechanics. *J Biomechanics.* 1987; **20**: 1025–1034

Rubin CT, Lanyon LE. Regulation of bone mass by mechanical strain magnitude. *Calcif Tissue Int.* 1985; **37**: 411–417

Rubin C, Gross T, Qin YX, Fritton S, Guilak F, McLeod K. Differentiation of the bone-tissue remodeling response to axial and torsional loading in the turkey ulna. *J Bone Jt Surg.* 1996; **78A**; 1523–1533

Vernon-Roberts B, Pirie CJ. Healing trabecular microfractures in the bodies of lumbar vertebrae. *Ann Rheum Dis.* 1973; **32**: 406–412

Wolff J. *Das Gesetz der Transformation der Knochen.* Berlin: Hirschwald; 1892

Wright TM. Hayes WC. Tensile testing of bone over a wide range of strain rates: effects of strain rate, microstructure and density. *Med Biol Engng.* 1976; **14**: 671–680

15 Mechanical Aspects of Skin

Skin has several functions, only part of which are mechanical. Save for forces acting on the teeth, external forces on the locomotor system are transmitted exclusively via the skin. Strain and deformation of the soft tissues distribute the effect of these forces over larger areas of contact. In addition, deformation and shifting of the skin assists in attenuating peak forces. The ability of the skin to be readily elongated is extremely important to the functioning of joints. Any noticeable force required to elongate the skin on the convex aspect of a joint would make joint movement strenuous and decrease the range of motion. One example is the limited range of motion experienced in a case of a swollen joint. Here the skin is already strained by the swelling and tolerates only minor additional elongation. Another example is the decreased range of motion in the presence of scars close to a joint, as scar tissue is less extensible than normal skin.

Grasping and holding objects effects relatively high pressures and shear forces on the palm of the hand. Pressure distribution, with peak pressure values in characteristic locations, also exists under the sole of the foot. When a person is sitting or lying down, the skin is subjected to less pressure, because the gravitational force acts on a larger area of contact. In contrast to hand and foot, where we usually experience pressurization and unloading in rapid succession, the pressure on skin when sitting or lying may persist for longer periods. This may have undesirable consequences. Knowledge of the effects of pressure, tension, and shear on the skin is required for the construction and fitting of prostheses and orthoses. Deformation characteristics of the skin are of interest when planning surgical incisions and optimizing wound closure.

In addition to its mechanical functions, skin has a protective function. First and foremost, its external layer, the stratum corneum, acts as a microbial and chemical barrier. Receptors in the skin register touch, pressure, strain, and temperature. Strain effects a sensation of tension; above a certain limit, this sensation is transformed into pain. Skin plays an important role in maintaining the correct body temperature by controlling the blood flow in the skin and by regulating the production of sweat.

▨ Anatomical basics

The following description of the anatomy and architecture of skin is confined to items of importance for an understanding of its mechanical properties. For comprehensive information the reader is referred to textbooks of anatomy and physiology. Skin is composed of several distinct layers: epidermis, dermis, and subdermis (Fig. 15.1). The epidermis is an avascular cellular layer. Its thickness at different locations of the body is typically 0.1 mm; on the palms of the hands or the soles of the feet a thickness of up to 1.0 mm may be encountered. Cells originate at the basement membrane, at the borderline between epidermis and dermis. Within a period of approximately one month these cells migrate towards the skin surface. In the course of

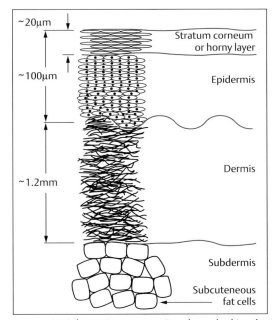

Fig. 15.1 Schematic cross section through skin, depicting the epidermis and its external stratum corneum layer, the dermis, and the subdermis. Typical thickness dimensions are quoted; at certain locations the thickness of one or more layers may be substantially higher. (adapted from Payne, 1991)

the migration they gradually assume a flat form, lose their nuclei and finally die.

During the migration the cells synthesize keratin, a fibrous protein. The keratin from the dead cells, reinforced by additional chemical bonding, remains at the surface of the skin and forms the stratum corneum (horny layer). At body locations that are only rarely loaded, if at all, the horny layer has a thickness of the order of 0.02 mm; at frequently and highly loaded locations, the thickness can be substantially greater. During everyday life the surface of the stratum corneum is subject to continuous wear and tear. The fact that its thickness is maintained in the long run is clear proof of the continuous cellular renewal of the epidermis.

The primary function of the dermis is to provide nourishment and mechanical support to the epidermis, as its thin cellular layer is of limited mechanical strength. In terms of volume, the dermis is composed of approximately 35 % collagen, 0.5 % elastin, and 65 % water, with small admixtures of cells and intercellular substances. The collagen fibers are identical with the tension-resistant fibers employed in tendons and ligaments. The collagen fibers form a two-dimensional mesh; in part they are arranged in preferred directions. In the unloaded state, the fibers are not straight but assume a spiral, wavy form. The form of the fibers, and their arrangement in the mesh, determine the elongation properties and tensile strength of the dermis. The elastin fibers form a second mesh. It is hypothesized that the elastin mesh is responsible for the elongation properties of skin under low stress. The intercellular substances are held responsible for the viscoelastic properties of skin.

Material properties

Tensile properties of skin can be determined *in vivo* or *in vitro*. Studies in vivo, documenting the change in distance of markers glued on to the skin under the influence of a tensile force, measure the strain of the skin connected to the underlying muscle or fat tissue. Such studies are appropriate for documenting changes in the tensile properties due to disease or radiation exposure, for example. It is not possible, however, to extract numerical values for moduli of elasticity from such data, because the thickness of the tissue layers involved is not known. Studies *in vitro* are not subject to this restriction. However, the extent to which the data obtained from skin samples are representative of the behavior of skin *in vivo* deserves examination.

Fig. 15.**2** shows the stress-strain diagram of a skin sample *in vitro*. Starting from the unloaded

state, the sample is elongated by more than 50 % of its initial length under tensile stress of small magnitude (region A). After a transitional zone (region B), the strain exhibits only a small further increase in relation to the increase in stress (region C). When the strain approaches the value 1.0 (i.e. 100 % elongation with respect to the initial length), the sample eventually ruptures.

The shape of the stress-strain curve in Fig. 15.**2** is qualitatively explained by the fact (Daly, 1982) that in region A of the diagram (Fig. 15.**3**) the wavy, unordered collagen fibers offer virtually no resistance to elongation. In the transitional region B, the fibers straighten out and become more and more aligned in the direction of the tensile force. The more the fibers are straightened and aligned, the steeper is the slope of the stress-strain curve, i.e. the higher is the modulus of elasticity. With all fibers aligned, the strain can increase only by a small amount before rupture occurs. In regions B and C, the stress-strain curve of skin resembles stress-strain curves of tendons. Tendons, however, do not exhibit the large initial strain (region A) under low stress, which is characteristic of skin.

Fig. 15.**4** shows the initial part of the stress-strain curve of Fig. 15.**2** drawn to a stress scale enlarged

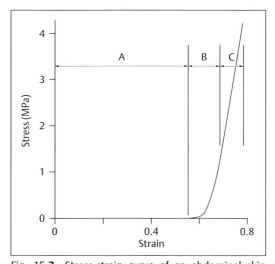

Fig. 15.**2** Stress-strain curve of an abdominal skin sample *in vitro*. A: region of high strain under comparatively low tensile stress, i. e. low stiffness region. (Between the origin of the diagram and strain equal to approx. 0.6, the stress increases, though only by a small amount. This increase is so small that in this graph the curve seems to coincide with the horizontal axis.) B: transitional region. C: high stress region exhibiting high stiffness. (adapted from Daly, 1982)

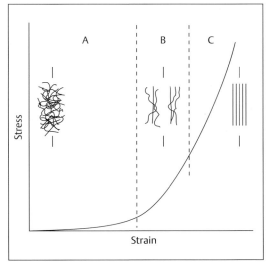

Fig. 15.**3** Qualitative explanation for the shape of the stress-strain curve depicted in Fig. 15.**2**. In region A, the collagen fibers assume a wavy form and are not aligned in preferred directions. The collagen fibers carry no tensile load. In the transitional region B, the fibers begin to straighten and gradually align in the direction of the tensile force. In region C all collagen fibers are aligned. Measured tensile stiffness is now determined by the material properties of collagen fibers. (adapted from Daly, 1982)

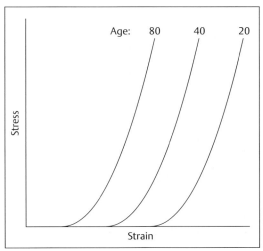

Fig. 15.**5** Effect of age on the stress-strain relation of human skin *in vitro* (schematic). With increasing age, the initial region of high strain under low stress decreases. The shape of the curve in the high stress region (high stiffness region) is left unchanged. Note: the origin of a stress-strain curve is defined as that point where the tissue begins to exhibit resistance to elongation. Plastic elongation, effected virtually without application of a tensile force, is disregarded in this type of experiment. (adapted from Daly and Odland, 1979)

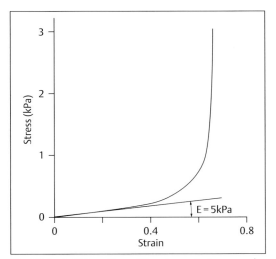

Fig. 15.**4** Initial portion of the stress-strain curve depicted in Fig. 15.**2**, though enlarged with respect to the stress scale by a factor of 100. Between zero strain and a strain equal to 0.4 there is a linear relation between stress and strain. The modulus of elasticity (slope of the curve) amounts typically to 5 kPa. (adapted from Daly, 1982)

by a factor of approximately 100. It can be noted that, in the strain range between $\varepsilon = 0$ and $\varepsilon = 0.4$, there is a virtually linear relation between stress and strain. In this region the modulus of elasticity of skin (the slope of the curve) typically amounts to 5 kPa (Daly, 1982). This modulus is approximately 100 times lower than that of soft rubber. The elastic behavior of skin in the initial region of large strain is assumed to be determined not by the collagen but by the elastin mesh. In this region, where the collagen fibers are completely relaxed, elastin is responsible for the mechanical properties of skin. The strain at the rupture limit, on the other hand, is not influenced by the elastin (Oxlund *et al.*, 1988).

When strain properties of skin samples from subjects of varying age are tested, it is noted (Daly and Odland, 1979) that the initial region of high strain, region A in Fig. 15.**2**, decreases with increasing age (Fig. 15.**5**). In the region of higher stress, the shape of the stress-strain curves appears not to depend on age. The authors conclude from this finding that the stiffness of the collagen fibers of the dermis shows no age dependence. At first sight the measured, age-related decrease of the initial high-strain region seems to contradict practical experience. This apparent contradiction can, however, be explained by age-dependent disintegration of the elastin mesh. Deprived of elastin, a skin sample will not return to its initial length after having been stretched. Upon unloading, a plastic deformation will persist. When testing skin samples, the starting point of the stress-strain curve is given by that length of the sample, where the sample is just beginning to exhibit resistance to elongation. Thus, if there is plastic deformation under zero stress, the strain interval between the starting point of the curve and that region where the collagen fibers begin to straighten and align decreases, even if in reality the total range of strain of the sample is increased. This accounts for the apparent contradiction between the results shown in Fig. 15.**5** and the qualitative findings from the skin of elderly subjects. The disintegration of the elastin mesh is thought to be associated with the development of wrinkles.

As one example of changed mechanical properties of skin, the tensile properties of scar tissue are reported. So-called hypertrophic scars develop at deep wounds, especially after burns. Scar tissue is characterized by its hardness and its red color. Compared with normal skin, it contains a much higher percentage of collagen fibers (Dunn *et al.*, 1985, Clark *et al.*, 1996). Fig. 15.**6** shows the stress-strain curve of hypertrophic scar tissue compared with normal skin. The initial region of high strain under low stress, which is characteristic of normal skin, is absent in scar tissue. The maximum strain of scar tissue is thus less than that of normal skin. The maximum stiffness (the slope of the curves in their end region) exhibits no difference between scar tissue and skin. It is assumed that, in scar tissue, the collagen fibers are already aligned preferentially in the longitudinal direction of the scar. For this reason, an initial region of the stress-strain curve, where the collagen fibers align, is missing. Under high stress, the collagen fibers determine the shape of the curve, both for scar tissue and for skin.

It has to be added that a uniaxial tensile test, i.e. a test stretching a sample in only one single direction, and the modulus of elasticity determined from such a test, describe the mechanical properties of skin only in an approximate fashion. It can readily be imagined that, in a uniaxial tensile test imposing high strain, the width of a sample in its middle portion will decrease substantially. If this decrease in width were to be hindered by additional tensile stress directed perpendicular to the original stress direction, this would certainly influence the measured stress-strain curve. As collagen and elastin form planar meshes, and since imposed strains are high, a precise description of skin properties necessitates pulling a sample simultaneously in two directions (biaxial test) and observing the related stresses and strains (Lanir and Fung, 1974). Strictly speaking, the behavior of a two-dimensional, anisotropic material, i.e. a material with orientation-dependent properties, should be described by six elastic constants (see, for example, Reihsner *et al.*, 1995). Determination of the complete set of constants is, however, laborious. For many practical applications their precise knowledge is not of importance, so that one can continue to rely on data from simple, uniaxial tensile tests. If, on the other hand, the architecture of the collagen mesh or the mechanical foundation of surgical incision planning or suture techniques are to be investigated, the complications involved in a comprehensive description of the mechanical properties cannot be avoided (see, for example, Reihsner and Menzel, 1998).

Skin is viscoelastic. If the strain of a sample is kept constant, the stress will decrease in time (stress relaxation). If the stress is kept constant, the strain will increase in time (creep deformation). The viscoelastic properties of skin are assumed to be regulated by the ground substance of the dermis. The ground substance influences the internal friction between the collagen fibers and the potential shift of fluid within the dermis.

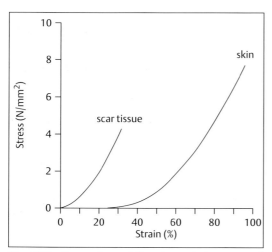

Fig. 15.**6** Comparison of the stress-strain curves of skin and hypertrophic scar tissue. In contrast to skin, hypertrophic scar tissue exhibits only low strain under low stress. The slopes of the scar and skin curves in the high stress (high stiffness) regions are similar. The observed difference in stress-strain behavior is assumed to be due to the ordered alignment of collagen fibers in scar tissue. (adapted from Dunn *et al.*, 1985)

Aside from the uniaxial test *in vitro* or *in vivo*, a number of other test procedures for documenting changes in skin properties, caused for example by X-ray exposure, sunlight, or specific diseases, has been proposed (Edwards and Marks, 1995). In order to observe shear deformation, adjacent skin areas are rotated against one another. A so-called compression test determines the non-invasive indentation of a probe into the skin and underlying tissue. This method bears some resemblance to the determination of Shore hardness, as employed for characterizing technical materials.

▨ Reaction of the skin to mechanical factors

Pressure. In the past, a number of experiments on animals and humans have been conducted to explore the effect of short- or long-term pressure on the skin with respect to blood flow, inflammation, and the development of ulcers. For an overview see, for example, Sanders *et al.*, 1995. These experiments show that very high pressures induce direct injury to skin and underlying muscles. Pressure acting over longer periods of time may cause ischemia and inflammatory reactions, potentially resulting in further damage (Brand *et al.*, 1999).

Pressure above a limit of approximately 35 mm Hg (approximately 4650 Pa) reduces, and eventually stops, the blood flow. The consequences are oxygen deficiency (hypoxia) and accumulation of waste products in the tissue. If the blood flow is stopped for too long, the outcome is tissue necrosis and ulcer formation. The tolerance of the skin with respect to ischemia, i.e. the length of time for which the blood flow can be interrupted without resulting in permanent damage, depends on the magnitude of the pressure and the duration of pressure application. High pressure is tolerated only for short, and lower pressure for longer, periods. The study by Reswick and Rogers (1976) gives an impression of the tolerance limits (Fig. 15.7). It has to be kept in mind, however, that, the tolerance range depends not only on pressure and time but also strongly on the location of the skin, and on additional factors such as temperature, humidity, and intermittent unloading (recovery) periods. Thin skin located directly over bones exhibits a reduced tolerance. Increased temperature and a humid environment lead to reduced tolerance. These findings are the rationale for practical measures for preventing pressure ulcers (bedsores, decubitus): reduced pressure through increased contact areas, temporary pressure relief to allow for recovery, control of temperature and humidity.

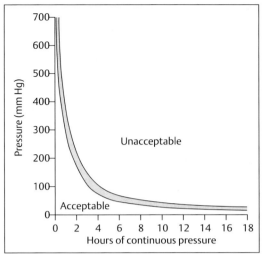

Fig. **15.7** Tolerance limit of skin under bony prominences with respect to pressure magnitude and time of pressure application. High pressures are tolerated only for short periods; low pressures are acceptable for longer periods. The shaded zone indicates that, aside from pressure magnitude and time of duration, additional factors such as temperature and humidity modify the location of the borderline between acceptable and unacceptable regions. (adapted from Reswick and Rogers, 1976)

If the pressure loading stays within the tolerance limits with respect to magnitude and duration, all blood vessels re-open upon load relief and the tissue swells. If there is too little recovery time up to a subsequent loading episode, the tolerance limits for the next pressure loading are lowered. Intermittent loading with excessively short recovery intervals can thus lead to a 'zero tolerance' state. This can be observed, for example, in the case of poorly designed or fitted orthoses, splints, or shoes, which are permanently discarded by patients after some brave attempts to wear them according to the doctor's prescription.

The accumulation of metabolites caused by blockage of the blood flow causes pain. This pain signals the urgent need for a change of body posture or adjustments to orthoses, splints, or shoes. Subjects with a decrease or complete loss of sensitivity of the skin are at an increased risk, because their physiologic 'warning system' is impaired. This is the case, for example, in diabetes patients with reduced sensitivity of the skin on the sole of the foot, or in paraplegic or tetraplegic patients suffering a complete loss of the sensitivity of the skin. As there is no warning of a potential violation of the tolerance limits, the risk of developing pressure ulcers is particularly high in this cohort. (In addition, in diabetics a change in physiology of the skin plays a role.) Subjects with low muscle force are at risk, as well. They sense the warnings but may not be able to react appropriately. Reduced motion of elderly subjects while sleeping, furthered by (excessive) sleeping medication, may be responsible for the increased risk of bedsores in the back and hip region.

Shear deformation. A force acting parallel to the surface of the skin induces tensile strain and shear deformation. Shear deformation occurs due to static or gliding friction acting on the skin. Static friction exists, for example, between the skin and the handle of a screwdriver. Gliding friction exists, for example, between the hind foot and the shoe. Shear deformation of the skin also occurs at the periphery of an area exposed to pressure. It seems that shear deformation of the kind occurring in everyday life has a greater potential to produce damage than pressure loading.

Excessively high or excessively frequent shear deformation damages the epidermis and the dermis. Under repeated deformation the skin assumes a red color and flaking of the stratum corneum occurs. Finally, accompanied by sharp pain, the epidermis ruptures. At locations with a thin stratum corneum, open wounds are likely to develop in response to gliding friction. Alternatively, blisters may be formed, preferentially at locations where the stratum corneum is relatively thick, i.e. on the palms of the hands or the soles of the feet. The tendency for blisters to develop shows large inter-individual differences. Humid skin tends more to blister formation than does dry skin. The reason may be that humid skin permits higher moments to be transmitted (for example, to the handle of a screwdriver), which subject the tissue to higher shear deformation.

As an adaptive response to shear deformation, a so-called callus is produced, a plane layer of stratum corneum with increased thickness. Sweat can still pass through the callus covering the skin of hands or feet because the openings of the sweat glands pass through the callus layer. This is of importance not only in maintaining a certain level of humidity on the skin surface, but because humidity keeps the callus material (keratin) compliant. Dehydrated callus is brittle. For this reason, dry skin tends to develop superficial fissures. This is the biomechanical rationale for keeping the skin suitably humid.

If a pressure pad with surface A is pressed on to the skin with force **F**, the mean pressure p_{mean} = F/A is produced at the interface. While the tissue under the central part of the pad is exposed to pressure (Fig. 15.**8**), the indentation of the pad into the surface exposes the tissue in the region of the periphery to tensile stress and shear deformation. In Fig. 15.**8** this is illustrated by the deformation of the unloaded 'rectangular elements' of the skin tissue into trapezoids. Shear deformation is especially conspicuous at deep indentations and around sharp edges of the pressure-transmitting surface. Similarly, a bone with sharp edges or ridges produces shear deformation of the adjacent soft tissue. If the bone is highly loaded, the tissue may be subject to damage or injury by excessive shear. The effect of shear deformation of the skin can be readily demonstrated by pressing a small plane object with sharp edges for some minutes on to the skin. After relief, the recovery reaction (redness, swelling) can easily be seen with the naked eye to concentrate on the edge region, where shear deformation has predominantly occurred. For these rea-

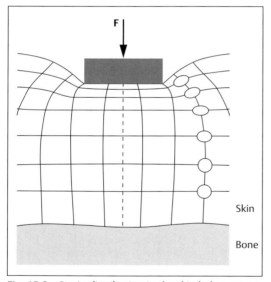

Fig. 15.**8** Strain distribution in the skin below a pressure pad and in the region of its edges. The force **F** effects a mean pressure F/A at the interface where A designates the contact area of the pad. Below the central part of the pad the tissue is compressed. This is indicated (in grossly exaggerated fashion) by the decreased height of the tissue volume elements. Due to the pad pressing into the tissue, the tissue is subject to tensile stress and shear deformation in the region of the edges of the pad. This is illustrated by the trapezoid deformation of the volume elements in the edge region as well as by the deformation of a circular cross section (representing a vessel) into a narrow, elliptic cross section in the edge region. (adapted from Brand *et al.*, 1999)

sons, efforts are made to avoid sharp edges or ridges on contact areas of orthoses or splints.

Further Reading

Textbooks and review papers

Brand PW, Hollister AM, Giurintano D, Thompson DE. External stress: effect at the surface. In: Brand PW, Hollister AM (eds). *Clinical mechanics of the hand.* 3rd ed. St.Louis: Mosby, 1999

Payne PA. Measurement of properties and function of skin. *Clin Phys Physiol Meas.* 1991; **12**, 105–129 [review paper, 94 references]

Scientific papers, cited in the text or the figures

Clark JA, Cheng JCY, Leung KS. Mechanical properties of normal skin and hypertrophic scars. *Burns.* 1996; **22**: 443–446

Daly CH. Biomechanical properties of the dermis. *J Invest Dermatol.* 1982; **79**: 17s–20s

Daly CH, Odland GF. Age-related changes in the mechanical properties of human skin. J Invest Dermatol. 1979; **73**: 84–87

Dunn MG, Silver FH, Swann DA. Mechanical analysis of hypertrophic scar tissue: structural basis for apparent increased rigidity. *J Invest Dermatol.* 1985; **84**: 9–13

Edwards C, Marks R. Evaluation of biomechanical properties of human skin. *Clinics in Dermatology.* 1995; **13**: 375–380

Lanir Y, Fung YC. Two dimensional mechanical properties of rabbit skin I. Experimental system. *J Biomechanics.* 1974; **7**: 29–34

Oxlund H, Manschott J, Viidik A. The role of elastin in the mechanical properties of skin. *J Biomechanics.* 1988; **21**: 213–218

Reihsner R, Balogh B, Menzel EJ. Two-dimensional elastic properties of human skin in terms of an incremental model at the in vivo configuration. *Med Eng Phys.* 1995; **17**: 304–313

Reihsner R, Menzel EJ. Two-dimensional stress-relaxation behavior of human skin as influenced by non-enzymatic glycation and the inhibitory agent aminoguanidine. *J Biomechanics.* 1998; **31**: 985–993

Reswick JB, Rogers JE. Experience at Rancho Los Amigos hospital with devices and techniques to prevent pressure sores. In: Kenedi RM, Cowden JM, Scales JT (eds). *Bed sore biomechanics.* London: Macmillan; 1976

Sanders JE, Goldstein BS, Leotta DF. Skin response to mechanical stress: adaptation rather than breakdown – a review of the literature. *J Rehabil Res Develop.* 1995; **32**: 214–226

Appendix

A1 Loading of the Lumbar Spine when Sitting or Standing

Without generation of muscle forces the posture of the body when sitting or standing would be unstable. A minor external perturbation would suffice to tilt the trunk forwards, backwards, or to the side. Postural stability is achieved by antagonistic activation of the trunk musculature. The co-contraction of the muscles ensures that the remaining postural sway stays below certain limits. This guarantees that the center of mass of the body remains positioned above the area of support, thus preventing the person from falling over. Antagonistic activation of the trunk muscles increases spinal loading; this is the price to be paid for preserving postural stability.

In the erect posture of the upper trunk, the load on the lumbar spine in standing or sitting assumes a minimum value when the force of the trunk musculature is minimized. In the sitting posture, the muscles of the lower extremity are, to a large extent, relaxed. It is indisputable that the loading of the joints of the lower extremity is lower in sitting than in standing. Whether the forces generated by the trunk musculature, and thus the loading of the lumbar spine, are lower in sitting or standing is not clear from the very outset. This issue cannot be solved by reasoning but only by measurement.

Knowledge of the load on the lumbar spine in the sitting and standing postures has been obtained in the past a) from measurements of intradiskal pressure, b) from precision measurements of stature change and, c) recently also from model calculations. From measurements of intradiskal pressure, the load on the lumbar spine was concluded to be higher in sitting than in standing. The advice given to patients with problems of the lumbar spine to stand rather than to sit, is based on these measurements. In contrast, precision measurements of stature change indicated that the load on the spine was generally lower in sitting than in standing. In view of the importance of this issue to clinical and ergonomic applications, this chapter discusses the measurement methods, including potential error influences, with the aim of resolving the issue.

Loading of the lumbar spine determined by measurement of intradiskal pressure

The method of determining the load on the lumbar spine by measuring intradiskal pressure was discussed in detail in Chapter 11. Nachemson (1960) determined *in vitro* the relation between intradiskal pressure, axial load and cross-sectional area of the intervertebral disk:

$$\text{pressure} = (1.5 \pm 0.1) \cdot \text{load} / \text{disk cross-sectional area [Pa]}$$

In these experiments, the angle between the endplates of the motion segments investigated corresponded to the angle of lordosis observed *in vivo* with the subject standing (called by Nachemson the 'in situ reference position'). When the load was kept constant and the angle between the endplates deviated from its *in situ* reference value, deviations from the above relation between pressure and force were observed (Nachemson, 1963). If a spec-

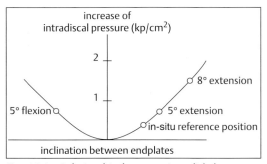

Fig. A1.**1** Relationship between intradiskal pressure measured *in vitro* and the angle of lordosis (adapted from Nachemson, 1963; 1 kp/cm² = 9.81 N/cm²). The intradiskal pressure depends not only on the axial load but also on the angle between the endplates of the neighboring vertebral bodies. With the load kept constant, the intradiskal pressure increases when the specimen is moved from the 'in situ reference' position, adjusted to the average angle of lordosis in erect standing, into maximum extension or flexion. This effect was not originally allowed for when converting measured pressure data *in vivo* into spinal load data *in vivo*.

Table A1.1   Load on segment L3/L4 determined from measurement of intradiskal pressure during standing, sitting erect without a backrest, and sitting with a 5 cm lumbar support and a backrest inclined backward. n: number of subjects in the cohorts investigated. The angle of the backrest quoted in the table is specified with respect to the horizontal. The loads quoted from Nachemson 1985 and 1992 stem from the intradiskal pressure measurements of Nachemson and Elfström (1970); the loads quoted from Chaffin *et al.* (1999) stem from the intradiskal pressure measurements of Andersson *et al.* (1974a)

	Nachemson 1985 n = 7	Nachemson 1992 n = 7	Chaffin *et al.* 1999 n = 4
Standing	700 N	500 N	330 N
Sitting, erect without backrest	1000 N	700 N	410 N
Sitting, angle of backrest 90°	–	–	370 N
Sitting, angle of backrest 100°	–	450 N	300 N
Sitting, angle of backrest 120°	–	–	150 N

imen (under constant axial load) was moved from the *in situ* reference angle farther into extension, the intradiskal pressure increased. If the specimen was moved into flexion, the intradiskal pressure first decreased and then increased again (Fig. A1.**1**). The underlying reason for the observed change of pressure is that, near the limits of the range of motion, the ligaments crossing the disk space, as well as the outermost layer of the annulus fibrosus, are subjected to tensile stress either ventrally (in extension) or dorsally (in flexion). To maintain the equilibrium of forces, the compressive stress in the central region of the disk must rise accordingly.

Nachemson and Elfström (1970) instrumented volunteers with a miniature pressure transducer at the center of disk L3/L4 and recorded the pressure during standing or sitting. The cross-sectional area of the disks was determined from radiographs. The relation between pressure, load, and area, previously obtained *in vitro*, was subsequently used to calculate the compressive force *in vivo* on disk L3/L4. As factor of proportionality between pressure and the product of force and area, Nachemson and Elfström, and in later investigations Andersson *et al.* (1974a), always employed the value 1.5. The fact that this factor actually varied with the angle of lordosis, i.e. that different factors of proportionality should have been used for different postures, was explicitly disregarded. Table A1.**1** contains the load (axial compressive force) on the disk L3/L4, averaged over the cohort (n = 7) investigated by Nachemson and Elfström (quoted from Nachemson, 1985, 1992).

Following the protocol of Nachemson and Elfström, Andersson *et al.* (1974a, 1975) conducted additional measurements of intradiskal pressure in different postures, with the subject sitting on a chair without a backrest, and on a chair with a vertically oriented as well as a backward inclined backrest. This chair was equipped with a 5 cm wide lumbar support. The average values of the load on segment L3/L4 of the cohort investigated (n = 4) are also quoted in Table A1.**1**.

It is seen that, according to Nachemson and Elfström as well as to Andersson and colleagues, the load on the lumbar spine was higher during erect sitting without a backrest than during standing. The magnitude of the load, however, differs substantially between the two series. Potentially these differences may be due to differences in body mass, differences in actual posture, or random fluctuations in the antagonistic activation of the trunk musculature of the subjects. The discrepancy between the values quoted by Nachemson in 1985 and in 1992 remains unexplained. According to Nachemson (1992) as well as to Chaffin *et al.* (1999), measurement of intradiskal pressure showed that the load on segment L3/L4 was lower when the subjects were sitting on a chair with a small backward inclination of the backrest (angle between seat and backrest 100°) than when they were standing. Increasing the backward inclination of the backrest resulted in a further decrease in spinal loading (Andersson, 1974a; Chaffin *et al.*, 1999).

The influence of a backrest on the load on the lumbar spine may be due a) to relaxation of the trunk musculature and b) to the fact that a backward inclined backrest supports a fraction of the body weight. It is hypothesized that the fear of falling backward from the chair disappears in the presence of a backrest; thus the trunk muscles are allowed to relax. This hypothesis is supported by the observation that, even when sitting on a chair with vertically aligned backrest, spinal loading decreases in relation to standing (see Table A1.**1**) although a vertical backrest cannot support any fraction of the body weight. Only a backward inclined backrest supports a fraction of the body weight, proportional to the sine of the angle α of the inclination (measured with respect to the vertical). The load on the lumbar spine is then decreased by the weight of the upper trunk multiplied by the factor (1.0 –cosα). This formula shows that for small angles α, load relief is small as well; for example, for α = 10°, cosα amounts to 0.98 and (1.0 –cosα) = 0.02, corresponding to 2 %. In fact, a decrease in the antagonistic activity of the trunk musculature is observed in the presence of a vertically aligned backrest (Corlett and Eklund, 1984; Bendix et al., 1996). A further decrease in EMG activity occurs when the backrest is inclined backward (Andersson et al., 1974a).

In addition to intradiskal pressure, Andersson et al. (1974b) measured the myoelectric activity of 11 muscle groups of the trunk, partially with surface and partially with needle electrodes. It was found that, when the posture was changed from standing to erect sitting, the amplitude of the EMG signal decreased in five of the muscle groups investigated and increased in six groups. Since the amplitude of the EMG signal does not allow conclusions to be drawn on muscle force, these data do not permit conclusions to be drawn on the change in spinal loading when changing from standing to sitting. A decision on the problem discussed here would have been possible only if the activity of all muscle groups in one of the two postures had been very small or zero. In this case it could have been concluded that the spinal load reached a minimum value in the posture with a small or zero signal amplitude.

In short, according to the studies by Nachemson and Elfström and by Andersson and colleagues, erect sitting on a chair without a backrest loads the lumbar spine more than erect standing. The two studies, however, differ considerably with respect to the magnitude of the spinal load and to the relation of the load in standing versus sitting. The presence and backward inclination of a backrest influence spinal loading. When sitting on a chair with a vertical backrest, spinal loading, according to Andersson and colleagues, is only marginally higher than when standing. If the backrest is inclined backward by 10° (or more), the load when sitting is lower than when standing.

Loading of the lumbar spine, determined from measurement of stature change

The method of determining spinal loading by measuring stature change was described in Chapter 11. The method is based on the observation that intervertebral disks lose height under increased load, due to viscoelastic deformation and diffusion of water from the disk into the surrounding space. During phases of lower loading, relaxation of the viscoelastic deformation and diffusion of water in the reverse direction occur. As result the disk height increases in such phases. The height changes of the disks result in a measurable change of stature.

Althoff et al. (1992, 1993) investigated the stature change in subjects sitting in a variety of postures on a variety of chairs. Fig. A1.**2** shows an example of the recorded stature data of subjects sitting 30 min in erect posture on a chair without a backrest. In a pre-test phase lasting about 30 min, the stature of the test subject, instructed to stand or walk slowly in the laboratory without any additional external load, was repeatedly measured at 3 min intervals (open circles in Fig A1.**2**). An exponential function was mathematically fitted to these data points. This function is employed to predict what the future time course of stature would be if standing were continued. It is seen that stature decreased slightly in the pre-test phase. The sitting phase that followed was interrupted every 5 min for a stature measurement (solid squares). A second exponential was fitted to these data points. This example shows that 30 min sitting resulted in an increase in stature (difference between the two exponentials at the end of the sitting phase) of approximately 0.5 mm.

Fig. A1.**3** shows the measurement record for 30 min comfortable sitting (solid squares) on an office chair with armrests and backward inclined backrest. The increase in stature observed in this example at the end of the sitting phase amounted to approximately 3.5 mm. During subsequent standing (open squares) stature decreased rapidly. Althoff and colleagues, who investigated a cohort of 10 subjects in the age range between 20 and 52 years, invariably observed an increase in stature when the subjects were sitting, irrespective of the type of chair used and the posture assumed (Fig. A1.**4**).

Previous data published by Althoff and colleagues proved that any additional loading of the spine invariably resulted in a decrease in stature. The comparison of stature decrease under load increase, and stature increase during sitting, thus leads to the conclusion that sitting unloads the spine relative to standing. The results of Althoff and colleagues with respect to change of stature when sitting or standing comply with those of Drerup and Granitzka (1994) and of Leivseth and Drerup (1997), but not with those of Magnusson et al. (1990). The protocol of these latter authors provided, however, for the test persons to lie down in a

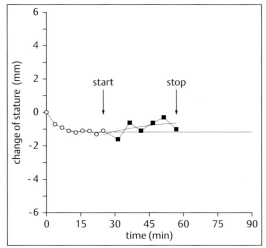

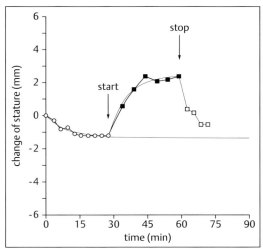

Fig. A1.2 Example of the change of stature during 30 min of erect sitting on a chair without a backrest (adapted from: Althoff *et al.* 1992, 1993). Open circles: stature data of the test subject while standing or slowly walking in the laboratory; solid squares: stature data while sitting. To reduce random errors and to predict the time course of stature if pre-test standing and walking were continued, exponential functions are fitted to the data. The stature change quoted is the difference between these functions at the end of the sitting phase. In the example shown, stature increased by approximately 0.5 mm.

Fig. A1.3 Example of the change of stature during 30 min of comfortable sitting on an office chair with backward inclined backrest (adapted from: Althoff *et al.*, 1992, 1993). Open circles: stature data of the test subject while standing or slowly walking in the laboratory; solid squares: stature data while sitting; open squares: stature data while standing subsequent to the sitting period. To reduce random errors and to predict the time course of stature if standing and walking were continued, exponential functions are fitted to the data. The stature change quoted is the difference between these functions at the end of the sitting phase. In the example shown, stature increased by approximately 3.5 mm. While standing subsequent to the sitting period, stature decreased rapidly and approached its initial value.

Fig. A1.4 Change of stature after 30 min of sitting on a variety of chairs in a variety of postures in relation to standing (adapted from Althoff *et al.*, 1992, 1993)

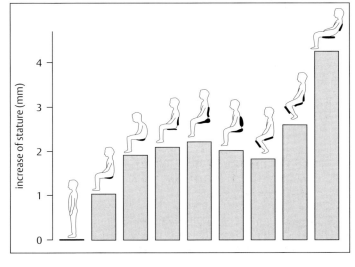

relaxed state for 15 min before beginning the sitting phase. In the supine posture, stature increases markedly due to the considerable unloading of the spine. This increase regresses in the subsequent sitting phase, which accounts for the decrease in stature observed by Magnusson and colleagues in sitting subjects. Thus, the results of that study do not allow conclusions to be drawn on the difference in spinal loading between standing and sitting.

Loading of the lumbar spine, determined by an EMG-assisted model calculation

The method to determine joint loading from model calculations has been described in Chapter 8. Callaghan and McGill (2001) determined the load on the segment L4/L5 during standing and unsupported sitting, using an EMG-assisted, detailed biomechanical model that incorporated 104 muscles, passive ligaments and intervertebral disks. Eight subjects were tested for sitting periods of 2 hours in forward bent postures. When sitting, forward bending varied between 30% and 80% of the lumbar spine range of motion (determined as the difference between maximum flexion and extension). Under these conditions, loading when sitting (on average 1698 ± 467 N) was considerably higher compared with standing (on average 1076 ± 243 N). The authors conclude that the increase in joint compression when sitting was due to increased force generation of the extensor muscles and passive forces from strains of the soft tissues.

Biomechanical model comparing spinal loading in sitting and standing

The load on a motion segment of the lumbar spine in standing or sitting depends on a) the gravitational force of the body mass cranial to the segment in question, b) the (passive) elastic tension of muscles and ligaments crossing the segment, c) muscle forces required (in dependence on the position of the center of mass) to keep the trunk upright and, potentially, d) additional forces resulting from co-contraction of the trunk muscles.

If we compare a simplified model of the body in standing and in erect sitting posture (Fig. A1.**5**), we expect no differences in relation to the gravitational force of the body mass located cranially to the segment in question, and negligible differences

with respect to the elastic tension of muscles or ligaments. If the distance of the center of mass of the cranial body with respect to the center of the disk (the center of rotation) is equal in sitting and standing, there will be no difference between the two postures in the force of the extensors of the back. If furthermore, we assume antagonistic muscle activation to be negligibly small, we expect virtually no difference in spinal loading between the two postures.

A closer look, however, reveals a number of subtle differences between standing and sitting, which may have effects on spinal loading as well as on the interpretation of the experiments cited above. When a subject is sitting down, the angle of lordosis of the lumbar spine changes. When he is standing, the angle is practically at its maximum value.

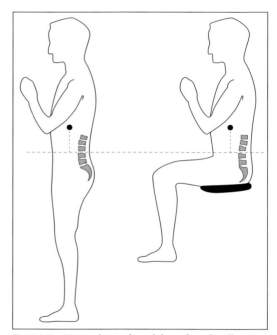

Fig. A1.**5** Biomechanical model employed to illustrate the difference in spinal loading between sitting and standing. The load on the lumbar spine depends a) on the gravitational force of the body mass cranial to the segment in question, b) the (passive) elastic tension of muscles and ligaments crossing the segment, c) muscle forces required (in dependence on the position of the center of mass) to keep the trunk upright and, potentially, d) additional forces originating from co-contraction of the trunk muscles. The full circle designates the location of the center of body mass cranial to segment L3/L4. The angle of lordosis may differ between standing and sitting.

During sitting without a backrest, the angle varies in a wide range, according to the posture attained. In relaxed sitting, the angle of lordosis approaches zero, or the lordosis is even transformed into a kyphosis. During forcibly erect sitting, the angle of lordosis may be greater than during standing. The measurements recorded *in vivo* by Nachemson (see Fig. A1.1) showed that the intradiskal pressure rises under constant load, either when the lordosis increases with respect to standing, or when the lordosis is transformed into a marked kyphosis. This effect was explicitly not taken into account at the time by Nachemson and Elfström, or by Andersson and colleagues. It is thus possible that the pressure increase recorded by these two groups was due to changes in shape of the lumbar spine and not to differences in spinal loading. In retrospect, however, it is impossible to specify the magnitude of this potential error, because the shape of the lumbar spine adopted by the test subjects at that time is unknown.

Antagonistic activation of the trunk musculature has a great influence on spinal loading. While the load on the disk L3/L4 in erect standing was 700 N according to Nachemson (1985), it rose to 1200 N when the trunk musculature was activated (still while standing) to create intra-abdominal pressure. This increase (1200 N compared to 700 N) exceeds the difference recorded between standing and sitting (1000 N compared to 700N). It is therefore possible that uncontrolled co-activation of the trunk musculature confounded the measurement of spinal loading. The extent to which the test subjects instrumented with intradiskal pressure transducers stood or sat in a relaxed state at that time cannot be reconstructed in retrospect.

Sitting permits a broader variation in the posture of the trunk than standing, because the location of the center of gravity can be varied in a wider region during sitting without the risk of falling. Especially during sitting without a backrest, differences in posture (i. e. differences in the location of the center of gravity of the body mass cranial to the segment in question) might influence the intradiskal pressure as well as the stature change. Althoff and colleagues, for example, observed a small average increase in stature for erect sitting without a backrest (i. e. the posture comparable with that studied by Nachemson and Elfström and by Andersson and colleagues). The individual data, however, were subject to substantial scatter. The stature of some test subjects actually decreased when they were sitting erect without a backrest. The presence of a backrest allows the trunk muscles to relax. Incidentally, crossing the legs when sitting allows for a further muscle relaxation, specifically of the oblique abdominals (Snijders et al., 1995).

Wilke *et al.* (1999) succeeded in reproducing the experiment of Nachemson and Elfström in one single test subject. This study showed the intradiskal pressure during erect sitting without a backrest to be lower than that recorded during standing. This single-subject result is not in accordance with results of previous intradiskal pressure studies. It is, however, compatible with the results of stature change measurements and with the qualitative conclusions drawn from the model quoted above.

▨ Conclusions

Compared with standing, stature increases when sitting erect or in a relaxed state on a chair without a backrest. This finding suggests that sitting unloads the spine compared with standing. This result contradicts results of previous studies, which determined spinal loading by measuring intradiskal pressure and concluded that spinal loading was higher during erect sitting than during standing. The conclusions from stature measurement studies are not contradictory to the model calculation by Callaghan and McGill, resulting in higher load when sitting, because the cohort they investigated adopted a forward flexed posture when sitting, i.e. definitely different from an erect or relaxed posture.

The fact that one fixed factor (and not a factor varying in relation to the angle of lordosis) has been used to convert intradiskal pressure into force, challenges the conclusion drawn from the intradiskal pressure observations, i.e. that spinal loading is higher when sitting erect without a backrest than when standing. In addition, uncontrolled variations of posture, and episodes of antagonistic trunk muscle activation, may have influenced the magnitude of the intradiskal pressure in the comparatively small cohorts investigated. Circumstantial evidence upholding this conjecture is provided by Wilke *et al.* (1999) whose results differed from those of previous intradiskal pressure studies.

There is no contradiction between the results of stature and intradiskal pressure measurements with respect to sitting on chairs with a backward inclined backrest. According to all studies employing one of these two methods, spinal loading when sitting on a chair with a backrest inclined backward by at least 10° is lower than when standing.

The advice given to patients not to sit down because the spine might be overloaded appears not to be justified in the light of recent studies and in consideration of the potential, systematic errors inherent in studies based on intradiskal pressure measurement. With respect to a chair with a backrest inclined by at least 10° (the usual situation, as there are only few chairs with vertically aligned backrests), this recommendation was never justified. i.e. definitively not in view of the studies performed by Nachemson and Elfström and by Andersson and colleagues between 1970 and 1974.

It must be stressed that the results of the study by Althoff and colleagues, according to which spinal loading during sitting is lower than during standing, is valid only for short-term sitting episodes. This result cannot simply be generalized to cover situations where constrained or rigid postures or long periods of sitting are involved. Rigid postures are encountered, for example, at workplaces requiring high concentration or high working speed. Constrained sitting can be encountered in too well customized seats for handicapped persons. In both cases spinal loading may reach high values due to antagonistic activation of the trunk musculature. For quantification of spinal loading in such situations, the stature-change measurement provides a unique and unrivalled tool.

▒ Scientific papers, cited in the text or the figures

Althoff I, Brinckmann P, Frobin W, Sandover J, Burton K. An improved method of stature measurement for quantitative determination of spinal loading. Application to sitting postures and whole body vibration. *Spine.* 1992; **17**: 682–693

Althoff, I., Brinckmann, P., Frobin, W., Sandover, J., Burton, K. *Die Bestimmung der Belastung der Wirbelsäule mit Hilfe einer Präzisionsmessung der Körpergröße. Schriftenreihe der Bundesanstalt für Arbeitsschutz Fb 683.* Bremerhaven: Wirtschaftsverlag NW; 1993

Andersson BJG, Örtengren R, Nachemson A, Elfström G. Lumbar disc pressure and myoelectric back muscle activity during sitting. Studies on an experimental chair. *Scand J Rehab Med.* 1974a; **6**: 104–114

Andersson BJG, Jonsson B, Örtengren R. Myoelectric activity in individual lumbar erector spinae muscles in sitting. A study with surface and wire electrodes. *Scand J Rehab Med.* 1974b; Suppl **3**: 91–108

Andersson BJG, Örtengren R, Nachemson AL, Elfström G, Broman H. The sitting posture: An electromyographic and discometric study. *Orthop Clin North Am.* 1975; **6**: 105–120

Bendix T, Poulsen V, Klausen K, Jensen CV. What does a backrest actually do to the lumbar spine? *Ergonomics.* 1996; **39**: 533–542

Callaghan JP, McGill SM. Low back joint loading and kinematics during standing and unsupported sitting. *Ergonomics.* 2001; **44**: 280–294

Chaffin DB, Andersson GBJ, Martin BJ. *Occupational Biomechanics.* 3rd ed. Wiley: New York; 1999

Corlett EN, Eklund JAE. How does a backrest work? *Applied Ergonomics.* 1984; **15**: 111–114

Drerup B, Granitzka M. *Bestimmung des Schädigungsgrades von Bandscheiben nach langjähriger Ganzkörpervibrations-Exposition mit Hilfe der Stadiometrie. Schriftenreihe der Bundesanstalt für Arbeitsmedizin Fb 10.002.* Bremerhaven: Wirtschaftsverlag NW, 1994

Leivseth G, Drerup B. Spinal shrinkage during work in a sitting posture compared to work in a standing posture. *Clin Biomechanics.* 1997; **12**: 409–418

Magnusson M, Hult E, Lindström I, Lindell V, Pope M, Hansson T. Measurement of time-dependent height loss during sitting. *Clin Biomechanics.* 1990; **5**: 137–142

Nachemson A. Lumbar intradiscal pressure. Experimental studies on post mortem material. *Acta Orthop Scand.* 1960; Suppl. **43**: 1–104

Nachemson A. The influence of spinal movements on the lumbar intradiscal pressure and on the tensile stresses in the annulus fibrosus. *Acta Orthop Scand.* 1963; **33**: 183–207

Nachemson A, Elfström G. Intravital dynamic pressure measurements in lumbar discs. A study of common movements, maneuvers and exercises. *Scand J Rehab Med.* 1970; **Suppl 1**: 1–40

Nachemson, A. Lumbar intradiscal pressure. In: Jayson MIV (ed). *The lumbar spine and back pain.* 2nd ed. London: Pitman; 1985, 341–358

Nachemson, A. Lumbar mechanics as revealed by lumbar intradiscal pressure measurements. In: Jayson MIV (ed). *The lumbar spine and back pain.* 4th ed. Edinburgh: Churchill Livingstone; 1992, 157–172

Snijders CJ, Slagter AHE, van Strik R, Vleeming A, Stoeckart R, Stam HJ. Why leg crossing? The influence of common postures on abdominal muscle activity. *Spine.* 1995; **20**: 1989–1993

Wilke HJ, Neef P, Caimi M, Hoogland T, Claes LE. New *in vivo* measurements of pressures in the intervertebral disc in daily life. *Spine.* 1999; **24**: 755–762

A2 What do we know about Primary Mechanical Causes of Lumbar Disk Prolapse?

A lumbar disk prolapse occurs when a separate tissue fragment extrudes or sequestrates through a complete tear of the anulus. By definition, then, a prolapse requires both a fissure and a fragment. The temporal sequence of these events has yet to be established. There are two hypotheses, the first that the prolapse is an isolated event, and the second that the prolapse is the final episode in a degenerative process.

The high axial compressive loading of lumbar disks (often in combination with side-bending or rotation of the trunk), as well as case reports from patients, seem to suggest that lumbar disk prolapse has a primary mechanical cause. The designation 'primary' is chosen to make it clear that we are discussing the causal event(s) at the very outset of the process ending in a disk prolapse. This is in contrast to a 'secondary' mechanical contribution leading to prolapse of a disk already impaired by other, non-mechanical factors. Direct experiments *in vivo* aimed at proving or disproving hypotheses on the etiology of lumbar disk prolapse are not feasible in view of potentially irreversible consequences. Knowledge can only be derived indirectly from experiments *in vitro* on specimens, from biomechanical model calculations, and from epidemiological investigations.

Studies *in vitro*

Laboratory studies have attempted to answer the question by modeling disk prolapse *in vitro*. Under axial overload of a motion segment, vertebral body fracture invariably occurs first (Perey, 1957; Hutton *et al.*, 1979; Brinckmann *et al.*, 1989). Injury of the anulus fibrosus or a prolapse of disk tissue have not been observed in overload experiments. This holds for single overload episodes, as well as for fatigue fractures (Brinckmann *et al.*, 1988).

Only in flexion beyond the physiological limit ('hyperflexion') will the posterior anulus rupture, or sometimes tear from the vertebral endplate. In a pioneering experiment, Adams and Hutton (1982) demonstrated that hyperflexion combined with high axial load can sometimes produce a prolapse *in vitro*. Investigations on bovine caudal disks (Simunic *et al.*, 2001) suggest that full hydration of

the disk may make the disk more susceptible to injury in such situations. The mechanism simulated by Adams and Hutton may account for the prolapse occasionally seen in athletes, sometimes in combination with a fracture of the posterior rim of the vertebral body (e. g. Epstein and Epstein, 1991). A typical event in this respect is a faulty landing from a horizontal bar (or similar), in a posture flexed too far forward. It is, however, unlikely that such events are responsible for the majority of incidents of lumbar disk prolapse.

The potential influence of tears ('fissures') of the anulus fibrosus in triggering disk prolapse has been investigated in specimens with artificial, radially directed fissures (Brinckmann, 1986). Starting from the center of the disk, these incisions divided the complete anulus save for an outermost, peripheral layer of 1–2 mm thickness. Axial overloading of these impaired specimens resulted in fractures of the vertebral bodies but not in disk prolapse.

The influence of axial rotation in the etiology of disk prolapse has been investigated experimentally, as well as by means of biomechanical model calculations (Ahmed *et al.*, 1990, Duncan and Ahmed, 1991). These studies concluded that, without facet damage, axial rotation (approximately 2° in the lumbar spine) is insufficient to cause disk injury leading to prolapse.

It must be pointed out that present knowledge derived from experiments *in vitro* and model calculations is severely limited. It is not yet possible to preserve disk specimens for long periods (i. e. essentially for longer than 1 day) in a state suitable for biomechanical experimentation. This is due to the enzymatic decomposition of the tissue, which cannot be halted without its mechanical properties being changed. Thus, we see at present no possibility of investigating the effects of long-term static or cyclic loading in the laboratory. The interpretation of relevant experiments employing cyclic loading (Gordon *et al.*, 1991; Callaghan and McGill, 2001) is difficult. In addition it must be kept in mind that long-term processes are always in competition with physiologic tissue repair. At present such repair (if such exists for disk tissue) cannot be reliably simulated in experiments *in vitro* nor in model calculations.

Extruded disk tissue obtained in surgical interventions has been investigated in a number of studies aimed at determining the origin of such fragments, nucleus pulposus or anulus fibrosus (Reimers, 1961; Brock *et al.*, 1992). The vast majority of these fragments proved to consist of disk tissue together with pieces of hyaline endplate cartilage. There is no conclusive argument for a primary mechanical process leading to fragmentation of the disk tissue and its detachment from the bony vertebral endplates. In flexion, extension, side-bending, or axial rotation, strain on the tissue is minimal in the central volume of the disk. If straining of the tissue were to play a role, fragmentation of the disk should thus be initiated at its periphery. These findings, as well as the results of an experiment *in vitro* simulating tissue fragmentation in the central volume of the disk (Brinckmann and Porter, 1994), rather suggest that the actual prolapse is preceded by an unknown process not of a primary mechanical nature.

Influence of posture on disk bulge and prolapse

In flexion or lateral bending, the vertebral endplates approach each other unilaterally and the disk space assumes a wedge form. As the tissue is virtually incompressible, parts of the anulus fibrosus and the nucleus pulposus must move within the disk space in the direction of the opening of the wedge. Some authors concluded that this shift causes the radial bulge of the disk to increase in flexion, and that such an increase might encourage the development of disk prolapse. Loading of the spine in forward bent posture of the trunk was thus regarded as an unfavorable condition for the disk tissue.

The postulated increase in the dorsal bulge of an otherwise normal disk in flexion, however, does not comply with measurements of disk bulging from specimens of motion segments (see Chapter 11) nor with observations *in vivo* in patients injected with a contrast medium in the spinal canal ('myelography'). In contrast to the above reasoning, the dorsal bulge of the disk decreases in flexion while a bulge increase is seen ventrally. To date, epidemiological studies have failed to substantiate the hypothesized relation between the occurrence of disk prolapse and loading of the lumbar spine in flexion.

The increased incidence of disk prolapse in the caudal segments of the lumbar spine, as compared with the cranial segments, appears to support the hypothesis of a mechanical cause of prolapse. Specifically, in the forward bent posture these segments are most highly loaded in compression. It is, however, unclear whether the caudal segments have the highest incidence of disk prolapse or merely the highest incidence of symptomatic disk prolapse (not the same thing!). In addition, it must be taken into account that, in the erect posture (in contrast to forward bending), lifting and carrying results in approximately uniform compressive loading of all segments of the lumbar spine (see Chapter 11). Due to the smaller dimensions of the disks in the cranial region, the resulting stress on the tissue is greater here than in the caudal region. If prolapse had a mechanical cause, disk prolapse should not be rare in segments T12/L1 to L3/L4.

Epidemiological studies of the relation between heavy physical exertions and the prevalence of lumbar disk prolapse

Epidemiological studies (Braun, 1969; Kelsey, 1975; Kelsey *et al.*, 1984a, b; Heliövaara, 1987) have demonstrated an increased risk of being hospitalized for symptomatic lumbar disk prolapse in a number of cohorts, exposed to long-term physical exertions. As lumbar disk prolapse is a rare disease, these studies had been designed as case-control studies. Cohorts of subjects hospitalized due to symptomatic disk prolapse were compared with gender- and age-adjusted control cohorts. Thus, the results of these studies are (inevitably, as are all case-control studies) subject to systematic errors stemming from the selection and cooperation of the patient and the control cohort.

According to Braun, males with highly loaded spines have a significantly increased risk of being hospitalized for the treatment of disk prolapse. The author puts this result into perspective by referring to the surprisingly small risk of females with highly loaded spines being hospitalized for the treatment of disk prolapse. For an explanation the author considers unknown, confounding factors, which in his study shifted the probability of being hospitalized, but not the probability of suffering a symptomatic disk prolapse, to higher values in males than in females.

In the studies by Kelsey and coworkers, too, lifting and carrying of heavy loads entails a higher risk of disk prolapse. These studies, however, have methodological shortcomings. To classify spinal loading, data collection comprised only the weight of the objects handled but not the moment (product of weight and distance) exerted in relation to the lumbar spine. In addition, the selection of subjects for the patient and control cohorts may have been confounded by the substantial fraction (> 20%) of all cases and controls not interviewed successfully (Kelsey *et al.*, 1984b). The difficulty in conducting and interpreting case–control studies is also evident from the fact that, with respect to sitting as a risk factor, the results reported by Kelsey and colleagues in their 1975 and 1984a studies were contradictory.

According to Heliövaara, the risk of being hospitalized due to disk prolapse is significantly increased for males performing physically demanding work, whereas (in conformity with Braun) highly loaded females exhibit only a slight increase in this risk. Farm workers exhibit a moderately increased risk. Subjects with sedentary occupations exhibit no increased risk. In the light of these findings, Heliövaara urges that the results of his study be interpreted with caution. The risk factors established might be confounded by differences in opportunity and willingness to undergo hospital treatment. According to the author, the results of the study should not be interpreted as proof of a relation between spinal loading and the development of disk prolapse.

Heliövaara et al., proposed that prospective studies should be conducted to clarify the issue. In such a prospective study, two cohorts, e. g. a cohort with normal, everyday loading and a cohort with maximum loading of the spine, would be observed for a specific period of time. If the incidence of disk prolapse in the highly loaded cohort were significantly higher than in the normal control cohort, this would support the hypothesis of a causal relation between spinal loading and the development of disk prolapse. However, prospective studies in this field have yet to be published.

The incidence (number of new cases) of symptomatic, treatment requiring lumbar disk prolapse ranges between 6 and $8 \cdot 10^{-4}$ per year and person (Heliövaara *et al.*, 1987; Berney *et al.*, 1990). The follow-up of such a rare disease in a prospective study would, if it were to produce statistically significant results, require large cohorts and long follow-up times, while spinal loading conditions remained essentially unchanged. Thus, there is little hope of such studies actually being conducted. A numerical example is given to illustrate the problem:

It may be assumed that a) the incidence of lumbar disk prolapse is 10^{-3} per year and person (rounded value to facilitate calculation) and b) heavy spinal loading by physically demanding work doubles the incidence of prolapse (a drastic effect). Under these assumptions we would expect 2 cases of prolapse in the control cohort (10^{-3} per year and person x 10 years x 200 subjects) and 4 cases in the heavily loaded cohort in a prospective study comprising two cohorts of 200 subjects each

Table A2.1 A 2 by 2 contingency table of a (hypothetical) study of the relation between high spinal loading and the incidence of lumbar disk prolapse. 200 subjects in each of the cohorts with highly and normally loaded spines.

	disk prolapse yes	disk prolapse no	n
heavy spinal loading yes	4	196	200
heavy spinal loading no	2	198	200

Table A2.2 A 2 by 2 contingency table of a (hypothetical) study of the relation between high spinal loading and the incidence of lumbar disk prolapse. 2000 subjects in each of the cohorts with highly and normally loaded spines.

	disk prolapse yes	disk prolapse no	n
heavy spinal loading yes	20	980	1 000
heavy spinal loading no	10	990	1 000

and covering a 10-year follow-up period (Table A2.1).

The statistical significance of this result (the extent to which we tend to believe the result) would, however, be low. The *chi* square test tells us that, with a probability of over 40 %, this numerical result might have been obtained by chance, with no relationship existing in reality between heavy spinal loading and disk prolapse. To increase the statistical significance, either the size of the cohorts or the follow-up period would have to be increased. In a study surveying 2000 subjects over 10 years we would expect, under the above assumptions, 10 cases of prolapse in the control cohort and 20 cases in the heavily loaded cohort (Table A2.2). The probability of obtaining such a result by chance would still range between 5 % and 10 % (*chi* square test). In other words, such a result would support the hypothesis of a relation between spinal loading and disk prolapse, but still with an appreciable probability of error. The number of subjects involved (n = 2000) and the required follow-up period (10 years) suggest that such a study is most unlikely ever to be conducted.

Conclusions and outlook

At present, the issue of the relationship between heavy spinal loading and the incidence of lumbar disk prolapse is unresolved. Up to now, experiments *in vitro* have failed to identify a primary mechanical cause of prolapse. The exceptions are traumatic episodes with simultaneous hyperflexion and high axial loading of the spine. Knowledge derived from laboratory studies is fragmentary, as simulation of long-term or cyclic loading of disk specimens is not yet possible. There is no doubt that disks can be 'conditioned' or loaded in such a fashion (see the studies mentioned above) that they finally have no other chance than eventually to extrude. The question remains, which (if any) of the models pursued in the different studies *in vitro* simulates non-traumatic lumbar disk extrusion in middle-aged humans.

Epidemiological studies indicate that subjects in certain work places have an increased probability of being hospitalized for lumbar disk prolapse. These case-control studies were subject to error influences so that their results do not necessarily support the hypothesis of a relationship between high spinal loading and increased incidence of lumbar disk prolapse (rather than hospitalization due to disk prolapse). The results of the epidemiological studies, and of the experiments *in vitro*, comply with the conjecture that mechanical influences can trigger prolapse of a disk already damaged by an unknown process. There may be a familial disposition favoring the development of disk prolapse (Videman and Battié, 1999).

As demonstrated by previous searches for the causes of other rare diseases, progress might be made along two paths. The possibility of future experiments, or model calculations, leading to a model for the origin and progress of mechanically induced lumbar disk prolapse cannot be ruled out. Alternatively, medical history provides examples of the causes of rare diseases being revealed by ingenious investigators who first noted an increased incidence of a disease under very special circumstances. Related to disk prolapse: it is conceivable that it is not heavy spinal loading in general but rather special (as yet unspecified) loading modes that are responsible for the development of prolapse. In all events, it is easier to prove (or disprove) a well specified supposition than a vaguely formulated conjecture.

The search for causes is, however, impeded by difficulties in specifying work-related and leisure-time spinal loading, and in describing degenerative alterations of lumbar disks (Videman and Battié, 1999). In addition, it has been suggested that irritation of the nerve roots is caused, not by mechanical pressure, but by a biochemical agent (Olmarker *et al.*, 1995; Harrington *et al.*, 2000). If this were the case, we would expect a certain time (say, some days or weeks) to elapse between the actual prolapse and the occurrence of clinical symptoms. This would complicate the relating of special loading modes (postures or activities) to the prolapse event.

With increasing refinement of diagnostic methods (computed tomography and magnetic resonance imaging) a high prevalence of pathologic alterations of disks, e. g. protrusions and extrusions, is noted in studies *in vivo* and *post mortem*, while these alterations had not been linked with clinical symptoms (McRae, 1956; Jensen *et al.*, 1994; Wood *et al.*, 1995). Protrusions (local increases in radial disk bulge) seem to be frequent, while extrusions (tissue fragments almost or completely separated from the rest of the disk) seem to be rare. If the alterations observed in these studies were not pathologic but part of the normal ageing process, one might be inclined to replace the question 'How does disk prolapse develop?' with the question 'Why do so few prolapsed disks generate clinical symptoms?'

Stages in the process (if it is a long-term process and not one single event) leading finally to extrusion of a fragment of disk tissue could, as yet, not be documented, because the disease is rare, and up to the appearance of magnetic resonance imaging (MRI) radiographic follow-up of healthy subjects was inadmissible for reasons of radiation exposure. Little is known, for example, on whether or not local increases in disk bulge (protrusions), which are not rare in healthy subjects, are precursors of prolapse. Wood *et al.*, (1997) noted virtually no change of the existing protrusions in 48 subjects with asymptomatic thoracic disk herniations, in a follow-up study employing magnetic resonance imaging. A recently published, five-year follow-up study (Boos *et al.*, 2000), on 46 asymptomatic subjects using magnetic resonance imaging, confirmed the high prevalence of asymptomatic pathologic findings, but observed virtually no change in the severity of the protrusions in the observation period. Only in one subject was a change from a protrusion to an extrusion documented. In view of the low incidence of disk prolapse, the cohort size of these studies was possibly too small and follow-up time too short to obtain hard evidence on the stages of development of prolapse.

Suggestions for further reading

Textbooks

Krämer J. *Bandscheibenbedingte Erkrankungen. Ursachen, Diagnose, Behandlung, Vorbeugung, Begutachtung.* 2nd ed. Stuttgart: Thieme; 1986

Postacchini F. *Lumbar disc herniation.* Wien: Springer; 1999

Original papers cited in the text

Adams MA, Hutton WC. Prolapsed intervertebral disc. A hyperflexion injury. *Spine.* 1982; **7**: 184–191

Ahmed AM, Duncan NA, Burke DL. The effect of facet geometry on the axial torque-rotation response of human lumbar motion segments. *Spine.* 1990; **15**: 391–401

Berney J, Jeanpretre M, Kostli A. Facteurs épidémiologiques de la hernie discale lombaire. *Neurochirurgie.* 1990; **36**: 354–365

Boos N, Semmer N, Elfering A, Schade V, Gal I, Zanetti M, Kissling R, Buchegger N, Hodler J, Main CJ. Natural history of individuals with asymptomatic disc abnormalities in magnetic resonance imaging. Predictors of low back pain-related medical consultation and work incapacity. *Spine.* 2000; **25**: 1484–1492

Braun W. *Ursachen des lumbalen Bandscheibenvorfalls. Wirbelsäule in Forschung und Praxis 43.* Stuttgart: Hippokrates; 1969

Brinckmann P. Injury of the annulus fibrosus and disc protrusions. An in vitro investigation on human lumbar discs. *Spine.* 1986; **11**: 149–153

Brinckmann P, Biggemann M, Hilweg D. Fatigue fracture of human lumbar vertebrae. Clinical Biomechanics. 1988; **3** Suppl 1: S1–S23

Brinckmann P, Biggemann M, Hilweg D. Prediction of the compressive strength of human lumbar vertebrae. *Clinical Biomechanics.* 1989; **4** Suppl 2, S1–S27

Brinckmann P, Porter RW. A laboratory model of lumbar disc protrusion. *Spine.* 1994; **19**: 228–235

Brock M, Patt S, Mayer HM. The form and structure of the extruded disc. *Spine.* 1992; **17**: 1457–1461

Callaghan JP, McGill SM. Intervertebral disc herniation. Studies on a porcine model exposed to highly repetitive flexion/extension motion with compressive force. *Clinical Biomechanics.* 2001; **16**: 28–37

Duncan NA, Ahmed AM. The role of axial rotation in the etiology of unilateral disc prolapse. An experimental and finite-element analysis. *Spine.* 1991; **16**: 1089–1098

Epstein NE, Epstein JA. Limbus lumbar vertebral fractures in 27 adolescents and adults. *Spine.* 1991; **16**: 962–966

Gordon SJ, Yang KH, Mayer PJ, Mace AH, Kish VL, Radin EL. Mechanism of disc rupture. A preliminary report. *Spine.* 1991; **16**: 450–456

Harrington FJ, Messier AA, Bereiter D, Barnes B, Epstein MH. Herniated lumbar disc material as a source of free glutamate available to effect pain signals through the dorsal root ganglion. *Spine.* 2000; **25**: 929–936

Heliövaara M, Knekt P, Aromaa A. Incidence and risk factors of herniated lumbar intervertebral disc or sciatica leading to hospitalization. *J Chron Dis.* 1987; **40**: 251–258

Heliövaara M. Occupation and risk of herniated lumbar intervertebral disc or sciatica leading to hospitalization. *J Chron Dis.* 1987; **40**: 259–264

Hutton WC, Cyron BM, Stott JRR. The compressive strength of lumbar vertebrae. *J Anat.* 1979; **129**: 753–758

Jensen MC, Brant-Zawadzki MN, Obuchowski N, Modic MT, Malkasian D, Ross JS. Magnetic resonance imaging of the lumbar spine in people without back pain. *New Engl J Med.* 1994; **331**: 69–73

Kelsey JL. An epidemiological study of the relationship between occupations and acute herniated lumbar intervertebral discs. *Int J Epidemiol.* 1975; **4**: 197–205

Kelsey JL, Githens PB, White AA, Holford TR, Walter SD, O'Connor T, Ostfeld AM, Weil U, Southwick WO, Calogero JA. An epidemiologic study of lifting and twisting on the job and risk for acute prolapsed lumbar intervertebral disc. *J Orthop Res.* 1984a; **2**: 61–66

Kelsey JL, Githens PB, O'Conner T, Weil U, Calogero JA, Holford TR, White AA, Walter SD, Ostfeld AM, Southwick WO. Acute prolapsed lumbar intervertebral disc. An epidemiologic study with special reference to driving automobiles and smoking. *Spine.* 1984b; **9**: 608–613

McRae DL. Asymtomatic intervertebral disc protrusions. *Acta Radiol.* 1956; **46**: 9–27

Olmarker K, Blomquist J, Strömberg J, Nannmark U, Thomsen P, Rydevik B. Inflammatogenic properties of nucleus pulposus. *Spine.* 1995; **20**: 665–669

Perey O. Fracture of the vertebral end-plate in the lumbar spine. *Acta Orthop Scand Suppl.* 1957; **25**: 1–101

Reimers C. Untersuchungen zur Entstehung der lumbalen Bandscheibenhernie. *Wirbelsäule in Forschung und Praxis.* 1961; **25**: 89–106

Simunic DI, Broom ND, Robertson PA. Biomechanical factors influencing nuclear disruption of the intervertebral disc. *Spine.* 2001; **26**: 1223–1230

Videman T, Battié MC. The influence of occupation on lumbar degeneration. *Spine.* 1999; **24**: 1164–1168

Wood KB, Garvey TA, Gundry C, Heithoff KB. Magnetic resonance imaging of the thoracic spine. *J Bone Jt Surg.* 1995; **77A**: 1631–1638

Wood KB, Blair JM, Aepple DM, Schendel MJ, Garvey TA, Gundry CR, Heithoff KB. The natural history of asymptomatic thoracic disc herniations. *Spine.* 1997; **22**: 525–530

A3 Influence of Physical Activity on Architecture and Density of Bones. An Overview of Observations in Humans

There are numerous reports on increase in density of trabecular bone and increase in thickness of cortical bone following greater mechanical loading. In contrast, reduction in loading is often accompanied by a loss of bone mineral. In view of the severe problems resulting from the impaired strength of bones of osteoporosis patients, it seems reasonable to try to increase the strength of bones through increased physical activity or purpose-designed exercise program. Two questions are then of focal interest:
- The natural history of bone density in man shows a continuous decrease with age. Is it possible to slow down the rate of decrease, or even to reverse the process into an increase, by means of appropriate mechanical influences?
- Is it possible to make provision, when young or middle-aged, for the loss of bone strength resulting from the osteoporosis to be expected in old age?

Resorption of old and depositing of new bone are ultimately performed by specialized cells (osteoclasts and osteoblasts). To answer the above questions it is thus necessary to study mechanical influences on these cells (Lanyon, 1993; MacDonald and Gowen, 1993; Jones et al., 1995; McLeod et al., 1998). A number of mechanical signals that could potentially trigger and control the activity of the bone resorbing and depositing cells are under discussion and investigation: strain, strain rate, strain gradients, hydrostatic pressure of the water component of bone, and electrical fields originating from the deformation of the bone mineral.

In the past, animal experiments have provided important data on the effect of mechanical influences on the cortical and trabecular bone of long bones. Experiments quantifying the mechanical loading showed that remodeling of bones is induced, not by static (or only very gradually changing) strain but by dynamic strain, which changes rapidly with time (Lanyon, 1992). Strain of less than 0.001 or complete immobilization results in bone resorption (Rubin and Lanyon, 1985; Gross and Rubin, 1995; Qin et al., 1998). Strains of more than 0.004, unusual (as compared with normal physiologic use) strains, rapid change of strain (high strain rate) and differences in strain between

neighboring volume elements of a bone (strain gradients) stimulate bone deposition (Lanyon, 1996; Mosley et al., 1997; Gross et al., 1997).

Apart from mechanical stimuli, the activity of cells in the human body is subject to a large number of additional influences. For this reason, we cannot reasonably expect mechanical stimuli that produce certain effects with isolated cells to produce identical effects with respect to the remodeling of bones in our bodies. In addition to studies in the field of cell biology and animal experiments, observations in humans are thus indispensable sources of information, specifically on long-term and long-lasting effects of mechanical stimuli on bones.

Methods for measuring bone density and bone mineral content

To quantify the effects of mechanical stimuli on density and architecture of bone, the following methods are employed:
- measurement of the calcium balance (difference between uptake and excretion of calcium);
- measurement of the thickness of cortical bone layers from radiographs;
- determination of bone mineral density from the absorption of γ- or roentgen radiation; and
- determination of the density of the trabecular bone by quantitative computed tomography (see Chapter 14).

If the calcium content of a diet is known, a measurement of calcium excretion can be employed to determine whether there is a net calcium uptake or loss. Excretion of calcium occurs via urine, stools, and sweat. The quantity of calcium excreted per day normally amounts to about 200 mg, approximately 22% of which is excreted in the urine, 76% in feces, and 2% in sweat (Donaldson et al., 1970). A difference between calcium uptake and excretion – a calcium balance not equal to zero – indicates a change in the activity of the osteoclast and osteoblast cells. Due to the physiologic, temporal delay between the activity of osteoclasts and osteoblasts, short-term observation of the calcium balance does not allow conclusions to be drawn on whether more bone is resorbed, or more newly produced bone deposited, in the long term.

Where the magnification is known, the thickness of layers of cortical bone can be measured from radiographic images. The density of bone mineral can be determined from the absorption of γ- or roentgen radiation (SPA, DPA, DEXA, see Chapter 14). The density, called bone mineral density (BMD), is quoted in units of g/cm^2 or g/cm. The bone mineral content (BMC) quantifies the mineral content of an entire organ and is quoted in units of grams (g). Computed tomography measures spatial densities (g/cm^3). In quantitative computed tomography (QCT) calibration devices are scanned together with the object of interest and the measured density is transformed into an equivalent density, given in units of mg/cm^3 K_2HPO_4.

▪ Effects of increased mechanical loading

Effects of increased loading have been documented in athletes from a variety of disciplines, in participants in exercise programs designed for the elderly, and in subjects exposed to high physical exertions in the workplace. Observations in athletes usually reveal drastic effects. This finding may be due to the loading of bones in the various athletic disciplines differing substantially from normal, everyday loading.

Jones *et al.* (1977) measured the thickness of the cortical bone of the humerus of professional tennis players, using anterior-posterior and lateral radiographic views of the dominant and non-dominant arms. The comparison showed the thickness of the cortical bone to be significantly greater on the dominant side compared with the control side (Table A3.1). In addition, the outer diameter of the humerus, measured in the dorsoventral as well as in the mediolateral direction, was shown to be about 10 % larger on the dominant, as compared with the non-dominant, side.

Nilsson and Westlin (1971) investigated the bone mineral density of the distal femur in four cohorts: top rank athletes at international and at national level, physically active subjects, and subjects with subnormal physical activity (Table A3.2). The athletic disciplines comprised hammer throwing, running, football, and swimming. Bone density was measured by SPA; the dimensions of the femur were measured as well, so that the bone mineral density could be given in units of g/cm^3. The results showed a marked increase in bone mineral density in the cohorts with high physical activity.

Granhed *et al.* (1987) investigated the bone mineral density of the vertebral body L3 of weightlifters in relation to training intensity. The results (Fig. A3.1) show impressively that bone density increased with increasing training intensity, i. e. with increasing mass lifted per year for training purposes. The bone mineral density of the cohort investigated ranged between 6.5 and 8.5 g/cm while that of subjects not engaged in this athletic discipline ranges between 2.0 and 5.0 g/cm (Hansson *et al.*, 1980).

Suominen (1993) collected data from 23 studies on athletes performed in the years 1988 to 1991. According to this compilation, young athletes with

Table A3.1 Thickness of the cortical bone of the humerus of tennis players, measured 11 cm proximally from the elbow joint. Numbers in parentheses ± 1 SD (Jones *et al.*, 1977)

	n	gender	dominant arm [cm]	control arm [cm]
anterior	44	m	0.76 (0.09)	0.55 (0.06)
	23	f	0.61 (0.07)	0.49 (0.07)
posterior	43	m	0.71 (0.10)	0.51 (0.07)
	22	f	0.58 (0.08)	0.46 (0.06)

Table A3.2 Bone mineral density in the distal femur. Numbers in parentheses ±1 SD. (Nilsson and Westlin, 1971)

	n	bone mineral density [g/cm^3]	mean age [y]
elite athletes	9	0.252 (0.049)	22.3
athletes	55	0.236 (0.049)	22.2
controls, active	24	0.213 (0.031)	22.5
controls, inactive	15	0.168 (0.037)	22.8

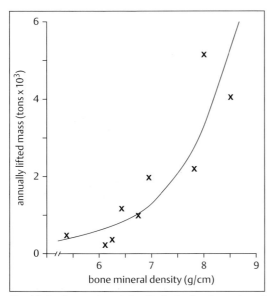

Fig. A3.**1** Bone mineral density in the lumbar spine of weight lifters in relation to the mass lifted per year for training purposes. The curve in the diagram is inserted only to guide the eye; it does not illustrate a functional relation (adapted from Granhed *et al.*, 1987). For comparison, the bone mineral density of the normal population ranges between 2 and 5 g/cm (Hansson *et al.*, 1980).

power and force training, e.g. in the disciplines weightlifting and wrestling, exhibit maximally increased bone mineral density. In general, the increase differs among bones and depends on the athletic discipline pursued. The increase with respect to non-athletes amounts typically to between 5% and 20%. Endurance training, however, for example in sports such as swimming and long-distance running, results in a decrease of between 1% and 10% in bone mineral density. A decrease of up to 20% is observed in cases of intense training and amenorrhea. Men and women in the age range 40 to 60 years with a history of long-term athletic training have a moderately increased bone mineral density compared with controls. Suominen draws attention to the problem that comparisons between athletes and subjects not engaged in athletic training may be confounded because the cohorts of athletes and of controls may differ with respect to general health status, standard of living, medication, and smoking.

It is of great interest to learn whether the increased bone mineral density observed in some disciplines is retained in later years, specifically beyond the age of 65. Düppe *et al.* (1996) investigated

the bone mineral density in the lumbar spine and the proximal femur of active and formerly active female football players. Active players exhibited a density increase of about 11% in the femur in relation to a control population; in the lumbar spine this increase was about 5%. No dependence on training intensity was observed. The mean age of the former football players was 40 years, and termination of their athletic activity occurred approximately 10 years previously. Former players exhibited a bone mineral density marginally higher than normal in the femur, but not in the lumbar spine.

Etherington *et al.* (1996) investigated the bone mineral density in the lumbar spine of female ex-elite athletes in the age range 40 to 65 years and of control cohorts with different degrees of physical activity. The study showed a 10% increase in bone mineral density in the lumbar spine of former athletes and very active controls, compared to relatively or totally inactive controls.

Granhed *et al.* (1988) investigated the bone mineral density in the lumbar spine of active wrestlers and weightlifters in the age ranges 12–20 years and 20–40 years, as well as of formerly active athletes and of controls (subjects who never engaged in athletics) between 40 and 70 years of age. The bone mineral density of active athletes showed a steep rise in the age range between 12 and 20 years (Fig. A3.**2**). This is thought to be due to skeletal maturation as well as to high loading of the lumbar spine. During the period of active elite performance between 20 and 40 years, bone mineral density stayed at a high level. Following termination of athletic activity, the bone mineral density decreased, exhibiting, in the age range between 40 and 60 years, no difference from controls who had never been engaged in athletics. Thus a permanent effect persisting in old age was not observed. This result agrees with that of a study by Karlsson *et al.* (1995) of former weightlifters, who exhibited no increased bone density compared with controls, in the age range above 65 years.

Encouraged by the observations in athletes, which undoubtedly demonstrate a relation between increased physical activity and increased bone density, a number of studies have been performed, with the aim of increasing the bone density of subjects aged above 55 years by means of purpose-designed, age-appropriate exercise programs. One example of such a study is that by Dalsky *et al.* (1988). These authors compared the bone mineral density in vertebral bodies L2–L4 of a cohort of 17 subjects, aged between 55 and 70 years, taking part in an exercise program composed of walking, jogging, and stair climbing, with that of a non-exercising control cohort of 18 subjects. After 9 months the mineral density of the exercising co-

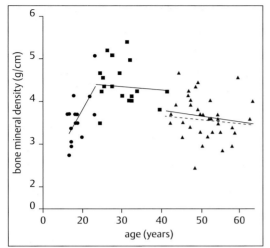

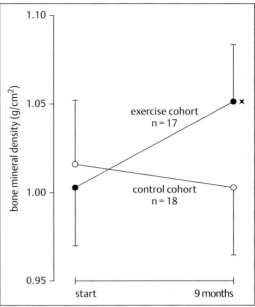

Fig. A3.**2** Age dependence of bone mineral density in vertebra L3 of weightlifters and wrestlers in the starting phase of high intensity training (solid circles), in the active phase (solid squares) and after cessation of the active phase (solid triangles). Also shown are the regression lines of bone density versus age for the three cohorts. The dashed line characterizes the average bone density of subjects who never engaged in athletic training (adapted from Granhed et al., 1988).

Fig. A3.**3** Effect of an exercise program, composed of jogging, walking on a moving belt, and stair climbing, on bone mineral density in the lumbar spine of a cohort aged between 55 and 70 years. The bone mineral density of the exercise group was increased significantly after 9 months of exercise by approximately 5%; in the control group no significant change in bone mineral density was observed (adapted from Dalsky et al., 1988).

hort had increased by 5.2% while that of the control cohort exhibited no significant change (Fig. A3.**3**). Part of the exercise cohort continued the training for a further 13 months, while the remaining part terminated the training. After this additional 13 months, the bone mineral density had increased by 6.1%, in relation to its initial value, in those subjects who had continued the training, but by only 1.1% in those who had terminated the training. The bone density of the non-exercising subjects showed no change in the 27-month observation period.

The result of the study by Dalsky and colleagues agrees with those of comparable studies of elderly subjects by other authors (Krølner et al., 1983; Bloomfield et al., 1993; Need et al., 1995; Ernst, 1998; for an overview see Chilibeck et al., 1995). Moderate physical exercise programs regularly result in a 2 to 4% increase in bone mineral density; no further increase is observed (Mosekilde, 1995). The amount of density increase depends on the type of training, i.e. on whether endurance training, walking, or resistance training is performed (Chilibeck et al., 1995, Pruitt et al., 1995). If the training intensity of elderly subjects is set too high, a decrease in bone density is occasionally observed (Michel et al., 1989).

It might be very interesting to compare observations made in long-term athletic training and in ex-

ercise programs for the elderly with observations in subjects involuntarily exposed to long-term 'high level physical training' at certain physically demanding workplaces. Surprisingly, very few studies have focused on this topic. Karlsson et al. (1993) determined the bone mineral density in the spine and the extremities of professional ballet dancers. The training program of male and female dancers induces high loading of the trunk and the lower extremities. The study showed that the bone mineral density of dancers compared with controls is higher in the hip and femur, but not in the spine. After termination of the career, bone density decreased more rapidly compared with controls.

Drerup et al. (1999) employed QCT to measure the trabecular bone density in the central volume of vertebra L3 of 14 subjects who had been exposed to whole body vibration for 19.9 years on average. This cohort was composed of drivers of earthmoving machinery in an opencast lignite mine. Their spines were exposed to vibration in the frequency range between 1 and 15 Hz and, in addition, to shock loading when dredging or driving on uneven

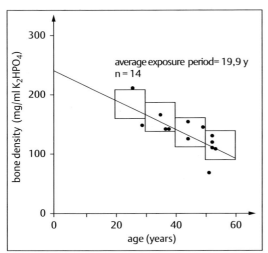

Fig. A3.**4**   Trabecular bone density of vertebra L3 after long-tem exposure to whole-body vibration and shock loading. The straight line indicates the normal value of bone density in relation to age; the rectangles show the normal age-related ranges of bone density (Felsenberg *et al.*, 1988). Adapted from Drerup *et al.*, 1999.

ground. Fig. A3.**4** shows the measured bone density in relation to the age of the subjects. For comparison purposes, the gender- and age-related standard bone density values (Felsenberg *et al.*, 1988) are indicated by the rectangles. Within the statistical error limits, the bone density of the exposed cohort showed no difference from that of non-exposed subjects.

Effects of reduced mechanical loading

Donaldson *et al.* (1970) observed the calcium balance of three male volunteers, aged 21 to 22 years, during a 30- to 36-week period of bed rest. This period had been preceded by 1 week of normal activity during which the volunteers were on a diet with a known calcium content. This served to determine reference values of calcium excretion. The diet was then left unchanged for the entire duration of the study. During the one-week pre-test phase, daily urine samples were taken. In the course of the bed rest period urine, sweat, and stool samples were taken every seven days for analysis of their calcium content. Starting from the 12th week of bed rest, the bone mineral density of the calcaneus was measured every six weeks by SPA (with correction for the soft tissue portion). After the ending of bed rest, the bone density was monitored for a further 30 weeks.

Throughout the bed-rest period, the amount of calcium excreted daily exceeded the intake (Fig. A3.**5**). The total amount of calcium lost during the bed-rest period was estimated to amount to approximately 4 % of the total calcium content of the body. From the 12th week of bed rest, the bone mineral density of the calcaneus decreased by between 25 % and 45 % up to the 18th or 24th week respectively. After the bed-rest period, the mineral density increased again, exceeding its initial value after 36 weeks (Fig. A3.**6**). The authors hypothesize the effects of unloading to be especially pronounced in those bones that are normally subject to high loading.

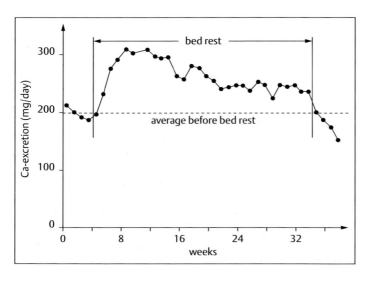

Fig. A3.**5**   Calcium excretion in the urine of a healthy volunteer during 30 weeks of bed rest (adapted from Donaldson *et al.*, 1970).

Fig. A3.**6** Bone mineral density in the os calcis of three healthy volunteers during (solid symbols) and after (open symbols) 30 to 36 weeks of bed rest (adapted from Donaldson *et al.*, 1970).

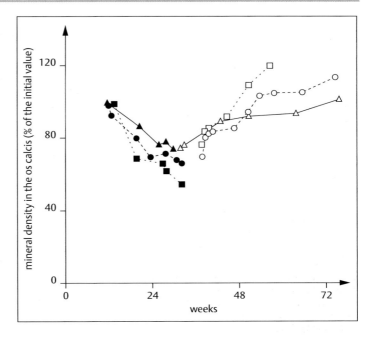

Parfitt (1981) compared the calcium balance and the change in bone mineral density of the calcaneus of the Skylab II, III, and IV astronauts (1973/74) with the data recorded by Donaldson *et al.* (1970) during prolonged bed rest. He noted that values for negative calcium balance and mineral loss in the calcaneus (Fig. A3.**7**) were comparable in the astronauts and the bed rest volunteers. According to Parfitt, the negative calcium balance and the mineral loss allow no conclusion to be drawn on whether more bone is deposited than resorbed in the long run. A negative calcium balance initially indicates an increased turnover of bone tissue, because a bone remodeling process always starts with resorption before new bone is (possibly) deposited. Despite the initial increase seen in calcium excretion, it is quite possible that, after a certain time in weightlessness, normal balance may be restored. If this were the case, we would not expect harmful effects to be induced by a long-term stay in weightlessness, and after the return from the journey the bone mineral density should be restored to its initial value. Alternatively, an irreversible loss of bone mineral might persist after a longer stay in weightlessness. This would result in a higher fracture risk.

Whedon (1984) reported on calcium excretion data recorded during the 84-day Skylab IV mission (Fig. A3.**8**). According to these results, calcium excretion increases during weightlessness in a fashion very similar to that seen during long-term bed rest (Donaldson *et al.*, 1970). After the return from

the mission, the excretion was restored to normal within three weeks. Parallel to the loss of calcium, the astronauts suffered a loss of muscle tissue. Exercise programs during the flight failed to prevent this loss. The author concludes that losses during 8- to 10-month space flights can still be tolerated.

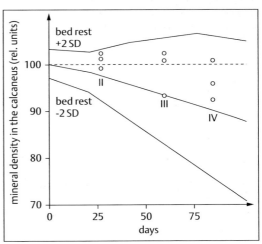

Fig. A3.**7** Change of the bone mineral density in the calcaneus of three Skylab astronauts in relation to the initial value and to the change in mineral density observed during bed rest. The middle curve shows the average mineral loss during bed rest; in addition the curves for average loss ± 2 SD are shown (adapted from Parfitt, 1981).

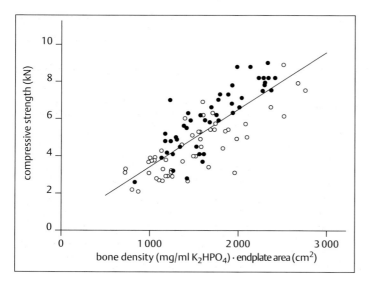

Fig. A3.**8** Calcium excretion in the urine of an astronaut before, during, and after an 84 day flight in Skylab IV (adapted from Whedon, 1984).

Longer missions might well give rise to serious problems if no preventive measures were taken.

Grigoriev *et al.* (1998) communicated data on bone mineral density in the lumbar spine of 18 astronauts who had spent between 4.5 and 14.5 months in the space module. At the end of the flights bone mineral density in the lumbar spine was 5.6 % lower, on average, than at the start. However, the mineral density in the cranial part of the skeleton remained unchanged. Similar observations were reported by Miyamoto *et al.* (1998). During the mission the astronauts under investigation lost 3 % of the bone mineral in the lumbar spine (L2–L4), while the mineral density of the skull increased in this period. Overall, it can be concluded that the stay in weightlessness affects bone mineral density in the same fashion as strict bed rest. A mineral decrease of between 1 % and 2 % per month is observed in single bones (Holick, 1998).

The result of an experiment *in vitro* measuring the strength of human lumbar vertebrae (Brinckmann *et al.*, 1989) indicates that the decrease in strength observed after periods of unloading or inactivity is probably not due to decreased bone density alone. Fig. A3.**9** shows the compressive strength of vertebrae in relation to the product of trabecular bone density and endplate area. In addition, the graph includes the regression line giving the average statistical relationship between strength and the product of density and area. Strength data of specimens from donors who had been bedridden for at least 4 weeks, or who had been severely restricted in their physical activity for more than 2 years prior to death are marked with open circles. It is striking that the strength of

Fig. A3.**9** Compressive strength of lumbar vertebrae *in vitro* in relation to the product of bone density and endplate area. The regression line shows the mean relationship of strength to the product of density and area. Open symbols designate specimens from donors who were either bedridden for more than 4 weeks prior to death, or maximally restricted in their physical activity during their last two years of life. The strength of such specimens is significantly lower than that predicted from the product of trabecular density and endplate area. (Adapted from Brinckmann *et al.*, 1989).

these specimens was generally lower than that of the rest of the study material. We conclude that, in addition to loss of bone density (already allowed for in this graph), another process, as yet unknown, induces a further reduction in compressive strength during the period of inactivity. Hypothetically, changes in the architecture of the trabecular bone could occur (Palle *et al.*, 1992). Alternatively, the material properties of the organic component of bone might undergo changes eventually leading to reduced bone strength.

Summary and outlook

High loading of the skeleton by athletic power training increases bone mineral density. The recorded increase is specific to the athletic discipline pursued. Typically, the relative gain ranges between 5 % and 20 % at maximum. Only in cases of exceptionally high athletic loading is an increase beyond these limits observed. In addition to the increase in mineral density, an increase occurs in the thickness of the cortical bone in the long bones of highly loaded extremities. In contrast, endurance training, or high training intensity combined with amenorrhea, results in a 1 % to 20 % loss of bone mineral.

In the age range of 40 to 65 years, bone mineral density of ex-elite athletes stays slightly higher than normal or returns to normal. Above 65 years of age, bone mineral density in the lumbar spine of former athletes exhibits no difference from that of subjects of the same age who had never engaged in any athletic activity whatsoever.

In elderly subjects, age-appropriate exercise programs increase the bone density in the lumbar spine by 2 % to 6 %, at most, after 1 to 2 years of exercise. Continuation of the exercises induces no further increase in mineral density. In view of this marginal increase, offering such programs for the elderly appears hardly to be worthwhile, because we can expect the compressive strength of the vertebral bodies to be increased by only the same percentage, at most. While conventional exercise programs thus have virtually no influence on the strength of vertebral bodies, their positive effect on muscle force and regulation of the circulation is indisputable.

Only few studies have explored the effects of long-term physical loading at the workplace on bone mineral density or trabecular bone density. Intensive training of professional dancers induces a minor increase in mineral density; this gain is not sustained after cessation of the training. Long-term exposure to whole-body vibration and shock loading, producing a mechanical stimulus broadly comparable to exercise programs for the elderly, does not increase the trabecular bone density in the lumbar spine.

Inactivity due to a prolonged period of bed rest or of weightlessness leads to a decrease in bone mineral density. There are indications that the trabecular architecture and the mechanical properties of the organic component of bones might be altered as well. In general, a decrease in mineral density, of the order of 1 %–2 % per month, in the weight-bearing bones of the skeleton is observed. The mechanism underlying the rapid excretion of calcium occurring under such circumstances is not yet fully understood (Holick, 1998). After bed rest for 6 months, or a stay in weightlessness of up to three months, the mineral loss appears to be reversible. However, observations in astronauts currently allow no prediction of the time course of bone mineral density loss and its regression during, and after, longer stays in weightlessness.

The modest increase in bone mineral density resulting from intense athletic training (i. e. <20 % gain), and the surprising and unexplained absence of an increase in bone density during long-term exposure at the workplace, raise little hope of exerting a positive influence on the bone mineral density of the elderly with the exercise programs currently in use. It appears that completely new paths will have to be pursued, and new procedures tested, if this aim is to be realized.

Further reading

Review papers

Duncan RL, Turner CH. Mechanotransduction and the functional response of bone to mechanical strain. *Calcif Tissue Int.* 1995; **57**: 344–358 [review paper, 225 references]

Original papers cited in the text or the figures

Bloomfield SA, Williams NI, Lamb DR, Jackson RD. Nonweightbearing exercise may increase lumbar spine bone mineral density in healthy postmenopausal women. *Am J Phys Med Rehab.* 1993; **72**: 204–209

Brinckmann P, Biggemann M, Hilweg D. Prediction of the compressive strength of lumbar vertebrae. *Clinical Biomechanics.* 1989; **4** Suppl 2: S1–S27

Chilibeck PD, Sale DG, Webber CE. Exercise and bone mineral density. *Sports Med.* 1995; **19**: 103–122 [review paper, 162 references]

Dalsky GP, Stocke KS, Ehsani AA, Slatopolsky E, Lee WC, Birge SJ. Weight-bearing exercise training and lumbar bone mineral content in postmenopausal women. *Ann Int Med.* 1988; **108**: 824–828

Donaldson CL, Hulley SB, Vogel JM, Hattner RS, Bayers JH, McMilllan DE. Effect of prolonged bed rest on bone mineral. *Metabolism.* 1970; **19**: 1071–1084

Drerup B, Granitzka M. Assheuer J, Zerlett G. Assessment of disc injury in subjects exposed to long-term whole body vibration. *Eur Spine J.* 1999; **8**: 458–467

Düppe H, Gärdsell P, Johnell O, Ornstein E. Bone mineral density in female junior, senior and former football players. *Osteoporosis Int.* 1996; **6**: 437–441

Ernst E. Exercise for female osteoporosis. A systematic review of randomised clinical trials. *Sports Med.* 1998; **25**: 359–368 [review paper, 78 references]

Etherington J, Harris PA, Nandra D, Hart DJ, Wolman RL, Doyle DV, Spector TD. The effect of weight-bearing exercise on bone mineral density: a study of female ex-elite athletes and the general population. *J Bone Min Res.* 1996; **11**: 1333–1338

Felsenberg D, Kalender WA, Banzer D, Schmilinsky G, Heyse M, Fischer E, Schneider U. Quantitative computertomografische Knochenmineralgehaltsbestimmung. *Fortschr Röntgenstr.* 1988; **148**: 431–436

Granhed H, Jonson R, Hansson T. The loads on the lumbar spine during extreme weight lifting. *Spine.* 1987; **12**: 55–58

Granhed H, Jonson R, Keller T, Hansson T. *Short and long-term effects of vigorous physical activity on bone mineral in the human lumbar spine.* Thesis. Göteborg: University of Göteborg; 1988

Grigoriev AL, Oganov AV, Bakulin AV, Poliakov VV, Voronin LI, *et al.* Clinical and physiological evaluation of bone changes among astronauts after long-term space flights. *Aviakosm Ekolog Med.* 1998; **32**: 21–25

Gross TS, Rubin CT. Uniformity of resorptive bone loss induced by disuse. *J Orthop Res.* 1995; **13**: 708–714

Gross TS, Edwards JL, McLeod KJ, Rubin CT. Strain gradients correlate with sites of periostal bone formation. *J Bone Min Res.* 1997; **12**: 982–988

Hansson T, Roos B, Nachemson A. The bone mineral content and ultimate compressive strength of lumbar vertebrae. *Spine.* 1980; **5**: 46–55

Holick MF. Perspective on the impact of weightlessness on calcium and bone metabolism. *Bone.* 1998; **22** (5 Suppl): 105S–111S

Jones HH, Priest JD, Hayes WC, Tichenor CC, Nagel DA. Humeral hypertrophy in response to exercise. *J Bone Jt Surg.* 1977; **59A**: 204–208

Jones D, Leivseth G, Tenbosch J. Mechano-reception in osteoblast-like cells. *Biochem Cell Biol.* 1995; **73**: 525–534

Karlsson MK, Johnell O, Obrant KJ. Bone mineral density in professional ballet dancers. *Bone Mineral.* 1993; **21**: 163–169

Karlsson MK, Johnell O, Obrant KJ. Is bone mineral density advantage maintained long-term in previous weight lifters? *Calcif Tissue Int.* 1995; **57**: 325–328

Krølner B, Toft B, Nielsen SP, Tøndevold E. Physical exercise as prophylaxis against involutional vertebral bone loss: a controlled trial. *Clinical Science.* 1983; **64**: 541–546

Lanyon LE. Control of bone architecture by functional load bearing. *J Bone Min Res.* 1992; **7** Suppl 2: S369–S375

Lanyon LE. Osteocytes, strain detection, bone modeling and remodeling. *Calcif Tiss Int.* 1993; **53** Suppl 1: S102–S107

Lanyon LE. Using functional loading to influence bone mass and architecture: objectives, mechanisms, and relationship with estrogen of the mechanically adaptive process in bone. *Bone.* 1996; **18** Suppl: 37S–43S

MacDonald BR, Gowen M. The cell biology of bone. *Bailliere's Clin Rheumatol.* 1993; **7**: 421–443 [review paper, 93 references]

McLeod KJ, Rubin CT, Otter MW, Qin YX. Skeletal cell stresses and bone adaption. *Am J Med Sci.* 1998; **316**: 176–183

Michel BA, Bloch DA, Fries JF. Weight-bearing exercise, over-exercise, and lumbar bone density over age 50 years. *Arch Intern Med.* 1989; **149**: 2325–2329

Miyamoto A, Shigematsu T, Fukunaga T, Kawakami K, Mukai C, *et al.* Medical baseline collection on bone and muscle change with space flight. *Bone.* 1998; **22** (5 Suppl): 79S–82S

Mosekilde L. Osteoporosis and exercise. *Bone.* 1995; **17**: 193–195

Mosley JR, March BM, Lynch J, Lanyon LE. Strain magnitude related changes in whole bone architecture in growing rats. *Bone.* 1997; **20**: 191–198

Need AG, Wishart JM, Scopacasa F, Horowitz M, Morris HA, Nordin BEC. Effect of physical activity on femoral bone density in men. *BMJ.* 1995; **310**: 1501–1502

Nilsson BE, Westlin NE. Bone density in athletes. *Clin Orthop Rel Res.* 1971; **77**: 179–182

Palle S, Vico L, Bourrin S, Alexandre C. Bone tissue response to four-month antiorthostatic bedrest: a bone histomorphometric study. *Calcif Tissue Int.* 1992; **51**: 189–194

Parfitt AM. Bone effects of space flight. Analysis by quantum concept of bone remodelling. *Acta Astronautica.* 1981; **8**: 1083–1090

Pruitt LA, Taaffe DR, Marcus R. Effects of a one year high-intensity versus low-intensity resistance training program on bone mineral density in older women. *J Bone Min Res.* 1995; **10**: 1788–1795

Qin YX, Rubin CT, McLeod KJ. Nonlinear dependence of loading intensity and cycle number in the maintenance of bone mass and morphology. *J Orthop Res.* 1998; **16**: 482–489

Rubin CT, Lanyon LE. Regulation of bone mass by mechanical strain magnitude. *Calcif Tiss Int.* 1985; **37**: 411–417

Suominen H. Bone mineral density and long term exercise. An overview of cross-sectional athlete studies. *Sports Medicine.* 1993; **16**: 316–330 [review paper, 72 references]

Whedon GD. Disuse osteoporosis: physiological aspects. *Calcif Tiss Int.* 1984; **36**: S146–S150

B1 Mathematical Description of Translation and Rotation in a Plane

Cartesian coordinates

The description of translation and rotation in a plane was given in Chapter 4 in a graphical fashion without the aid of algebraic tools. This allowed the basic concepts to come across vividly without any calculations having to be performed. If, however, the motion of more than one single object is to be monitored, or if high precision is required, it is advisable to use a coordinate-based calculation instead of attempting a graphic solution. This chapter introduces a simple concept, one dispensing with vectors and matrices, for the mathematical description of motion in a plane. In the last section of this chapter it is shown that all equations can be formulated in matrix notation as well. Matrix notation is shorter and more to the point than coordinate notation.

If the motion of an object is documented, for example by a series of photographic images, geometric information extracted from the images has to be mathematically processed. Relations between each single image and the recording device (camera) on the one hand, and between consecutive images on the other, have to be established. Coordinate systems are used for this purpose. Within each image the location of an image point can be unequivocally described, for example by an ordered pair of numbers designating the distance of the point from the lower and left edges of the image. In this case the edges of the image represent the coordinate system; the distances are the relevant point coordinates.

To introduce a geometric reference system into what is, in principle, an infinitely extended plane, we draw a horizontal and a vertical line (Fig. B1.1). The intersecting lines form the xy coordinate system. The horizontal axis (x-axis) is termed the 'abscissa'; the vertical axis (y-axis) is termed the 'ordinate'. The point of intersection of the axes is termed the 'origin' of the coordinate system. The axes bear scales whose zero point coincides with the origin of the coordinate system. Positive values of the scale of the x-axis are usually plotted to the right of the origin, and negative values to the left. Positive values of the scale of the y-axis are usually plotted upwards, and negative values downwards.

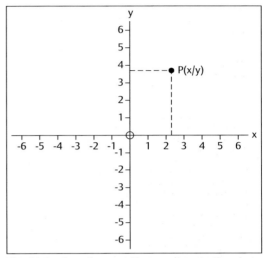

Fig. B1.1 Cartesian coordinate system in the plane. The location of a point P(x/y) in a plane is unequivocally described by two numbers (x/y). If a perpendicular is drawn from P to the horizontal axis, the perpendicular intersects the axis at a distance of x units from the origin of the coordinate system. Likewise, the intersection of the perpendicular from P on the vertical axis occurs at a distance of y units from the origin.

The location of a point is described by its coordinates x,y. The coordinates are those scale values where a perpendicular from the point intersects the coordinate axes. Conversely, the location of a point P can be constructed when its coordinates x,y are known. In the example shown in Fig. B1.1, point P has the coordinates x = 2.3 and y = 3.7 (in units of the scales on the axes).

Translation

A point P (x/y) is translated (Fig. B1.2). The shifted point is designated P'(x'/y'). In general, point P' is designated the geometric 'image' of point P; x' and y' are the image coordinates. Imaging is described by the mathematical relation between the initial and the image coordinates. In case of a translation

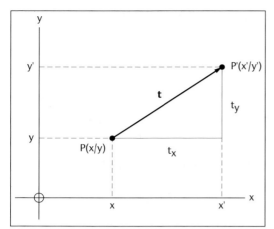

Fig. B1.**2** Plane translation. A point P with coordinates x/y is linearly shifted by t_x, in the x-direction, and by t_y, in the y-direction, to its final location with coordinates x'/y'. P'(x'/y') is termed the image of point P(x/y).

the shifts t_x and t_y are to be added to the initial coordinates

(1)
$$x' = x + t_x$$
$$y' = y + t_y$$

The shifts t_x and t_y may bear positive or negative signs. Conversely, with known coordinates for the initial point P(x/y) and the shifted point P'(x'/y'), the shifts t_x and t_y can be calculated

(2)
$$t_x = x' - x$$
$$t_y = y' - y$$

▨ Rotation

To describe a rotation, a center of rotation and an angle of rotation have to be specified. In the simplest case, a rotation can occur around the origin of the coordinate system (Fig. B1.**3**). Let us consider point P(x/y). Its distance from the origin amounts to $r = \sqrt{x^2 + y^2}$. The line OP is inclined by an angle α with respect to the x-axis. For the coordinates of P it holds that

(3)
$$x = r \cdot \cos\alpha$$
$$y = r \cdot \sin\alpha$$

Angles are counted from $-180°$ to $+180°$, or alternatively from $0°$ to $+360°$. Depending on the angle, the functions sine and cosine assume values between -1.0 and $+1.0$.

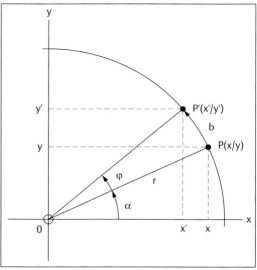

Fig. B1.**3**   Plane rotation of a point P(x/y) about the origin of the coordinate system. In the initial state the line OP is inclined by an angle φ with respect to the x-axis. During the rotational motion the point moves along a circle with radius r = OP. After the rotation along the arc b to the final location P', the line OP' is inclined at an angle $(\alpha + \varphi)$ with respect to the x-axis. In this diagram as well as in the following ones the arrowheads on the circular arcs show the direction of rotation. In the example shown, both α and φ are positive.

If point P is rotated by an angle φ, the image point P' (x'/y') is obtained. The line OP' is inclined by an angle $\alpha + \varphi$ with respect to the x-axis. Similarly to equation (3), the coordinates x',y' of the image point are obtained from

(4)
$$x' = r \cdot \cos(\alpha + \varphi)$$
$$y' = r \cdot \sin(\alpha + \varphi)$$

Using the addition formulae for sine and cosine functions

(5)
$$\cos(\alpha + \varphi) = \cos\alpha \cdot \cos\varphi - \sin\alpha \cdot \sin\varphi$$
$$\sin(\alpha + \varphi) = \sin\alpha \cdot \cos\varphi + \cos\alpha \cdot \sin\varphi$$

and employing (3), we obtain for the coordinates of the image point

(6)
$$x' = x \cdot \cos\varphi - y \cdot \sin\varphi$$
$$y' = x \cdot \sin\varphi + y \cdot \cos\varphi$$

In the general case a rotation is performed about a center of rotation C(x_m/y_m), see Fig. B1.**4**. The gen-

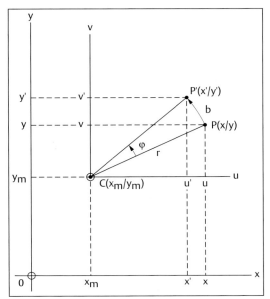

Fig. B1.4 Plane rotation of a point P(x/y) about an arbitrary center of rotation $C(x_m/y_m)$. The point moves along a circle with radius r = CP about an angle φ. By introducing relative coordinates $u = x - x_m$, $v = y - y_m$, this case is reduced to that illustrated in Fig. B1.3.

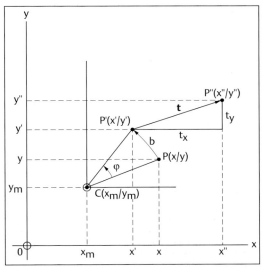

Fig. B1.5 Motion combined from translation and rotation. Point P(x/y) is rotated about the center of rotation $C(x_m/y_m)$ by an angle φ to point P' (x'/y'). P' is then shifted by t_x, t_y to point P'' (x''/y''). t_x and t_y define the translation vector **t**.

eral case can be reduced to that of a rotation about the origin (described above) by introducing an additional uv-coordinate system at point C. This coordinate system is shifted parallel with respect to the xy-coordinate system by x_m in x-direction and by y_m in y-direction. The coordinates u and v are given by the differences

$$(7) \qquad \begin{aligned} u &= x - x_m \\ v &= y - y_m \end{aligned}$$

If a rotation is performed in the uv-system, the coordinates of the image point P' read

$$(8) \qquad \begin{aligned} u' &= u \cdot \cos\varphi - v \cdot \sin\varphi \\ v' &= u \cdot \sin\varphi + v \cdot \cos\varphi \end{aligned}$$

In a last step a return is made to the xy-system by replacing the u,v with the x,y-based equation (7) and thus obtaining the image coordinates

$$(9) \qquad \begin{aligned} x' &= x_m + (x - x_m) \cdot \cos\varphi - (y - y_m) \cdot \sin\varphi \\ y' &= y_m + (x - x_m) \cdot \sin\varphi + (y - y_m) \cdot \cos\varphi \end{aligned}$$

Motion combining translation and rotation

With a given center of rotation $C(x_m/y_m)$ point P is rotated in a first step by an angle φ (Fig. B1.5). The intermediate image, calculated using equation (9), is designated P' (x'/y'). In a second step P' is shifted to the final location P'' (x''/y''). The coordinates of the final image (both steps combined) are

$$(10) \qquad \begin{aligned} x'' &= x_m + (x - x_m) \cdot \cos\varphi - (y - y_m) \cdot \sin\varphi + t_x \\ y'' &= y_m + (x - x_m) \cdot \sin\varphi + (y - y_m) \cdot \cos\varphi + t_y \end{aligned}$$

The equations (10) can be re-written as

$$(11) \qquad \begin{aligned} x'' &= x \cdot \cos\varphi - y \cdot \sin\varphi + a_x \\ y'' &= x \cdot \sin\varphi + y \cdot \cos\varphi + a_y \end{aligned}$$

with

$$(12) \qquad \begin{aligned} a_x &= x_m - x_m \cdot \cos\varphi + y_m \cdot \sin\varphi + t_x \\ a_y &= y_m - x_m \cdot \sin\varphi - y_m \cdot \cos\varphi + t_y \end{aligned}$$

Equation (11) describes the general case of plane motion, i. e. rotation about an arbitrary center of rotation $C(x_m/y_m)$ by an angle φ and shift (translation) by t_x, t_y, algebraically in the simplest fashion. From a formal point of view, equation (11) can also be interpreted as a description of a rotation about the origin of the coordinate system and a subsequent translation by a_x, a_y. Formulae (11) and (12) comprise the special cases of pure translation and pure rotation.

According to the theorem mentioned in Chapter 4, that a motion combining rotation and translation can also always be represented by a pure rotation (i. e. by a motion without a translation component), the parameters of this rotation should be deducible from equation (11). Unlike the graphical solution to this problem, the algebraic determination of the location of the center of rotation is not based on the construction of the perpendicular bisectors. Another algorithm (path of calculation) is better suited. Use is made of the knowledge that, in a pure rotation, the center of rotation is the only point that does not move. Such a point is termed the 'fixed point' of the image. Its coordinates may be x_F and y_F. As the coordinates of the fixed point are not changed (i. e. they remain identical after the imaging procedure to what they were before) it holds that

(13)
$$x_F = x_F \cdot \cos\varphi - y_F \cdot \sin\varphi + a_x$$
$$y_F = x_F \cdot \sin\varphi + y_F \cdot \cos\varphi + a_y$$

With a known angle of rotation φ, center of rotation x_m, y_m and translation t_x, t_y, the coordinates x_F, y_F of the fixed point can be determined from equation (13). The intermediate steps of the simple, but somewhat lengthy, conversion are omitted here; only the final outcome is stated

(14)
$$x_F = (a_x - a_y \cdot \cot(\varphi/2))/2$$
$$y_F = (a_y + a_x \cdot \cot(\varphi/2))/2$$

▨ **Determination of the imaging parameters from two points and their images**

We assume the coordinates of two points (x,y) and their images (x',y') to be known. The task is to determine the imaging parameters. For this purpose equations (11) are employed. The imaging parameters are the angle of rotation φ and the translations a_x, a_y. (The information on the intermediate image in the u,v coordinate system, see equations (8) and (9), is lost and cannot be retrieved subsequently.) The three parameters cannot be determined from one single point and its image because only two equations are available. If, however, co-

ordinates of two points and their images are available, the number of equations suffices to determine three unknowns. The calculation starts by inserting the coordinates of the points $P(x_1/y_1)$, $Q(x_2/y_2)$ and their images $P'(x_1'/y_1')$, $Q'(x_2'/y_2')$ into equation (11), thus obtaining 4 equations

(15)
$$x_1' = x_1 \cdot \cos\varphi - y_1 \cdot \sin\varphi + a_x$$
$$y_1' = x_1 \cdot \sin\varphi + y_1 \cdot \cos\varphi + a_y$$
$$x_2' = x_2 \cdot \cos\varphi - y_2 \cdot \sin\varphi + a_x$$
$$y_2' = x_2 \cdot \sin\varphi + y_2 \cdot \cos\varphi + a_y$$

(The double quotation marks in (11) are replaced with single quotation marks.) In a first step the angle of rotation is determined by calculating the differences between the coordinates

(16)
$$x_2' - x_1'$$
$$= (x_2 - x_1) \cdot \cos\varphi - (y_2 - y_1) \cdot \sin\varphi$$
$$y_2' - y_1'$$
$$= (x_2 - x_1) \cdot \sin\varphi + (y_2 - y_1) \cdot \cos\varphi$$

This yields an equation for the tangent of the angle of rotation

(17)
$$\tan\varphi = Z/N$$
$$\varphi = \operatorname{atan}(Z/N)$$

with

(18)
$$Z =$$
$$(x_2 - x_1) \cdot (y_2' - y_1') - (y_2 - y_1) \cdot (x_2' - x_1')$$
$$N =$$
$$(x_2 - x_1) \cdot (x_2' - x_1') + (y_2 - y_1) \cdot (y_2' - y_1')$$

If the angle φ equals zero, the motion considered is a pure translation. In this case it holds (as both points translate by the same amount) that

(19)
$$x_1' - x_1 = x_2' - x_2$$
$$y_1' - y_1 = y_2' - y_2$$

With a known angle of rotation, parameters a_x and a_y can be determined from equation (11). For this purpose we insert the coordinates of one point (either one of both points) into this equation. By choosing point P and its image P' we obtain

(20)
$$a_x = x_1' - x_1 \cdot \cos\varphi + y_1 \cdot \sin\varphi$$
$$a_y = y_1' - x_1 \cdot \sin\varphi - y_1 \cdot \cos\varphi$$

As a result all parameters of the motion (the imaging) are known from equations (17) and (20). If the motion is to be represented by a pure rotation, the coordinates of the relevant center of rotation can

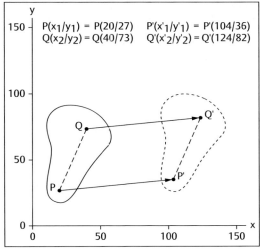

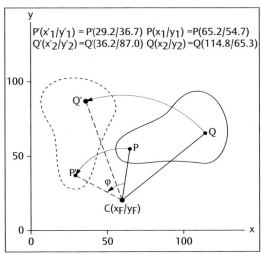

Fig. B1.6 Numerical example of a pure translation. As the differences between the x- and y-coordinates, $x'_1 - x_1 = x'_2 - x_2$ and $y'_1 - y_1 = y'_2 - y_2$, are equal, it follows that the motion did not contain a rotational component. In other words, the motion was a pure translation.

Fig. B1.7 Numerical example of a pure rotation. The angle of rotation and location of the center of rotation are to be determined. In a first step the angle of rotation is determined from the coordinate differences $x_2 - x_1$, $y_2 - y_1$ and $x'_2 - x'_1$, $y'_2 - y'_1$. In a second step the center of rotation $C(x_F/y_F)$ is obtained.

be calculated from equation (14) (the angle of rotation φ being identical in each case).

For the purpose of illustration, two problems solved graphically in Chapter 4 will now be solved algebraically. In the first example (Figs. 4.1 and B1.6) it will be shown that the motion is a pure translation. For this purpose, a coordinate system is introduced. $P(x_1/y_1)$ and $Q(x_2/y_2)$ are the landmarks of the body before the motion; $P'(x'_1/y'_1)$ and $Q'(x'_2/y'_2)$ are their images after the motion. Calculation of the differences between the coordinates yields

$$x'_1 - x_1 = 104 - 20 = 84 \text{ and}$$
$$y'_1 - y_1 = 36 - 27 = 9 \text{ (points P' and P)}$$
$$x'_2 - x_2 = 124 - 40 = 84 \text{ and}$$
$$y'_2 - y_2 = 82 - 73 = 9 \text{ (points Q' and Q)}$$

We see that the x- as well as the y-differences are equal. This means that points P and Q moved in an identical fashion. The motion was a pure translation with $t_x = 84$ and $t_y = 9$ (see equations 2 and 19). For the sake of completeness it is pointed out that, according to equation (17), the quantity Z and thus the tangent of the angle of rotation (and thus the angle of rotation as well) are equal to zero. This indicates again that a pure translation took place.

In the second example, the angle as well as the center of rotation are to be determined (Figs. 4.3a and B1.7). The differences between the coordinates are

$$x_2 - x_1 = 114.8 - 65.2 = 49.6 \text{ and}$$
$$y_2 - y_1 = 65.3 - 54.7 = 10.6 \text{ (points Q and P)}$$
$$x'_2 - x'_1 = 36.2 - 29.2 = 7.0 \text{ and}$$
$$y'_2 - y'_1 = 87.0 - 36.7 = 50.3 \text{ (points Q' and P')}$$

From this we calculate Z = 2420.7 and N = 880.4. According to equation (17) the angle of rotation is calculated as φ = 70.0°. With sinφ = 0.940 and cosφ = 0.342 we obtain from equation (20) $a_x = 58.3$ and $a_y = -43.3$. Finally we obtain with a_x, a_y, and $\cot(φ/2) = 1.43$, the coordinates of the fixed point (the center of rotation, assuming a pure rotation) from equation (14) as $x_F = 60.0$ and $y_F = 20.0$.

Matrix notation

Matrix and vector notation is frequently employed for a simplified, symbolic description of translation and rotation. A matrix is an arrangement of numbers; specific rules are defined for matrix addition, subtraction, and multiplication. Matrices employed to represent rotations in a plane contain $2 \cdot 2 = 4$ numbers. Matrices used to represent rotations in three-dimensional space (see the following chapter) contain $3 \cdot 3 = 9$ numbers. Points are represented by their radius vectors in column notation. A column vector representing a point in the plane contains two numbers; a column vector representing a point in three-dimensional space contains three numbers. Using matrix and column notation gives a unified representation for translation and rotation.

In column (vector) notation a translation (equation 1) is described by

$$(21) \qquad \begin{bmatrix} x' \\ y' \end{bmatrix} = \begin{bmatrix} x \\ y \end{bmatrix} + \begin{bmatrix} t_x \\ t_y \end{bmatrix} = \begin{bmatrix} x + t_x \\ y + t_y \end{bmatrix}$$

In this representation both equations (1) are symbolically merged into one single equation. A rotation about the origin of the coordinate system (equation 6) is described in matrix notation by

$$(22) \qquad \begin{bmatrix} x' \\ y' \end{bmatrix} = \begin{bmatrix} \cos\varphi & -\sin\varphi \\ \sin\varphi & \cos\varphi \end{bmatrix} \cdot \begin{bmatrix} x \\ y \end{bmatrix}$$

In this notation the columns represent the radius vectors before and after the rotation. To clarify the meaning of this notation, reference has to be made to the rule for multiplying a matrix **M** by a column vector **v**. For a 2 x 2 matrix and a column vector with two numbers this rule reads

$$(23) \qquad \begin{bmatrix} M_{11} & M_{12} \\ M_{21} & M_{22} \end{bmatrix} \cdot \begin{bmatrix} v_x \\ v_y \end{bmatrix} = \begin{bmatrix} M_{11} \cdot v_x + M_{12} \cdot v_y \\ M_{21} \cdot v_x + M_{22} \cdot v_y \end{bmatrix}$$

The reader can see that equation (22) is identical to equation (6) when the matrix is multiplied by the column vector according to this rule.

A matrix describing a rotation in a plane is composed of the matrix elements $M_{11} = \cos\varphi$, $M_{12} = -\sin\varphi$, $M_{21} = -M_{12}$, $M_{22} = M_{11}$. In the following this matrix is designated by the bold character **D**.

$$(24) \qquad \mathbf{D} = \begin{bmatrix} \cos\varphi & -\sin\varphi \\ \sin\varphi & \cos\varphi \end{bmatrix}$$

The description of a rotation about a center of rotation with the coordinates x_m, y_m (equation 9) reads in matrix notation

$$(25) \qquad \begin{bmatrix} x' \\ y' \end{bmatrix} = \begin{bmatrix} x_m \\ y_m \end{bmatrix} + \begin{bmatrix} \cos\varphi & -\sin\varphi \\ \sin\varphi & \cos\varphi \end{bmatrix} \cdot \begin{bmatrix} x - x_m \\ y - y_m \end{bmatrix}$$

The description of a motion composed of rotation and translation (equation 10) reads

$$(26) \qquad \begin{bmatrix} x' \\ y' \end{bmatrix} = \begin{bmatrix} x_m \\ y_m \end{bmatrix} + \begin{bmatrix} \cos\varphi & -\sin\varphi \\ \sin\varphi & \cos\varphi \end{bmatrix} \cdot \begin{bmatrix} x - x_m \\ y - y_m \end{bmatrix} + \begin{bmatrix} t_x \\ t_y \end{bmatrix}$$

Using the abbreviations

$$(27) \qquad \mathbf{r} = \begin{bmatrix} x \\ y \end{bmatrix}, \mathbf{r}' = \begin{bmatrix} x' \\ y' \end{bmatrix}, \mathbf{r}'' = \begin{bmatrix} x'' \\ y'' \end{bmatrix}, \mathbf{r}_m = \begin{bmatrix} x_m \\ y_m \end{bmatrix}, \mathbf{t} = \begin{bmatrix} t_x \\ t_y \end{bmatrix}$$

the equations can be written in an even more condensed format

(28) Translation: $\qquad \mathbf{r}' = \mathbf{r} + \mathbf{t}$

(29) Rotation about the origin:

$$\mathbf{r}' = \mathbf{D} \cdot \mathbf{r}$$

(30) Rotation about a center $\mathbf{r}_m$:

$$\mathbf{r}' = \mathbf{r}_m + \mathbf{D} \cdot (\mathbf{r} - \mathbf{r}_m)$$

(31) Rotation about a center $\mathbf{r}_m$ plus translation:

$$\mathbf{r}'' = \mathbf{r}_m + \mathbf{D} \cdot (\mathbf{r} - \mathbf{r}_m) + \mathbf{t}$$

Further reading

Textbooks

Lipschutz S. Beginning linear algebra. McGraw-Hill, New York 1997

Spiegel MR, Liu J. Mathematical handbook of formulas and tables. 2nd ed. McGraw-Hill, New York 1999

Spiegel MR. Vector analysis and an introduction to tensor analysis. McGraw-Hill, New York 1959

B2 Mathematical Description of Translation and Rotation in Three-Dimensional Space

This chapter deals with the mathematical description of the change of location and orientation of rigid bodies in three-dimensional space, i.e. the geometrical aspect of translation and rotation. The quantitative description of the change of location and orientation is of great importance in a variety of biomechanical investigations. This chapter aims to serve as a guide; it is not designed as a substitute for studying a textbook of analytical geometry. Two introductory sections on matrix notation, coordinates and vectors are followed by sections on coordinate transformations, translations, and rotations. Finally it is shown how, in principle, the parameters of the description of the motion of a body can be obtained if the initial and final locations of a set of reference points are known. It is expressly pointed out that calculation of the three-dimensional motion of rigid bodies under the influence of forces and moments is not dealt with. This aspect is extremely complex and far beyond the scope of this book. It is dealt with in textbooks on theoretical mechanics.

sense of rotation of the hand and the forefoot in the transverse plane. Some authors use the term eversion/inversion for the rotation of the hind foot in the transverse plane. (Other authors use these terms for the rotation of the foot around the subtalar axis.) In relation to abduction/adduction and internal/external rotation, it has to be kept in mind that these designations have different meanings for the right and left extremities. Internal rotation of the right leg is, for example, in an opposite direction to internal rotation of the left leg.

The description of motion 'in planes' is used not only for the whole body but also for body segments. Fig. B2.**3** shows a detail from Fig. B2.**1**. If we are interested only in movements of the hand, we imagine the three planes to be fixed at the lower arm and describe hand motion in these planes irrespective of whether the hand is positioned at the side, ventral to the body, or above the head.

In a mathematical description of rotations, reference is not usually made to rotations 'in a plane'

Is it really necessary to deal with the description of three-dimensional rotations in the context of orthopedic biomechanics?

To describe three-dimensional movements of the body segments in orthopedics and physiotherapy, motions are usually referred to in three mutually perpendicular planes: the sagittal, coronal, and transverse planes (Fig. B2.**1**). Forward bending of the trunk is thus a motion 'in the sagittal plane', lateral bending of the trunk a motion 'in the coronal plane', and rotation of the trunk around the long axis of the body a motion 'in the transverse plane'. The sense of rotation in these planes bears specific designations (Fig. B2.**2**). Extension/flexion designate the sense of rotation in the sagittal plane; abduction/adduction designate the sense of rotation in the coronal plane; internal/external rotation designate the sense of rotation in the transverse plane. Specific terms are used for the motion of hand and foot. Pronation/supination designate the

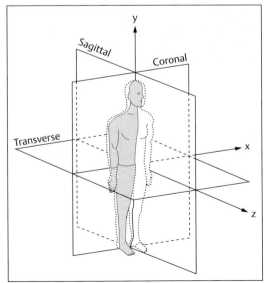

Fig. B2.**1**   Definition of the planes of motion and the xyz-coordinate system

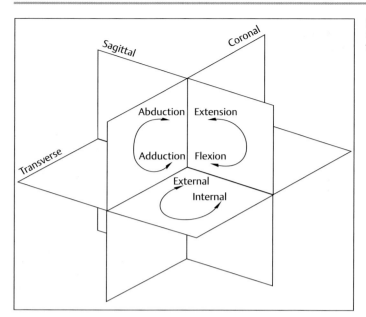

Fig. B2.2   Designation of the sense of rotation in the sagittal, coronal, and transverse planes

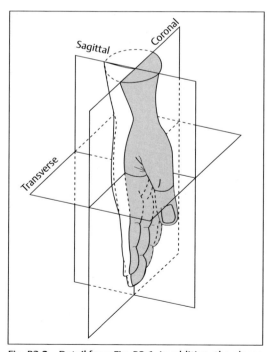

Fig. B2.3   Detail from Fig. B2.1. In addition, the planes are imagined to be fixed to the lower arm if movements of the hand are to be described, irrespective of the location of the hand.

but to spatial rotations 'about an axis of rotation'. An axis of rotation is directed perpendicular to the plane of interest. For the mathematical description of motions, a body-fixed, right-handed, Cartesian xyz-coordinate system is introduced (Fig. B2.1). Flexion/extension are thus rotations 'about the x-axis' (or about an axis parallel to the x-axis). Abduction/adduction (as well as pronation/supination of the foot) are rotations 'about the z-axis', internal/external rotation are rotations 'about the y-axis'.

For the majority of practical applications in orthopedics and physiotherapy the description of motion 'in the planes' shown in Fig. B2.1 suffices. What purpose, then, is served by the complicated description of three-dimensional rotations elaborated upon in this chapter? The simple description is inadequate in all those cases where motions are involved that are outside of the three planes shown in Fig. B2.1. In addition, it will be shown that three-dimensional rotations of a body can be represented in different fashions. From these different (but mathematically equivalent) representations, the one best suited to the biomechanical problem being worked on has to be selected. Some examples serve to illustrate the argument:

Example 1. The contributions of individual shoulder muscles to a motion of the upper arm are to be investigated. For this purpose the location and direction of the axis of rotation need to be known for calculation of the moment arms of the contributing muscles. (The location of this axis is not discussed at this point but is assumed to run through the center of the humeral head. The task is to determine the direction of the axis.) The motion of the upper arm can be measured with a commercially available device in which a sensor receives the magnetic field emitted by a transmitter located in the laboratory. The sensor is fixed on the upper arm. From the data received, the spatial coordinates of the sensor and its orientation are determined, specified by three Euler angles, with respect to the x'y'z'-coordinate system (Fig. B2.**4**) defined by the transmitter. A second sensor is fixed on the trunk (for example, on the thorax) so that its orientation coincides with that of the body-fixed xyz-coordinate system. The task is now a) to transform the motion measured in the x'y'z'-coordinate system into the translated and rotated xyz-coordinate system, and b) to calculate the direction of the axis of rotation from the angular orientation of the upper arm in its initial and final position.

Example 2. In the context of developing artificial joint replacements for the ankle joint, the question to be considered is which joints contribute to eversion/inversion of the hind foot (used here to designate a rotation of the hind foot about the long axis of the foot). The ankle joint and the subtalar joint are assumed to function like hinged joints with fixed axes. The axes of these joints are, however, not parallel (Fig. B2.**5**). While the axis of the ankle joint (in erect stance as in Fig. B2.**1**) runs broadly parallel to the x-axis, the axis of the subtalar joint runs obliquely from dorsally downwards to ventrally upwards. The question that arises is whether the rotation of the hind foot about the long axis of the foot can be explained by combined rotations about these two axes. The theory of three-dimensional rotations states that, in general, unlimited rotational motion can be achieved by combined rotations about three differently oriented axes, or by one single rotation about an axis with unrestricted orientation. It follows that combined rotations about only two fixed axes will restrict the range of motion.

In fact, the rotation of the hind foot discussed here requires, in addition to rotation about the ankle and subtalar axes, simultaneous rotation about the long axis of the tibia (the y-axis in Fig. B2.**1**). This rotation can be effected by rotating the whole tibia or by a 'loose fit' of the ankle joint. Combined rotations about these three axes now permit all rotations, as in a ball-and-socket joint. The range of motion in different directions is limited, however, because the participating joints have only small ranges of motion. In addition, due to the muscle attachments and ligamentous connections, rotations about the individual axes cannot be performed independently. The resulting composite motion thus

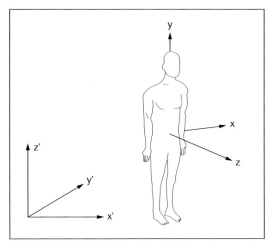

Fig. B2.**4** Body-related xyz-coordinate system and the laboratory x'y'z'-coordinate system, defined by the measuring equipment

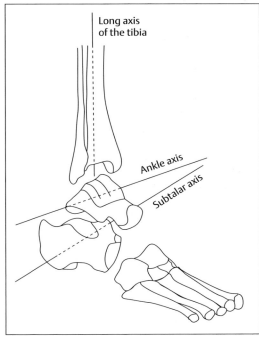

Fig. B2.**5** Axes contributing to the rotation of the hind-foot about the long axis of the foot: the ankle axis, subtalar axis, and long axis of the tibia. Adapted from Debrunner and Jacob, 1998.

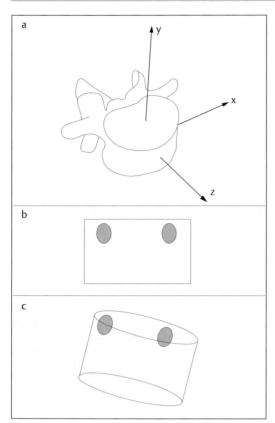

Fig. B2.**6 a** Body-related xyz-coordinate system of a lumbar vertebra. **b**: schematic drawing of the image of the physiologically oriented vertebra in the a-p radiographic view; outline of the vertebral body with insertions of the pedicles. **c**: schematic drawing of the image of a vertebra from a scoliotic spine in the a-p radiographic view; note the lateral and forward tilt about the body-related z- and x-axes as well as the rotation about the body-related y-axis. Adapted from Drerup, 1984.

bears some analogy to the motion of a technical gear.

Example 3. Fig. B2.**6a** shows a vertebra with a body-fixed coordinate system oriented parallel to the system shown in Fig. B2.**1**. In a simplified fashion, Fig. B2.**6b** shows the contours of the vertebral body in an anterior-posterior radiographic view, with the vertebra in its physiologic position and orientation. The contour of the vertebral body and the outlines of the dorsally located pedicles are clearly visible. Fig. B2.**6c** shows, again in a simplified fashion, the contours of a vertebra of a scoliotic spine in the anterior-posterior radiographic view. With the three-dimensional shape of a vertebra in

mind, we recognize qualitatively that, in relation to Fig. B2.**6b**, the vertebra is now tilted sideways and forward. In addition, the vertebra appears to be axially rotated. This is concluded from the asymmetric location of the pedicle outlines with respect to the contours of the vertebral body.

How can the pathologic deviation from the normal anatomical orientation best be characterized? One possibility is to construct the axis of rotation (helical axis), defining the observed motion, from the location of landmarks on the vertebra in its initial and final orientation. This, however, provides no vivid impression of the orientation of the scoliotic vertebra. It is an advantage to have an agreed sequence of three rotations about body-fixed axes of the vertebra. To describe the observed orientation of the scoliotic vertebra, it is assumed (Drerup, 1984) that the vertebra is first rotated about its z-axis (tilted sideways), then rotated about its x-axis (tilted forward), and then rotated about its y-axis. The 'vertebral rotation' about the y-axis is the parameter of primary medical interest because the deformation of the trunk of scoliosis patients seems to be due essentially to vertebral rotation.

It is pointed out that not only is this description based on three rotations on body-fixed axes (i.e. axes which move with the rotated body) but that the sequence of the rotations is of importance as well. This holds already for combined rotations about the z- and x-axes. For small angles, changing the sequence is of only minor effect (this is also true mathematically) but for larger angles the effect will be noticeable. We suggest that the reader might like to make a paper model of the upper endplate of a vertebra, to rotate this model through 90° about the z- and x-axes and then in reverse order about the x-and z-axes and observe the difference in the outcome.

If a rotation sequence differing from that proposed by Drerup were chosen, for example first the axial vertebral rotation and then the forward and sideways tilt, a different set of angles of rotation would be required to move the vertebra from its position in Fig. B2.**6b** to the final position in Fig. B2.**6c**. (Compare this with the small experiment proposed in the previous paragraph.) Specifically the vertebral rotation would assume a different value. The same holds for other possible sequences of the three rotations. Which one, then, is the true value of the vertebral rotation (Skalli *et al.*, 1995)? The answer is that all values are equally true, with respect to the rotation sequence selected. To make a choice, we should rather ask 'Which sequence of rotations is the most sensible one?' Here the answer definitely has to be 'That proposed by Drerup'. Any other sequence would result in the magnitude of the vertebral rotation measured from the radiograph depending on the forward and lateral tilt of the vertebra. This would probably not be a sensible way to describe the geometry of the scoliotic spine.

These examples show that, especially in the context of biomechanical research, conceptual and mathematical complications associated with three-dimensional rotations cannot always be evaded. These comprise coordinate transformations, calculation of a helical axis from a set of Euler angles, and theorems concerning combined rotations. All these items are treated in the following sections of this chapter, with the aim of providing the reader with an overview.

Matrix notation

As shown in the preceding chapter in the case of plane motion, it is also possible to represent three-dimensional motion by equations involving x-, y- and z-coordinates. Compared with this, a notation using vectors and matrices offers two advantages. Sets of equations for the three coordinates can be merged into one single equation and be more clearly set out. In addition, use can be made of established theorems concerning mathematical properties of matrices. For this reason, the rules of matrix and vector algebra are recapitulated below, at least to the extent to which they are referred in this chapter. To start with, we introduce a representation for vectors that is of advantage when dealing with matrix calculus. $\mathbf{e}_x$, $\mathbf{e}_y$, $\mathbf{e}_z$ are the unit vectors of a Cartesian coordinate system. In column representation, a vector $\mathbf{v}$

$$(1) \qquad \mathbf{v} = v_x \cdot \mathbf{e}_x + v_y \cdot \mathbf{e}_y + v_z \cdot \mathbf{e}_z$$

is represented by a column containing three numbers, termed 'coordinates' of the vector. Instead of (1) the vector is described by

$$(2) \qquad \mathbf{v} = \begin{bmatrix} v_x \\ v_y \\ v_z \end{bmatrix}$$

In such a representation the sum $\mathbf{c} = \mathbf{a} + \mathbf{b}$ of two vectors $\mathbf{a}$ and $\mathbf{b}$ is written as

$$(3) \qquad \begin{bmatrix} c_x \\ c_y \\ c_z \end{bmatrix} = \begin{bmatrix} a_x \\ a_y \\ a_z \end{bmatrix} + \begin{bmatrix} b_x \\ b_y \\ b_z \end{bmatrix} = \begin{bmatrix} a_x + b_x \\ a_y + b_y \\ a_z + b_z \end{bmatrix}$$

Besides the sum of two columns, the multiplication of a column by a factor can be defined (here column $\mathbf{v}$ by factor λ)

$$(4) \qquad \lambda \cdot \begin{bmatrix} v_x \\ v_y \\ v_z \end{bmatrix} = \begin{bmatrix} \lambda \cdot v_x \\ \lambda \cdot v_y \\ \lambda \cdot v_z \end{bmatrix}$$

The unit vectors $\mathbf{e}_x$, $\mathbf{e}_y$, $\mathbf{e}_z$, in the direction of the coordinate axes are represented by the columns

$$(5) \qquad \mathbf{e}_x = \begin{bmatrix} 1 \\ 0 \\ 0 \end{bmatrix}, \mathbf{e}_y = \begin{bmatrix} 0 \\ 1 \\ 0 \end{bmatrix}, \mathbf{e}_z = \begin{bmatrix} 0 \\ 0 \\ 1 \end{bmatrix}$$

Matrices employed for the description of motion in three-dimensional space are arrangements of nine elements, ordered in columns and rows. The nine elements, numbers or algebraic expressions, are enclosed (like columns) in rectangular brackets

$$(6) \qquad \mathbf{M} = \begin{bmatrix} M_{11} & M_{12} & M_{13} \\ M_{21} & M_{22} & M_{23} \\ M_{31} & M_{32} & M_{33} \end{bmatrix}$$

The position of each element of the matrix is designated by two indices. M_{23} (pronounced as 'M sub two three'), for example, designates the element in the second row and the third column. The multiplication of a matrix $\mathbf{M}$ by a column $\mathbf{v}$ results in a column and is performed according to the following scheme

$$(7) \qquad \begin{bmatrix} M_{11} & M_{12} & M_{13} \\ M_{21} & M_{22} & M_{23} \\ M_{31} & M_{32} & M_{33} \end{bmatrix} \cdot \begin{bmatrix} v_x \\ v_y \\ v_z \end{bmatrix} = $$

$$\begin{bmatrix} M_{11} \cdot v_x + M_{12} \cdot v_y + M_{13} \cdot v_z \\ M_{21} \cdot v_x + M_{22} \cdot v_y + M_{23} \cdot v_z \\ M_{31} \cdot v_x + M_{32} \cdot v_y + M_{33} \cdot v_z \end{bmatrix} = \begin{bmatrix} v'_x \\ v'_y \\ v'_z \end{bmatrix}$$

The new vector $\mathbf{v}'$ is termed the 'image' of the vector $\mathbf{v}$. The imaging is mediated by the matrix $\mathbf{M}$. The product of two matrices $\mathbf{A}$ and $\mathbf{B}$ is a matrix $\mathbf{M}$

$$(8) \qquad \mathbf{M} = \mathbf{A} \cdot \mathbf{B}$$

For calculation of the matrix product, i.e. of the nine elements of the matrix $\mathbf{M}$, rows of matrix $\mathbf{A}$ are multiplied by the columns of matrix $\mathbf{B}$. The general rule for the calculation of the elements of the matrix product $\mathbf{M} = \mathbf{A} \cdot \mathbf{B}$ is

$$(9) \qquad M_{ik} = \sum_s A_{is} B_{sk}$$

The Greek letter Σ (sigma) symbolizes summation. For each i and k between 1 and 3 the summation index s takes values from 1 to 3. For example, the matrix element in the first row and third column of the matrix $\mathbf{M}$ ($i = 1$, $k = 3$) is calculated as

(10) $M_{13} = A_{11} \cdot B_{13} + A_{12} \cdot B_{23} + A_{13} \cdot B_{33}$

Matrix multiplication is not commutative, i.e. in general (and unlike the multiplication of normal numbers) the result depends on the sequence of factors in the matrix product, for example

(11) $\mathbf{A} \cdot \mathbf{B} \neq \mathbf{B} \cdot \mathbf{A}$

This property is of importance in the context discussed below, where it is shown that three-dimensional imaging of vectors is mediated by matrices. The fact that the result of the product of two matrices depends on the sequence of the multiplication means that, in the case of successive rotations, the sequence of the rotations is of importance for the outcome.

Coordinates and vectors

To describe the location of points in space, a three-dimensional, right-handed coordinate system is introduced. Its axes are in pairs, perpendicular to each other; the axes are designated according to the 'right hand rule' (Fig. 3.**14**) as x (in the direction of the thumb), y (direction of the index finger), and z (direction of the middle finger of the right hand). The intersection of the axes is termed the 'origin' of the coordinate system. To describe the location of a point A, three numbers (coordinates) x_A, y_A, z_A, must be specified: $A(x_A/y_A/z_A)$. The spatial location of the point can be illustrated by a rectangular parallelepiped with side lengths x_A, y_A, z_A measured from the origin of the coordinate system. The point B is located on the spatial diagonal of the parallelepiped opposite the origin 0 (Fig. B2.**7**). Alternatively, in the diagram illustrating point B, an auxiliary point with coordinates x_B, y_B, 0, is constructed in the xy-plane. The point $B(x_B/y_B/z_B)$ is located above this point at a distance z_B. There is a close relation between pairs of points and vectors. It holds that for each pair of points A and B there exists exactly one vector $\mathbf{v}$. This vector is illustrated by an arrow beginning at A and ending with its arrowhead at B (Fig. B2.**7**). The vector from B to A is in the opposite direction to that from A to B and is designated by $-\mathbf{v}$.

Unit vectors in the direction of the coordinate axes (Fig. B2.**8**) are defined as follows

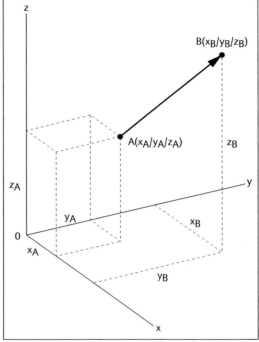

Fig. B2.7 Location of points and related vectors in a Cartesian coordinate system. Points are specified by three coordinates. Illustration of the location of a point by a rectangular parallelepiped (point A) or by three specified edges of a parallelepiped (point B). A vector $\mathbf{v}$ is assigned to the pair of points A,B (in that order) and shown as an arrow pointing from A to B.

$\mathbf{e}_x$ = vector,
       pointing from $O(0/0/0)$ to $P1(1/0/0)$
(12) $\mathbf{e}_y$ = vector,
       pointing from $O(0/0/0)$ to $P2(0/1/0)$
      $\mathbf{e}_z$ = vector,
       pointing from $O(0/0/0)$ to $P3 (0/0/1)$

$O(0/0/0)$ designates the origin of the coordinate system. The length of the unit vectors is one (in units of the scale of the axes). The unit vectors are in pairs, oriented perpendicular to each other. Any vector $\mathbf{v}$ can be represented by

(13) $\mathbf{v} = \mathbf{v}_x + \mathbf{v}_y + \mathbf{v}_z = v_x \cdot \mathbf{e}_x + v_y \cdot \mathbf{e}_y + v_z \cdot \mathbf{e}_z$

The reader should note the notation in equation (13). $\mathbf{v}_x$ is a component of vector $\mathbf{v}$ (i. e. a vector); v_x is its coordinate with respect to $\mathbf{e}_x$ (i.e. a number). The same holds for the y- and z-compo-

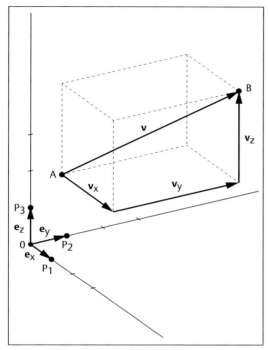

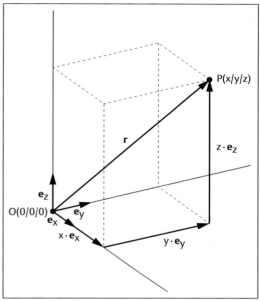

Fig. B2.9 Definition of the radius vector **r**. A vector pointing from the coordinate origin O(0/0/0) to a point P(x/y/z) is called a radius vector. There is an unequivocal relation between point coordinates x, y, z, and vector components $\mathbf{v}_x = x \cdot \mathbf{e}_x$, $\mathbf{v}_y = y \cdot \mathbf{e}_y$, $\mathbf{v}_z = z \cdot \mathbf{e}_z$.

Fig. B2.8 Unit vectors in the direction of the coordinate axes and representation of a vector by the sum of its components. Unit vectors $\mathbf{e}_x$, $\mathbf{e}_y$, $\mathbf{e}_z$, are vectors of length one, pointing from the origin 0 of the coordinate system in the direction of the coordinate axes. Using the unit vectors, a vector **v** is decomposed into three components $\mathbf{v}_x$, $\mathbf{v}_y$, $\mathbf{v}_z$, parallel to the coordinate axes.

For the purpose of illustration, the vector **v** (pointing from A to B) is depicted as a spatial diagonal of a rectangular parallelepiped with side lengths v_x, v_y, v_z. The vector components $\mathbf{v}_x = v_x \cdot \mathbf{e}_x$, $\mathbf{v}_y = v_y \cdot \mathbf{e}_y$, $\mathbf{v}_z = v_z \cdot \mathbf{e}_z$, of vector **v** point along the edges of the parallelepiped.

nents. The numbers v_x, v_y, v_z, apply only with respect to the base $\mathbf{e}_x$, $\mathbf{e}_y$, $\mathbf{e}_z$. If the coordinate system is changed, these numbers will change as well. Using the three unit vectors it is possible to reach any point in three-dimensional space. In mathematical terms, the three unit vectors form a base and span the three-dimensional space. As unit vectors have length one and are perpendicular to each other (in mathematical terms, orthogonal to each other), such a base is termed 'orthonormal'. For an orthonormal base, the scalar product of two vectors **a** and **b** is written as

$$(14) \qquad \mathbf{a} \cdot \mathbf{b} = a_x \cdot b_x + a_y \cdot b_y + a_z \cdot b_z$$

Using unit vectors, the vector product is written as

$$(15) \qquad \begin{aligned} \mathbf{a} \times \mathbf{b} = {} & (a_y \cdot b_z - b_y \cdot a_z) \cdot \mathbf{e}_x + \\ & (a_z \cdot b_x - b_z \cdot a_x) \cdot \mathbf{e}_y + (a_x \cdot b_y - b_x \cdot a)_y \cdot \mathbf{e}_z \end{aligned}$$

To illustrate the relation between point coordinates and vectors, we observe a point P(x/y/z) and a vector **r** pointing from the origin of the coordinate system O(0/0/0) to the point P. Vectors originating from the origin of the coordinate system are designated 'radius vectors'. In the following, such vectors are (usually) designated by the symbol **r**. It is obvious that a radius vector **r** can be decomposed (Fig. B2.**9**)

$$(16) \qquad \mathbf{r} = x \cdot \mathbf{e}_x + y \cdot \mathbf{e}_y + z \cdot \mathbf{e}_z$$

Obviously, the coordinates x, y, z, of a radius vector are identical with the point coordinates of its end point. Conversely, the coordinates of a radius vector are obtained by scalar multiplication by the unit vectors (for example, $x = \mathbf{r} \cdot \mathbf{e}_x$).

Coordinate transformations

The transformation of point coordinates from one coordinate system to another is a frequent task when evaluating experimental data. In gait analysis, for example, the coordinates of reference points measured in the laboratory system by means of film or video sequences must be converted to a reference system, imagined to be fixed to the skeleton of the test subjects. The laboratory system may be designated by xyz and the body reference system by uvw. The location of a point $P(u/v/w)$ in the body reference system is described by the radius vector $\mathbf{p} = u \cdot \mathbf{e}_u + v \cdot \mathbf{e}_v + w \cdot \mathbf{e}_w$. We imagine the body reference system to be embedded into the laboratory system. In the laboratory system the origin of the reference system is given by the radius vector $\mathbf{r}_m = x_m \cdot \mathbf{e}_x + y_m \cdot \mathbf{e}_y + z_m \cdot \mathbf{e}_z$. The location of $P(x/y/z)$ is to be expressed by the coordinates u, v, w. In the laboratory system the radius vector for point P

is given by the vector equation $\mathbf{r} = \mathbf{r}_m + \mathbf{p}$. In full (Fig. B2.**10**)

$$(17) \quad \begin{aligned} \mathbf{r} &= (x \cdot \mathbf{e}_x + y \cdot \mathbf{e}_y + z \cdot \mathbf{e}_z) = (x_m \cdot \mathbf{e}_x + y_m \cdot \mathbf{e}_y + \\ & \quad z_m \cdot \mathbf{e}_z) + (u \cdot \mathbf{e}_u + v \cdot \mathbf{e}_v + w \cdot \mathbf{e}_w) \end{aligned}$$

After some intermediate calculation (not given here) a set of transformation equations is obtained for the coordinates

$$(18) \quad \begin{aligned} x &= x_m + C_{11} \cdot u + C_{12} \cdot v + C_{13} \cdot w \\ y &= y_m + C_{21} \cdot u + C_{22} \cdot v + C_{23} \cdot w \\ z &= z_m + C_{31} \cdot u + C_{32} \cdot v + C_{33} \cdot w \end{aligned}$$

The coefficients C_{ik} in these equations are the scalar products of the unit vectors in the xyz and uvw systems. The value of the scalar products corresponds to the cosine of the angle between the coordinate axes of the two systems. For example, the coefficient C_{31} equals the cosine of the angle between the unit vectors $\mathbf{e}_z$ and $\mathbf{e}_u$: $C_{31} = \mathbf{e}_z \cdot \mathbf{e}_u$. The orientation of each unit vector in one system is defined by three 'direction cosines' with respect to the three unit vectors of the other system. Due to the unit length and orthogonality of the unit vectors there are six constraints on the nine direction cosines. Thus, we are left with three independent parameters describing the transformation. The transformation equation (18) can be written in column and matrix notation

$$(19) \quad \begin{bmatrix} x \\ y \\ z \end{bmatrix} = \begin{bmatrix} x_m \\ y_m \\ z_m \end{bmatrix} + \begin{bmatrix} C_{11} & C_{12} & C_{13} \\ C_{21} & C_{22} & C_{23} \\ C_{31} & C_{32} & C_{33} \end{bmatrix} \cdot \begin{bmatrix} u \\ v \\ w \end{bmatrix}$$

The following description of rotations in space reveals a close relationship between rotations and coordinate transformations. Coordinate transformations leave the objects unchanged but describe their location and orientation in a rotated (and possibly translated) coordinate system. If the relative spatial location and orientation of two coordinate systems is known, for example from a measurement, the relative translation of the two systems and the nine coefficients C_{ik} in (19) can be calculated. The coefficients C_{ik} contain all information on the relative rotation between the two coordinate systems.

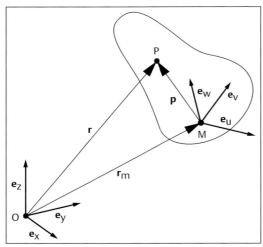

Fig. B2.10 Changing the coordinate system. A point P may be defined in the xyz-coordinate system (origin O; unit vectors $\mathbf{e}_x, \mathbf{e}_y, \mathbf{e}_z$) or in the uvw-coordinate system (origin M; unit vectors $\mathbf{e}_u, \mathbf{e}_v, \mathbf{e}_w$). The relative location of the coordinate systems is described by the vector $\mathbf{r}_m$ (pointing from O to M). The relative orientation is given by the set of direction cosines. The location of a point P may be described either by the vector $\mathbf{p}$ (in the uvw-system) or by the vector $\mathbf{r}$ (in the xyz-system). The (vector) relation $\mathbf{r} = \mathbf{r}_m + \mathbf{p}$ exists between these vectors. If the u,v,w coordinates of point P are to be transformed to x,y,z-coordinates, the uvw-unit vectors in the vector equation $\mathbf{p} = u \cdot \mathbf{e}_u + v \cdot \mathbf{e}_v + w \cdot \mathbf{e}_w$ have to be replaced by the xyz-unit vectors using the set of direction cosines.

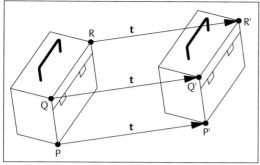

Fig. B2.11 Translation in three dimensions. A rigid body (suitcase) moves parallel to itself. A point P of the body moves to the point P' (difference vector **t**). One is dealing with a (pure) translation if the difference vectors PP', QQ', RR' of three points P, Q, R, which are not aligned on a line, are equal and identical with **t**. (Coordinate origin and radius vectors are not shown in this diagram.)

Translation in three-dimensional space

The motion of a point in a given coordinate system is considered here. A translation (motion along a straight line) shifts a point P(x/y/z) by the translation vector **t** to point P' (x'/y'/z'). The radius vectors from O to P and from O to P' are designated by **r** and **r'** (Fig. B2.**11**). It holds that

(20) $$\mathbf{r'} = \mathbf{r} + \mathbf{t}$$

or in column notation

(21) $$\begin{bmatrix} x' \\ y' \\ z' \end{bmatrix} = \begin{bmatrix} x \\ y \\ z \end{bmatrix} + \begin{bmatrix} t_x \\ t_y \\ t_z \end{bmatrix}$$

Like translation in a plane, a translation in three-dimensional space leaves the orientation of a body unchanged. All points are shifted by an identical distance along parallel lines. If two or more translations are performed consecutively, the result does not depend on the sequence of the translations.

Rotation in three-dimensional space

While translations in three-dimensional space are, in principle, quite similar to translations in a plane,

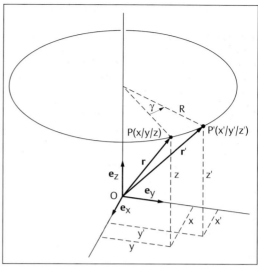

Fig. B2.12 Rotation of a point about the z-axis. The point P(x/y/z) moves in a plane, parallel to and located at a distance z from the xy-plane, along a circular arc through an angle of rotation γ to P'(x'/y'/z'). The related radius vector **r** moves on the surface of a cone with its tip at O, height = z and radius R = $\sqrt{x^2 + y^2}$.

rotations in three dimensions exhibit new, unexpected properties. One such property is that, if several rotations are performed consecutively, the sequence of the rotations is of importance, i.e. identical rotations, performed one after the other, will yield different results, depending on the order in which they are performed.

Rotations about the coordinate axes

A rotation in three-dimensional space is described by specifying an axis and an angle of rotation. An axis is described by its three-dimensional orientation and location. Depending on the sense of rotation, the angle of rotation is counted as positive (counterclockwise) or negative (clockwise). A rotation leaves all points on the axis unchanged; all other points move along circular arcs in planes oriented perpendicular to the axis. Fig. B2.**12** illustrates this with a rotation about the z-axis of the coordinate system. This rotation moves an arbitrary point P(x/y/z) in a plane with distance z from the xy-plane. The point moves along an arc with radius R = $\sqrt{x^2 + y^2}$ and angle γ. The center of the circle is located on the z-axis. This rotation changes the x- and y-coordinates; the z-coordinate is left unchanged. This permits the formulae describing rotation in a plane to be adopted for x and y:

$$\text{(22)} \quad \begin{aligned} x' &= \cos\gamma \cdot x - \sin\gamma \cdot y \\ y' &= \sin\gamma \cdot x + \cos\gamma \cdot y \\ z' &= z \end{aligned}$$

These equations can also be written as

$$\text{(23)} \quad \mathbf{r}' = \begin{bmatrix} x' \\ y' \\ z' \end{bmatrix} = \begin{bmatrix} \cos\gamma & -\sin\gamma & 0 \\ \sin\gamma & \cos\gamma & 0 \\ 0 & 0 & 1 \end{bmatrix} \cdot \begin{bmatrix} x \\ y \\ z \end{bmatrix} = \mathbf{D}_z(\gamma) \cdot \mathbf{r}$$

The matrix describing a rotation about the z-axis is designated $\mathbf{D}_z(\gamma)$. The matrices describing a rotation about the y-axis through angle β and about the x-axis through angle α are similar

$$\text{(24)} \quad \mathbf{r}' = \begin{bmatrix} x' \\ y' \\ z' \end{bmatrix} = \begin{bmatrix} \cos\beta & 0 & \sin\beta \\ 0 & 1 & 0 \\ -\sin\beta & 0 & \cos\beta \end{bmatrix} \cdot \begin{bmatrix} x \\ y \\ z \end{bmatrix} = \mathbf{D}_y(\beta) \cdot \mathbf{r}$$

$$\text{(25)} \quad \mathbf{r}' = \begin{bmatrix} x' \\ y' \\ z' \end{bmatrix} = \begin{bmatrix} 1 & 0 & 0 \\ 0 & \cos\alpha & -\sin\alpha \\ 0 & \sin\alpha & \cos\alpha \end{bmatrix} \cdot \begin{bmatrix} x \\ y \\ z \end{bmatrix} = \mathbf{D}_x(\alpha) \cdot \mathbf{r}$$

Combined rotation made up of a sequence of rotations

To illustrate the problems associated with combined rotations about body-fixed axes, we consider the example of two consecutive rotations of a suitcase. An xyz-system of coordinate axes is imagined to be fixed on the suitcase. We rotate the suitcase, first through +90° about its vertical axis and then through +90° about its longitudinal axis. After these two consecutive rotations the suitcase lies on its back (Fig. B2.**13**). Now, if we perform the same rotations, but in the reverse order, the final state of the suitcase is resting on one side (Fig. B2.**14**). This example illustrates the importance of the sequence of rotations. If the order is changed, the result changes as well. If several rotations are performed consecutively, not only must the rotations (axes and angles) be specified but also their sequence.

The rotations in Figs. B2.**13** and B2.**14** will now be analyzed mathematically. In the first case, the first rotation occurs about the z-axis of the suitcase. The rotation matrix related to the unit vectors $\mathbf{e}_x, \mathbf{e}_y, \mathbf{e}_z$ (compare equation 23) is

$$\text{(26)} \quad \mathbf{D}_z(\gamma = 90°) = \begin{bmatrix} 0 & -1 & 0 \\ 1 & 0 & 0 \\ 0 & 0 & 1 \end{bmatrix}$$

The second rotation occurs about the x'-axis, i.e. about a body-fixed axis of the suitcase (previously rotated about its z-axis). The rotation matrix relat-

ed to the unit vectors $\mathbf{e}'_x, \mathbf{e}'_y, \mathbf{e}'_z$ (compare equation 25) is

$$\text{(27)} \quad \mathbf{D}_{x'}(\alpha = 90°) = \begin{bmatrix} 1 & 0 & 0 \\ 0 & 0 & -1 \\ 0 & 1 & 0 \end{bmatrix}$$

Some intermediate calculation (not given here) provides for the combined rotation

$$\text{(28)} \quad \mathbf{r}'' = \mathbf{D}_z \cdot \mathbf{D}_{x'} \cdot \mathbf{r}$$

In this result, the sequence of the matrices deserves our attention, especially as this sequence differs from what one might expect. First, the matrix of the second partial rotation acts on the vector $\mathbf{r}$ and then, in a second step the matrix of the first partial rotation. If the sequence of the two partial rotations is interchanged, the combined rotation is described by

$$\text{(29)} \quad \mathbf{r}'' = \mathbf{D}_x \cdot \mathbf{D}_{z'} \cdot \mathbf{r}$$

For rotations about body-fixed axes it holds, in general, that the matrix of the last rotation in the sequence of rotations is the first one to be multiplied by the vector to be rotated. The matrix $\mathbf{M}$ describing the image resulting from n partial rotations about body-fixed axes is composed according to the rule

$$\text{(30)} \quad \mathbf{M}_{\text{body-fixed}} = \mathbf{D}_1 \cdot \mathbf{D}_2 \cdot \ldots \mathbf{D}_{n-1} \cdot \mathbf{D}_n$$

In this, as well as in the following formulae, the indices of the rotation matrices designate the sequence of the rotations: $\mathbf{D}_1$ is the first rotation, $\mathbf{D}_2$ the second rotation and $\mathbf{D}_n$ the nth rotation.

If, on the other hand, n rotations were to be performed about axes fixed in space (i. e. fixed in the laboratory) and not about body-fixed axes, the sequence of the matrices in the matrix product would be different (the proof of this theorem is not detailed here)

$$\text{(31)} \quad \mathbf{M}_{\text{space-fixed}} = \mathbf{D}_n \cdot \mathbf{D}_{n-1} \cdot \ldots \mathbf{D}_2 \cdot \mathbf{D}_1$$

For many applications in biomechanics, interpretation of motion by rotations about body-fixed axes is appropriate. In addition, rotations about such axes lend themselves more readily to visual perception. This may be illustrated by considering the spatial orientation of a vertebra of a scoliotic spine. As outlined earlier, the total rotation of the vertebra can be described by a sequence of three tations about body-fixed rotation axes. The first rotation effects sideways tilt about the body-fixed

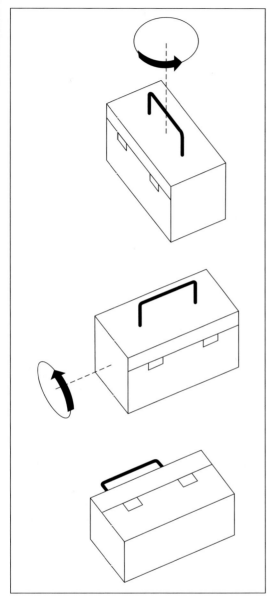

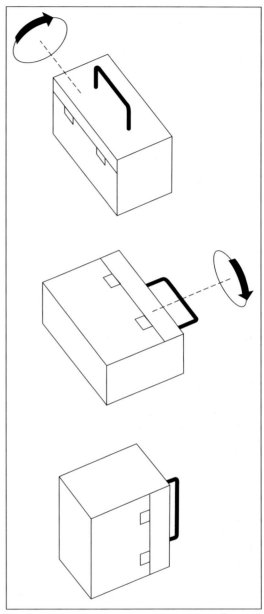

Fig. B2.**13** Two consecutive 90° rotations of a rigid body (suitcase) about its vertical and longitudinal axis. In step 1 the body is rotated about its vertical axis; in step 2 the body is rotated about its longitudinal axis. In the final state, the suitcase is lying on its back.

Fig. B2.**14** Two consecutive 90° rotations of a rigid body (suitcase) about its longitudinal and vertical axis. Axes and sense of rotation are identical with those in Fig B2.**13**; however, the sequence of the rotations is changed. The first rotation occurs about the longitudinal axis, the second about the vertical axis. In the final state the suitcase rests on its side.

z-axis (see Fig. B2.**6**), the second a forward tilt about the body fixed x-axis, and the third a rotation about the caudocranial (y-) axis of the vertebra (all three axes passing through the center of the vertebra). If an investigator communicates these three angles, we can vividly perceive the orientation of the vertebra. If, in contrast, three angles together with their sequence about space-fixed axes were reported, for example angles about axes defined by an x-ray apparatus in the laboratory, visual perception would be difficult, if not impossible. For this reason, the following paragraphs of this chapter deal exclusively with rotations about body-fixed axes.

Euler and Bryant-Cardan angles

Any desired orientation of a body can be obtained by performing rotations about three axes in sequence. There is, however, a multitude of possible ways of performing three such rotations. In principle, a choice from this multitude can be made at random, but two conventions are frequently used in the literature: Euler's and Bryant-Cardan's rotations. According to Euler, the general rotation is composed of three rotations about body-fixed axes as follows (Fig. B2.**15**)

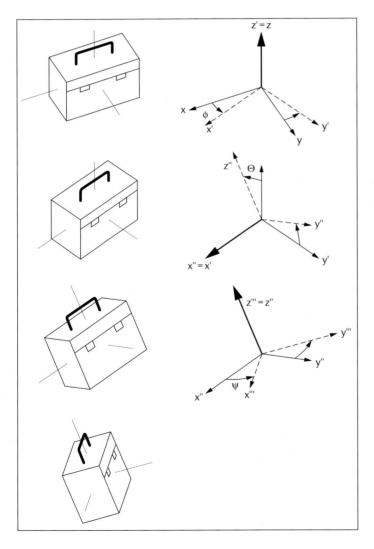

Fig. B2.**15** General rotation composed of three partial rotations. Selection of the axes and angles of rotation according to Euler. The coordinates of the initial state are designated x, y, z, those after the first rotation x', y', z', those after the second rotation x", y", z" and those after the third rotation x''', y''', z'''. The first rotation takes place about the z-axis (vertical axis of the suitcase) through an angle of $\phi = 20°$. The second rotation takes place about the x'-axis (longitudinal axis of the suitcase) through an angle $\theta = 30°$. The third rotation takes place about the z"-axis (vertical axis of the suitcase) through the angle $\psi = 40°$.

Rotation 1: about the z-axis through the angle ϕ; rotation matrix $\mathbf{D}_z(\phi)$

Rotation 2: about the x'-axis through the angle θ; rotation matrix $\mathbf{D}_{x'}(\theta)$

Rotation 3: about the z''-axis through the angle ψ; rotation matrix $\mathbf{D}_{z''}(\psi)$

The matrix describing Euler's combined rotation is given by the matrix product

(32) $\mathbf{M} = \mathbf{D}_z(\phi) \cdot \mathbf{D}_{x'}(\theta) \cdot \mathbf{D}_{z''}(\psi)$ (Euler)

According to both Bryant and Cardan, the general rotation is composed of three rotations about body-fixed axes as follows (Fig. B2.**16**)

Rotation 1: about the x-axis through the angle ϕ_1; rotation matrix $\mathbf{D}_x(\phi_1)$

Rotation 2: about the y'-axis through the angle ϕ_2; rotation matrix $\mathbf{D}_{y'}(\phi_2)$

Rotation 3: about the z''-axis through the angle ϕ_3; rotation matrix $\mathbf{D}_{z''}(\phi_3)$

The matrix of the combined rotation is given by the matrix product

$$\mathbf{M} = \mathbf{D}_x(\phi_1) \cdot \mathbf{D}_{y'}(\phi_2) \cdot \mathbf{D}_{z''}(\phi_3)$$
(33) (Bryant-Cardan)

Fig. B2.**16** General rotation composed of three partial rotations. Selection of the axes and angles of rotation according to the Bryant-Cardan convention. The coordinates of the initial state are designated x, y, z, those after the first rotation x', y', z', those after the second rotation x", y", z" and those after the third rotation x''', y''', z'''. The first rotation takes place about the x-axis (longitudinal axis of the suitcase) through an angle of $\phi_1 = 28.5°$. The second rotation takes place about the y'-axis (transverse axis of the suitcase) through an angle $\phi_2 = 9.8°$. The third rotation takes place about the z''-axis (vertical axis of the suitcase) through the angle $\phi_3 = 57.5°$. The angles of rotation in this diagram are selected in such a way that, when starting from an initial state identical with that of Fig. B2.**15**, the identical final state is reached. For this reason, the angles ϕ_1, ϕ_2, ϕ_3 are not integers.

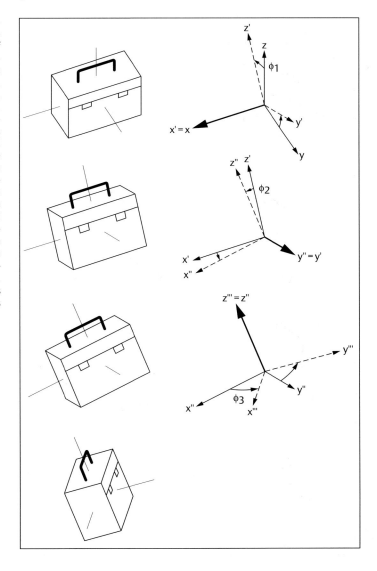

We recognize that each convention is based on three angles and a specified sequence of rotations to define the rotation matrix **M**. This bears some similarity to the transformation between two co-ordinate systems. The relative orientation of the unit vectors was similarly described there by three parameters.

Rotation about an arbitrary axis

For reasons of simplicity, we have dealt with single or combined rotations about coordinate axes up to this point. The concept is now to be broadened as we deal with rotations about arbitrary axes. For the moment, however, the discussion is confined to axes passing through the origin of the coordinate system. In Fig. B2.17 the axis of rotation is represented by the unit vector **n**. The radius vector of an arbitrary point P in space is designated by **r**. When rotated by an angle φ, P moves along a circular arc to P'. The related radius vector is termed **r'**. The relation between **r'** and **r** depends on the angle φ as well as on the axis **n** of rotation (the proof is not detailed here)

$$(34) \quad \begin{aligned} \mathbf{r'} = &\cos\varphi \cdot \mathbf{r} + \\ &(1 - \cos\varphi) \cdot \mathbf{n} \cdot (\mathbf{n} \cdot \mathbf{r}) + \sin\varphi \cdot (\mathbf{n} \times \mathbf{r}) \end{aligned}$$

The relation between **r'** and **r** can also be expressed in matrix notation. The coordinates of the unit vector **n** are designated u,v,w

$$(35) \quad \mathbf{n} = \begin{bmatrix} u \\ v \\ w \end{bmatrix}$$

With the abbreviations

$$(36) \quad \begin{aligned} C &= \cos\varphi \\ F &= 1 - \cos\varphi \\ S &= \sin\varphi \end{aligned}$$

the imaging equation can be written as

If we insert for **r** the vector **n**, we obtain

$$(38) \quad \mathbf{n'} = \mathbf{D_n}(\varphi) \cdot \mathbf{n} = \mathbf{n}$$

This means that the image vector **n'** is identical with the original vector **n** with respect to direction and magnitude. Points on the axis of rotation do not change their location (as is generally true of rotations). In mathematical terms, the vector **n** is called the 'eigenvector' of the matrix **D_n**. In general it holds that, if for a matrix **M** a vector **m** exists with the property $\mathbf{M} \cdot \mathbf{m} = \lambda \cdot \mathbf{m}$, **m** is the eigenvector of **M** and λ is the eigenvalue of **M**. Equation (38) states **n** to be an eigenvector of **D_n** with an eigenvalue equal to one.

The theorem holds that 'any rotation resulting from a series of consecutive rotations can also be described by one single rotation'. In other words, the product of rotation matrices is again a rotation matrix. The proof of this theorem, which is far from obvious, is not detailed here; it is furnished in the context of the theory of orthogonal matrices. The importance of this theorem in the context of biomechanics is in that any arbitrary sequence of consecutive rotations can be described by one single (combined) rotation about the Euler or Bryant-Cardan angles or as a rotation about one specific axis through a specific angle of rotation.

Motion in three-dimensional space, combined from rotation and translation. Chasles' Theorem.

Rotation and translation are now to be integrated into one single motion. To start with, the restriction that the axis of rotation runs through the coordinate origin is still maintained. In a first step the vector **r** is rotated about **n** through the angle φ. Its image **r'** is

$$(39) \quad \mathbf{r'} = \mathbf{D_n}(\varphi) \cdot \mathbf{r}$$

In a second step the image vector is translated by the translation vector **t**

$$(40) \quad \mathbf{r''} = \mathbf{r'} + \mathbf{t} = \mathbf{D_n}(\varphi) \cdot \mathbf{r} + \mathbf{t}$$

$$(37) \quad \mathbf{r'} = \mathbf{D_n}(\varphi) \cdot \mathbf{r} = \begin{bmatrix} C + F \cdot u^2 & F \cdot u \cdot v - S \cdot w & F \cdot u \cdot w + S \cdot v \\ F \cdot v \cdot u + S \cdot w & C + F \cdot v^2 & F \cdot v \cdot w - S \cdot u \\ F \cdot w \cdot u - S \cdot v & F \cdot w \cdot v + S \cdot u & C + F \cdot w^2 \end{bmatrix} \cdot \mathbf{r}$$

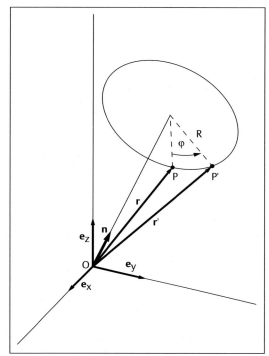

Fig. B2.**17** Rotation about an arbitrary axis passing through the coordinate origin. Rotation takes place about an arbitrarily oriented axis with unit vector **n** through an angle φ. The radius vector OP = **r** moves on the surface of a cone with its tip at the origin of the coordinate system to OP' = **r'**. The radius R of the base of the cone is equal to R = |**n** × **r**| (magnitude of the vector product).

We wish to discuss two special cases of this motion. In the fist case **t** is parallel to **n** (**t** = **t**$_p$). We consider a point P with radius vector **r**, at a distance R from the axis of rotation **n** (Fig. B2.**18**). When being rotated, the point P moves along a circle with radius R, in a plane perpendicular to **n**, to its intermediate image P'. Subsequently, it is translated from P', by the vector **t**$_p$ parallel to the axis of rotation, to P''. If we imagine a cylinder with radius R constructed around the axis of rotation, P, P' and P'', are located on the surface of that cylinder. The curve on which the point moves from its initial to its final position exhibits a sharp bend at P'. The alternative path, along a helix, would have been a smooth curve from P to P''. Despite the fact that equation (40) was formulated under the condition of consecutive rotation and translation, the motion is nevertheless termed 'helical motion'.

A motion that really does follow a helix is described similarly to equation (40). Along the helix, rotation and translation take place simultaneously.

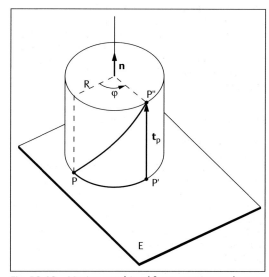

Fig. B2.**18** Motion combined from rotation and translation. Special case 1: Translation parallel to the axis of rotation. Rotation is performed through an angle φ about an arbitrarily oriented and located axis of rotation (unit vector **n**). For each given point P in space, there exists a plane E perpendicular to the axis of rotation **n**. The motion occurs on the (imagined) surface of a cylinder. The axis of the cylinder coincides with the axis of rotation, the base of the cylinder lies in the plane E, and the radius R of the cylinder is given by the length of the perpendicular from P to the axis of rotation. The first partial motion is a rotation where the point P moves along a circular arc (periphery of the cylinder base) to point P'. The second partial motion is a translation with translation vector **t**$_p$ parallel to **n**, by which the point P' moves to P'' on a straight generating line (generatrix) of the cylinder surface. In addition to the actual path P–P'–P'', the helix from P to P'' is shown in the diagram.

For this purpose, both angle and translation depend linearly and continuously on a parameter λ

$$(41) \quad \mathbf{r'}(\lambda) = \mathbf{D_n}(\lambda \cdot \varphi) \cdot \mathbf{r} + \lambda \cdot \mathbf{t}_p \quad (0 \leq \lambda \leq 1)$$

The initial and final location of the point are given by λ = 0 and λ = 1 respectively. Any intermediate position on the helix is described by 0 < λ < 1. In the final location, formula (41) is identical with (40).

In the second special case **t** is perpendicular to **n** (**t** = **t**$_q$). P is a point with radius vector **r**, at a distance R from the axis of rotation **n** (Fig. B2.**19**). The point P moves along a circular arc with radius R to its intermediate image P'. (The radius of the arc equals the magnitude of the perpendicular from P to the axis of rotation. A calculation of R would involve mathematical procedures beyond the scope

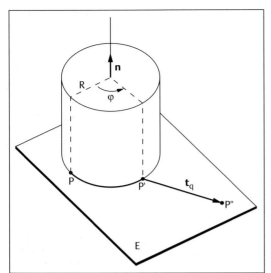

Fig. B2.19 Motion combined from rotation and translation. Special case 2: Translation perpendicular to the axis of rotation. Rotation is performed by an angle φ about an arbitrarily oriented and located axis of rotation (unit vector **n**). For comparison, the cylinder identical to that in Fig. B2.**18** is shown. The first partial motion is a rotation where the point P moves along a circular arc (periphery of the cylinder base) to point P'. The second partial motion is a translation with translation vector t_q perpendicular to **n**, by which the point P' is moved to P" in the plane E. Thus the combined motion occurs in a plane.

of this book.) Subsequently, point P' is translated by the vector t_q (in the identical plane) to P".

$$(42) \qquad \mathbf{r''} = \mathbf{D_n}(\phi) \cdot \mathbf{r} + \mathbf{t_q}$$

This situation is quite similar to the two-dimensional case. In two dimensions, there is a common movement of all points in the xy-plane. In the three-dimensional case discussed here, each point moves in a plane perpendicular to the axis of rotation and passing through the intersection of the perpendicular from the point to the axis. It has been shown in Chapter 4 and Appendix B1 that translation and rotation in a plane can be substituted by one single rotation about the fixed point of the imaging. We thus suspect that in three dimensions there might be a 'substitute' axis of rotation parallel to **n** with the properties equivalent to those of a fixed point (or better, a fixed line). We imagine the parallel planes appertaining to the points **r** projected on top of each other. The fixed

point determined in this plane is the point where the substitute axis intersects this plane. It can be shown (not detailed here) that a fixed line really does exist.

The discussion is now to be broadened as the rotation is performed through the angle φ about an axis of rotation with direction parallel to **n** and running through point $\mathbf{r_0}$. The image is then given by

$$(43) \qquad \mathbf{r'} = \mathbf{r_0} + \mathbf{D_n}(\phi) \cdot (\mathbf{r} - \mathbf{r_0})$$

This equation tells us that the origin of the coordinate system has been shifted to $\mathbf{r_0}$. The point **r** is rotated with respect to $\mathbf{r_0}$, i. e. the rotation is performed on the vector $\mathbf{p} = (\mathbf{r} - \mathbf{r_0})$. After the rotation the vector $\mathbf{r_0}$ is added to the image $\mathbf{p'} = \mathbf{D_n}(\phi) \cdot \mathbf{p}$ of the vector **p**. To combine translation and rotation, the (already rotated) point is shifted by the translation vector **t**

$$(44) \qquad \mathbf{r''} = \mathbf{r'} + \mathbf{t} = \mathbf{r_0} + \mathbf{D_n}(\phi) \cdot (\mathbf{r} - \mathbf{r_0}) + \mathbf{t}$$

If no restrictions are imposed on the direction of **t**, equation (44) describes the general motion in three-dimensional space. Equation (44) can be reformulated as

$$(45) \qquad \mathbf{r'} = \mathbf{D} \cdot \mathbf{r} + \mathbf{a}$$

and with **a** defined as (**r"** being replaced by **r'**)

$$(46) \qquad \mathbf{a} = \mathbf{r_0} - \mathbf{D_n}(\phi) \cdot (\mathbf{r_0} + \mathbf{t})$$

The **Chasles' theorem** states 'the general motion in three-dimensional space is helical motion', or 'the basic type of motion adapted to describe any change of location and orientation in three-dimensional space is helical motion'. The relevant axis of rotation is designated the 'helical axis'. The Chasles' theorem is also known as the 'helical axis theorem'. (The proof of this theorem is not detailed here.)

▨ Calculation of the parameters of rotation and translation in three-dimensional space from the coordinates of reference points and their images

If the parameters of the motion (rotation and translation) and of the initial location and orientation of a body are known, the formulae given in the previous section permit its final location and orientation to be calculated. In biomechanics, however, one is quite often confronted with the inverse problem. The coordinates of reference points on a body are known in the initial and final state and the parameters of the motion (the imaging) have to be determined. In the following, the solution to this problem is outlined under the assumption that measurement of the coordinates is performed with no experimental error (a condition never met in reality). The topic of how calculation procedures change when measurement errors are involved is briefly discussed in Appendix B3.

Parameters of the motion of a body observed in a laboratory coordinate system

To reconstruct the parameters of the motion of a rigid body in a laboratory coordinate system, the coordinates of three reference points fixed on the body but not lying on a straight line have to be known in the initial state A and the final state E (Fig. B2.**20**). To fit the parameters, the following equation is employed (compare equation 44)

$$(47) \qquad \mathbf{r'} = \mathbf{r}_S + \mathbf{D} \cdot (\mathbf{r} - \mathbf{r}_S) + \mathbf{t}_S$$

In this equation, $\mathbf{r}$ designates the locations of the reference points and $\mathbf{r}_S$ the location of the geometric center of the reference points in the initial state A. $\mathbf{r'}$ and $\mathbf{r'}_S$ designate the locations of the reference points and their geometric centers in the final state E. The steps of the calculation are then: 1) calculation of the translation vector $\mathbf{t}_S$ from A to E and reversal of the translation; 2) determination of the rotation matrix $\mathbf{D}$; 3) with $\mathbf{D}$ and the translation vector already determined in step 1 being known, the motion can be interpreted according to Chasles as helical motion; 4) alternatively, it is possible to select another interpretation for the rotation matrix, i. e. an interpretation according to Euler or to Bryant-Cardan.

1: Translation of the geometric centers. The geometric centers referred to in the following are the geometric centers of the reference points. From three reference points with radius vectors $\mathbf{r}_1, \mathbf{r}_2, \mathbf{r}_3$ the radius vector of their geometric center $\mathbf{r}_S$ is calculated as

$$(48) \qquad \mathbf{r}_S = 1/3 \cdot (\mathbf{r}_1 + \mathbf{r}_2 + \mathbf{r}_3)$$

(The geometric center of three points has nothing to do with a center of mass. Only if three equal masses were located at these points would both the geometric center and the center of mass be given by $\mathbf{r}_S$.) The translation vector $\mathbf{t}_S$ points from the geometric center in its initial location A to its final location E. Reversal of the translation

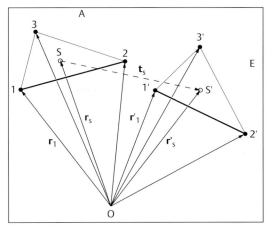

Fig. B2.**20** Motion of a rigid body: minimum configuration of three reference points in order to determine the parameters describing the spatial motion. Three reference points, which must not be aligned along a straight line, are fixed on the rigid body. In this diagram, the body itself is not shown; instead, we imagine the body to be replaced by the triangle formed by the three reference points. The initial state is designated A and the final state E. In addition to the corners of the triangle 1–3, their geometric centre S is shown. The spatial motion can be described as a rotation of the triangle about an axis passing through S and a subsequent translation of the rotated triangle by the translation vector $\mathbf{t}_S$. Points and vectors in the final state are designated by symbols with primes.

$$(49) \qquad \bar{\mathbf{r}} = \mathbf{r'} - \mathbf{t}_S$$

means that the geometric centers of the reference points are superimposed. We are now left with a difference in orientation (a rotation) of the body. **2: Determination of the rotation matrix.** After the translation has been reversed, the following equation is employed to obtain the rotation matrix

$$(50) \qquad \bar{\mathbf{r}}_i - \mathbf{r}_S = \mathbf{D} \cdot (\mathbf{r}_i - \mathbf{r}_S) \quad i = 1, 2, 3$$

The most commonly employed procedure for solving this equation for the rotation matrix $\mathbf{D}$ is trial and error by iteration. For example, we could insert formula (37) for the matrix $\mathbf{D}$ and, starting from rough estimates for the direction of the axis of rotation $\mathbf{n}$ and the angle of rotation φ, change both parameters in small steps until we finally arrive at a parameter set which satisfies equation (50). If the coordinates of the reference points are not known exactly, but only within certain error limits, it is not possible to find a set of parameters satisfying equation (50) exactly, but only a solution satisfying this equation as nearly as possible (a 'best possible fit'). Algorithms of iterative procedures have been adapted for use on computers; for details the reader is referred to textbooks on numerical methods. Alternatively we could have inserted formula (32) or (33) for **D** into equation (50) and determined the set of Euler or Bryant-Cardan angles by stepwise (iterative) searching for those sets of angles fulfilling the demands of equation (59) exactly (or, in the case of measurement errors, as nearly as possible).

3: Interpretation of the motion as helical motion. When the direction of the axis of rotation **n**, the angle of rotation φ, and the translation vector $\mathbf{t}_S = \mathbf{r}'_S - \mathbf{r}_S = \mathbf{r}_{S'} - \mathbf{r}_S$ are known, the motion is comprehensively described. In this description, the axis of rotation passes through the geometric center of the reference points on the body. The direction of the axis, the geometric center of the reference points and the translation vector are given in the laboratory coordinate system. If we wish to interpret the motion as helical motion, we conclude from the Chasles' theorem that this is always possible. The description as helical motion requires specification of the direction of the axis, of a point in space through which the axis passes, and of a translation vector along this axis. It can be shown (and this is far from being a matter of course) that the direction of the helical axis being searched for coincides with the direction **n** of the axis of rotation determined above. A point in space $\mathbf{r}_A$, through which the axis passes is calculated from

$$(51) \qquad \mathbf{r}_A = \frac{\mathbf{r}_S + \mathbf{r}'_S}{2} + \frac{1}{2} \cdot \cot\left(\frac{\varphi}{2}\right) \cdot \mathbf{n} \times (\mathbf{r}'_S - \mathbf{r}_S)$$

The translation vector $\mathbf{t}_p$ (parallel to **n**) is obtained from the projection of the translation vector $\mathbf{t}_S$ on to the direction of the helical axis

$$(52) \qquad \mathbf{t}_p = (\mathbf{t}_S \cdot \mathbf{n}) \cdot \mathbf{n}$$

Because of its importance in the interpretation of biomechanical measurements, the content of equations (51) and (52) is illustrated in Fig. B2.**21**. A comprehensive description of a helical motion requires specification of a point in space through which the axis of rotation passes. We recognize from the orientation of the suitcase in its initial and final position (Fig. B2.**21**) that the object was rotated about a vertical axis **n** by an angle φ. From these parameters and from the location of the center of the suitcase in its initial and final position $\mathbf{r}_S$, $\mathbf{r}'_S$, the location of a point A on the helical axis can be con-

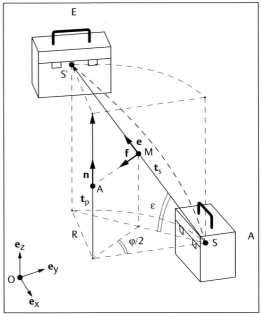

Fig. B2.**21** Motion of a rigid body: interpretation of the general motion as helical motion (Chasles' theorem). The required number of reference points is fixed on a rigid body (not shown in the diagram). From the spatial location of the reference points in the initial and final state, the locations of the geometric centres S ($\mathbf{r}_S$) and S' ($\mathbf{r}'_S$), as well as the rotation matrix **D** are determined. The change in location of the geometric centres is described by $\mathbf{t}_S = \mathbf{r}'_S - \mathbf{r}_S$. The axis of rotation **n** and the angle of rotation φ are determined from the rotation matrix. The translation $\mathbf{t}_p$ in direction of the helical axis is obtained by projection from **n** and $\mathbf{t}_S$. The location of the axis of rotation relative to the initial and final position of the suitcase is set by points A and M. M is the midpoint of the line SS'. The vector **f** directed from M to A is perpendicular to **n** and $\mathbf{t}_S$. The radius R and the radius vector $\mathbf{r}_A$ can be calculated by means of the unit vectors **e**, **n**, and **f**.

structed. $\mathbf{r}_S$ and $\mathbf{r}'_S$ are the locations of the center of the suitcase (used here to represent the geometric centers of the reference points on the suitcase), and M designates the midpoint of the line SS'. The relevant radius vector is $(\mathbf{r}_S + \mathbf{r}'_S)/2$. **e** is the unit vector in the direction of the difference vector $(\mathbf{r}'_S - \mathbf{r}_S)$. The line SS' and **n** are skew lines in space. M and A are those points where the distance between the two lines assumes a minimum value. The line connecting M and A is perpendicular to **n** as well as to SS'. **f** is a unit vector in the direction of MA. R is the radius of the cylindrical surface on which the suitcase moves. From the lines projected on to the base plane of the cylinder we deduce $|\mathbf{r}_A - \mathbf{r}_M| = R \cdot$ $\cos(\varphi/2)$ and $|\mathbf{r}_S' - \mathbf{r}_S| \cdot \cos(\varepsilon) = 2R \cdot \sin(\varphi/2)$. As A is the point of minimum distance between the lines, the unit vector $\mathbf{f}$ is oriented perpendicular to $\mathbf{n}$ and $\mathbf{e}$. Hence, $\mathbf{f}$ can be represented by the vector product $\mathbf{f} = (\mathbf{n} \times \mathbf{e})/\cos(\varepsilon)$. After some simple intermediate calculations, the result of equation (51) is reached.

4: Different interpretations of a rotation matrix D. Irrespective of how we whish to interpret the rotation, as rotation by one single angle about one single axis (37), as rotation sequence according to Euler about three axes (32) or as rotation sequence according to Bryant-Cardan about three axes (33), the matrix elements D_{ik} of the matrix **D** are numerically identical. These numbers are merely interpreted differently. From time to time one is confronted with the problem of switching from one interpretation to another. For example, the task may be to determine the helical axis and the angle of rotation when the three Euler angles are known, or to determine the set of Cardan angles when the helical axis and the appertaining angle of rotation are known. All of these tasks boil down to the problem of extracting the parameters of a three-dimensional rotation from the (known) elements of a rotation matrix **D**. This is possible, but in some cases there will prove to be no unequivocal solution to this problem.

Calculation of the Euler angles from the elements of a rotation matrix **D**. In the process of solving this, two cases have to be distinguished. Main case A (equations 53): for any given $\cos\theta$ there exist two sine values that differ by their sign. Consequently two sets of angles are obtained. For each of the three angles of each set the quadrant can be unequivocally determined from the sine and cosine functions by means of the atan2 function

(53)
$$\cos\theta = D_{33}$$
$$\sin\theta = \pm\sqrt{1 - (\cos\theta)^2}$$
$$\cos\psi = D_{32}/\sin\theta$$
$$\sin\psi = D_{31}/\sin\theta$$
$$\cos\phi = -D_{23}/\sin\theta$$
$$\sin\phi = D_{13}/\sin\theta$$

Special case B: if $\sin\theta = 0$, $\cos\theta$ can assume the values ± 1. Subcase 1 (equations 54): for $\cos\theta = +1$, θ has the value $0°$ or $\pm 360°$. In this case it is only the sum of the angles ϕ and ψ that can be obtained from

(54)
$$\cos(\phi + \psi) = D_{22}$$
$$\sin(\phi + \psi) = D_{21}$$

Subcase 2 (equations 55): for $\cos\theta = -1$, θ can assume the values $\pm 180°$. In this case it is only the difference between angles ϕ and ψ that can be obtained

(55)
$$\cos(\phi - \psi) = D_{11}$$
$$\sin(\phi - \psi) = D_{12}$$

Calculation of the Bryant-Cardan angles from the elements of a rotation matrix **D**. In the solving process, various cases have again to be distinguished. Main case A (equations 56): for any $\sin\phi_2 \neq \pm 1$ there exist two cosine values that differ in their sign. Accordingly, two sets of angles ϕ_1, ϕ_2, ϕ_3 are obtained. For each of the three angles of each set the quadrant can be unequivocally determined from the sine and cosine functions by means of the atan2 function

(56)
$$\sin\phi_2 = D_{13}$$
$$\cos\phi_2 = \pm\sqrt{1 - (\sin\phi_2)^2}$$
$$\cos\phi_1 = D_{33}/\cos\phi_2$$
$$\sin\phi_1 = -D_{23}/\cos\phi_2$$
$$\cos\phi_3 = D_{11}/\cos\phi_2$$
$$\sin\phi_3 = -D_{12}/\cos\phi_2$$

Special case B: $\cos\phi_2 = 0$. The relevant sine can assume the values ± 1. Subcase 1 (equations 57): $\cos\phi_2 = 0$, $\sin\phi_2 = +1$, corresponding to the angles $\phi_2 = -270°, +90°$. In this case it is only the sum of the other two angles $\phi 1$ and $\phi 3$ that can be determined

(57)
$$\cos(\phi_1 + \phi_3) = D_{22}$$
$$\sin(\phi_1 + \phi_3) = D_{32}$$

Subcase 2 (equations 58): $\cos\phi_2 = 0$, $\sin\phi_2 = -1$, corresponding to the angles. $\phi_2 = -90°, +270°$. In this case it is only the difference between the other two angles ϕ_1 and ϕ_3 that can be determined

(58)
$$\cos(\phi_1 - \phi_3) = D_{22}$$
$$\sin(\phi_1 - \phi_3) = D_{32}$$

Determination of the components of a unit vector u,v,w in direction of the axis of rotation **n** *as well as of the angle of rotation φ about this axis from the elements of a rotation matrix* **D**. As in the two problems discussed above, we need to distinguish between different cases. In the main case A we assume $\cos\varphi \neq 1$. The parameters searched for are calculated from

(59)
$$u^2 = \frac{D_{11} - C}{1 - C}$$
$$v^2 = \frac{D_{22} - C}{1 - C}$$
$$w^2 = \frac{D_{33} - C}{1 - C}$$

(60) $\qquad C = \cos\varphi = \dfrac{D_{11} + D_{22} + D_{33} - 1}{2}$

Square roots have to be extracted from the squares; the signs of u,v,w are determined by insertion in the eigenvalue equation (38). Once a valid combination of u,v,w-values and a φ-value has been established, the final choice is made by considering one of the valid relations between rotation matrices $\mathbf{D_n}(\varphi)$, i. e. $\mathbf{D(n, -360° + \varphi)} = \mathbf{D(n, \varphi)}$ or $\mathbf{D(-n, -\varphi)} = \mathbf{D(n, \varphi)}$. The first relation indicates that, with the direction of the axis of rotation unchanged, the rotation can also be explained by using an angle of rotation equal to $-360°+\varphi$. The second relation indicates that a change in the sense of direction of the axis of rotation requires the sense of the rotation to be changed as well. Depending on the problem being worked on, the investigator may be able to make a rough estimate of the axis and the angle of rotation; this will then permit a final choice to be made from the different mathematical solutions available.

Special case B: $\cos\varphi = 1$, corresponding to the angles of rotation $\varphi = 0°, \pm360°$. The rotation matrix then equals the unit matrix, i.e. the rotated points coincide with their images. Any direction can be chosen for the axis of rotation.

Parameters describing the relative motion of two bodies

In many cases of practical interest, the problem is not in describing the motion of a body in a laboratory coordinate system but in describing the relative motion of two bodies. One example of such relative motion is the motion of the lower leg relative to the motion of the thigh. If one succeeds in fixing a 'measurement coordinate system' on one of the bodies, for example on the thigh, the problem can be reduced to that discussed in the previous section. The motion of the lower leg would then be observed in the coordinate system of the thigh and interpreted according to one of the above conventions (Euler angles etc.). One measuring device employed in biomechanical research and defining its own coordinate system is a commercially available electromagnetic tracking device. Its transmitter is fixed on one body and its receiver on the other. The output data are the Euler angles of the transmitter with respect to the receiver and the distance coordinates between the two devices.

If, however, the locations of reference points fixed to the thigh and to the lower leg have been recorded simultaneously in a laboratory coordinate system (Fig. B2.**22**), a number of calculation steps

have to be performed before the relative motion between lower leg and thigh can be analyzed:

1. From the geometric centers of the reference points on the thigh, the translation of the thigh is calculated and reversed. The identical transformation is applied to the reference points of the lower leg.

2. An iterative procedure is used to determine the rotation matrix that images the already translated reference points of the thigh in the final state on to its reference points in the initial state. This rotation matrix is then applied to the already translated reference points of the lower leg. The effect of these transformations is that the reference points of the thigh in the initial and final state now coincide. The motion of the thigh in the laboratory system is thus compensated for.

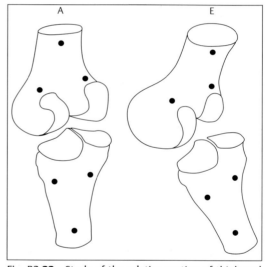

Fig. B2.**22** Study of the relative motion of thigh and lower leg (motion of the knee joint). The initial (A) and final (E) state are shown. Thigh and lower leg each bear three reference points. To obtain the parameters describing the relative motion, we assume the knee joint to be rigid in the initial as well as in the final state. By rotating and translating the (rigid) object we succeed in superimposing the reference points of the thigh in the final state E on to those in the initial state A. Thus the thighs are congruent. Position and orientation of the lower leg in both states still differ. This is the relative motion to be observed; it becomes evident after the movement of the thigh has been compensated for. This latter difference in position and orientation of the lower leg in states A and E serves to extract the parameters of the relative motion between lower leg and thigh.

3. The remaining differences in the locations of the reference points on the lower leg in the initial and the final state now characterize the relative motion of the lower leg with respect to the thigh. This motion can be analyzed, as described above, like the motion of a single body in a laboratory co-ordinate system. The direction and location of the helical axis and the related angle of rotation or, alternatively, the translation vector and the sets of angles, according to Euler or to Bryant-Cardan, can be determined.

Alternatively, a body-fixed coordinate system could be constructed from the radius vectors of the reference points fixed on the thigh. In three-dimensional space, three reference points are required for the definition of a coordinate system. These three reference points must not lie on a line but rather on the corners of a triangle. The radius vectors of the three reference points P_1, P_2, P_3 in the laboratory coordinate system are designated $\mathbf{r}_1$, $\mathbf{r}_2$, $\mathbf{r}_3$. To construct a body-fixed coordinate system, the first unit vector is obtained from the difference vector $\mathbf{a} = \mathbf{r}_2 - \mathbf{r}_1$ by dividing it by its magnitude

$$(61) \qquad \mathbf{e}_{k1} = \frac{\mathbf{a}}{|\mathbf{a}|}$$

Starting from the difference vector $\mathbf{b} = \mathbf{r}_3 - \mathbf{r}_1$, the vector $\mathbf{v} = \mathbf{b} - \mathbf{e}_{k1} \cdot (\mathbf{e}_{k1} \cdot \mathbf{b})$, which is perpendicular to $\mathbf{e}_{k1}$, is constructed. Dividing by its magnitude yields the second unit vector

$$(62) \qquad \mathbf{e}_{k2} = \mathbf{v}/|\mathbf{v}|.$$

The third unit vector $\mathbf{e}_{k3}$ is defined by the vector product

$$(63) \qquad \mathbf{e}_{k3} = \mathbf{e}_{k1} \times \mathbf{e}_{k2}$$

The geometric center $\mathbf{r}_s$ of the reference points P_1, P_2, P_3 at the thigh is chosen according to equation (48) as the origin of the coordinate system. The location of the reference points on the lower leg (with radius vectors $\mathbf{r}_j$ in the laboratory system) is now to be expressed in the thigh system. For this purpose the difference vectors $\mathbf{r}_j - \mathbf{r}_s$ given in the laboratory system are projected on to the unit vectors $\mathbf{e}_{k1}, \mathbf{e}_{k2}, \mathbf{e}_{k3}$. This provides the coordinates of the lower leg reference points in the system of the thigh. Any change in these coordinates directly reflects the relative motion between lower leg and thigh.

The description of the relative motion, for example as helical motion, is still unsatisfactory, because the location and orientation of the axis are given in the laboratory or, in the example discussed above, in the thigh-fixed, coordinate sys-

tem. If the motion of a joint is to be investigated, interest is usually focused on knowing the location and orientation of the axis in a coordinate system that is properly aligned with respect to the structures of our skeleton, and not with respect to a co-ordinate system that is dependent on the more or less randomly selected laboratory system or reference points on the moving object. A thigh coordinate system, sensibly adapted to visual interpretation of the results, would be a system aligned to the 'preferred directions' of the femur, i. e. with one axis pointing in a longitudinal direction and another in a mediolateral direction crossing the two condyles. The problem is that such anatomically preferred directions are not necessarily perpendicular to each other (as required for the definition of a normalized orthogonal coordinate system). In addition, a point must be selected where the coordinate axes intersect. Thus we have to choose a coordinate system not only adapted to the anatomical structures but also compatible with the mathematical requirements. The relative location and orientation of the laboratory system and of the anatomical system are determined from radiographs (imaging both the bones and the reference points) or from anatomical landmarks (points on the skin assumed to closely characterize the position and orientation of bones). When the relative orientation and translation between the landmarks and the anatomical system are known (again from iterative fitting as described above), the coordinates of the laboratory system can be transformed to the anatomical system.

In practice, additional problems arise from the fact that locations of reference points can never be measured exactly, but only with certain errors. It follows that there are no exact solutions for the rotation matrices but only best fits. Furthermore, reference points on biological objects are never rigidly fixed with respect to the bones, but may move slightly with respect to each other or with respect to the skeleton, for example, through movement and deformation of the skin.

Further reading

Textbooks and review papers

Goldstein H. *Classical Mechanics.* Addison Wesley 1980

Lipschutz S. *Beginning linear alegbra.* McGraw-Hill, New York 1997

Spiegel MR, Liu J. *Mathematical handbook of formulas and tables.* 2nd ed. McGraw-Hill, New York 1999

Wittenburg J. *Dynamics of Systems of Rigid Bodies.* Stuttgart: Teubner; 1977

Woltring HJ. Representation and calculation of 3-d joint movement. *Human Movement Science.* 1991; **10**: 603–616

Scientific papers cited in the text or in the figures

Debrunner HU, Jacob HAC. *Biomechanik des Fusses*. 2nd ed. Stuttgart: Enke; 1998

Drerup B. Principles of measurement of vertebral rotation from frontal projections of the pedicles. *J Biomechanics*. 1984; **17**: 923–935

Skalli W, Lavaste F, Descrimes JL. Quantification of three-dimensional vertebral rotations in scoliosis: what are the true values? *Spine*. 1995; 20: 546–553

B3 Dealing with Errors

There is virtually no problem in the field of biomechanics where there is no need to ponder over potential error influences, whether on the part of the investigator planning or conducting an experiment, or the reader making efforts to understand and interpret other investigators' data and conclusions. We distinguish between two types of error: systematic and random errors. Systematic errors always affect a result in the same fashion. For example, the distortion of an image caused by the lens of a camera is identical in every picture taken by that camera. Once we know the source of the error (here the distortion of the lens), the related systematic error can be corrected. But even if all systematic errors are corrected, repeated measurements taken from an identical object will exhibit different results. The data are scattered at random about the true, but unknown, value of the quantity to be measured.

This chapter is dedicated first and foremost to these random, 'statistical' errors. The fact that repeated measurements taken from the identical object do not give identical results may be due to the measuring apparatus or to the investigator. In addition, in medicine and biology we are confronted with the fact that objects 'of the same kind' are not identical in all their aspects and thus give rise to a scatter of measured data. Depending on the underlying cause, measuring equipment, investigator influence, or biological diversity, the interpretation of measurement errors will be different. However, the mathematical description and treatment of these three sources of error will prove to be largely similar.

To permit a mathematical approach to errors, the following assumptions are made. First, the measured data deviate at random from the true value in a positive or negative direction. Second, the deviations of any pair of measured data from the true value are not related to each other, they are 'uncorrelated'. Third, the magnitude of the deviations is quantified by the mean of the squares of the deviations. Under these assumptions, the influence of errors on the result of an experiment can usually be minimized by careful planning and use of appropriate mathematical tools. For example, the precision of a result can be increased by taking repeated measurements and averaging the data obtained. In this case, 'redundant' measurements (redundant, because in principle one single measurement could suffice) are employed to increase the precision of the result. This is also the concept underlying more complex tasks, for example when determining the functional relation between two quantities while both quantities are known only within certain error limits.

If the measurement errors of single physical quantities are known (for example, the errors of distance and time measurement), the laws of error propagation quantify the error to be expected for combined quantities (for example of the velocity as the quotient of distance and time). As an example (as mentioned in Chapter 4) the error of the measurement of an angle between two lines is determined below, with the errors of the coordinates of the end points of those lines, measured on a xy-digitiser table, being known.

Quite often the task with which one is confronted is to find a best fit of a mathematical function or a model to a set of data (inevitably) fraught with errors. This is done using the method of least squares. As examples, the fit of a regression line in two dimensions and the relative fit of two sets of points in three-dimensional space are dealt with below. The latter problem is mathematically demanding, but not infrequently encountered in the scientific literature. The aim is to provide the reader at least with an overview.

Mean and variance

Taking the average of a set of repeated measurements increases the precision. The true but unknown value searched for is designated x. x_k designates the results of repeated measurements from the identical object. Each x_k can be expressed as the sum of x and a random error ξ_k

$$(1) \qquad x_k = x + \xi_k \quad k = 1, 2, ..., n$$

The mean of the x_k is calculated from the arithmetic mean

$$(2) \qquad m_x = (x_1 + x_2 + ... + x_n)/n = x + m_\xi$$

where m_ξ designates the mean of the errors ξ_k. The mean quadratic deviation is defined as

(3)
$$s_x^2 = ((x_1 - m_x)^2 + (x_2 - m_x)^2 + \dots \\ + (x_n - m_x)^2)/(n - 1)$$

By introducing the differences $x_k - m_x$, x will be eliminated, resulting in

(4)
$$s_x^2 = s_\xi^2 = ((\xi_1 - m_\xi)^2 + (\xi_2 - m_\xi)^2 + \\ \dots + (\xi_n - m_\xi)^2)/(n - 1)$$

It is pointed out that, in the definition of the mean quadratic deviation, the sum of the squares of the single deviations is divided by n – 1, and not by n, as in calculation of the arithmetic mean.

Before we discuss what gain in precision is to be achieved by calculating m_x instead of using a single measured value x_k, the concept of an 'expectation value' is introduced. The expectation value designates the mean of a virtually infinite number of repeated measurements. An expectation value is enclosed in pointed brackets. The expectation value of the mean squared deviation is given (the proof is not detailed here) by

(5)
$$< s_x^2 > = < s_\xi^2 > = \sigma^2$$

or, expressed in words, the expectation value of s_x^2 is equal to σ^2. The quantity s_x^2, determined from a sample of size n, is accepted as an estimate of the unknown quantity σ^2. In the same sense, the sample mean m_x constitutes an estimate for the true but unknown value x. The mean squared deviation σ^2 is known as the 'variance'. The square root of the mean squared deviation, i. e. σ, is the 'standard deviation' and is usually abbreviated by the letters SD.

We can also ask for the expectation value of a single measurement. As no single measurement is distinguished with respect to any other measurement, it holds that the expectation value of the kth measurement x_k is equal to the expectation value of the pth measurement and to the true value x as well

(6)
$$< x_k > = < x_p > = x$$

For the expectation value of the square of the variable 'mean minus true value' the remarkable relation holds (the proof for the formula is not detailed here)

(7)
$$< (m_x - x)^2 > = \sigma^2/n$$

or

(8)
$$\sqrt{< (m_x - x)^2 >} = \sigma/\sqrt{n}$$

This means that the mean value m_x is closer to the true value x by a factor of $1/\sqrt{n}$ than a single value

x_k. Bearing in mind that σ^2 can be approximated by its estimate s_x^2, then the true value x can be approximately located within error limits

(9)
$$m_x - s_x/\sqrt{n} \leq x \leq m_x + s_x/\sqrt{n}$$

It follows that the confounding influence of measurement errors can be reduced by performing repeated measurements and averaging the data. How effective this proves to be (i. e. how narrow the error limits are), depends on the variance and on the number n of repetitions of the measurement.

Biological variance

Up to this point we have been concerned with random measurement errors and estimates of the deviation of the measured data from their true value. Biological statistics, too, deal with deviations from true or 'normal' values, but the results are interpreted differently. Data measured from biological objects exhibit individual variations. In contrast to random measurement errors, these variations are not to be interpreted as deviations from a true value but characterize biological diversity. If, for example, the stature of a cohort is measured, the individual stature measurements differ. This is due to the fact that stature really does differ among subjects and not to a faulty scale used. In addition, errors caused by the measurement device and, potentially, by the investigator as well, contribute to the diversity observed. Measurements from biological objects are thus influenced by biological diversity as well as by ordinary measurement errors.

For a number of investigations in the medical field it is important to know what portion of the observed variance is due to biological diversity or to measurement errors. The following example serves to illustrate the problem. The task is to test the effect of a hypotensive drug by intergroup comparison of the systolic blood pressure of two cohorts. To document a treatment effect, the mean values from samples of treated and non-treated test subjects are compared. Within each cohort the blood pressure does not assume identical values for all subjects but shows a natural diversity. Mean and variance (equations 2 and 3) are estimates of the population parameter 'systolic blood pressure' and its variance. Because all data are subject to measurement errors, both biological diversity and measurement errors contribute to this variance. It is obvious that the contribution from the measurement procedure must be small if samples with different features (here with and without medication) are to be discriminated. In other words, an imprecise measurement of blood pressure would seriously interfere with the aim of documenting the effect of the drug.

As biological diversity and measurement errors are not correlated, the total variance is the sum of the biological and measurement variances (the proof of this formula is not detailed here)

$$(10) \qquad \sigma_{total}^2 = \sigma_{biological}^2 + \sigma_{measurement}^2$$

The influence of the statistical measurement error on the total variance can be quantified by measuring the same sample twice. (To this end the sample has to be chosen at random and the size of the sample must not be too small. These requirements serve to ensure that the sample represents the biological diversity.) The sample may contain n objects. The results of the first measurement are designated x_k, while those of the second measurement y_k. m_x and m_y designate the means of the first and second measurement. R is the correlation coefficient of x and y; R is calculated from

$$(11) \qquad R = \frac{\sum\limits_{k=1}^{k=n}(x_k - m_x) \cdot (y_k - m_y)}{\sqrt{\sum\limits_{k=1}^{k=n}(x_k - m_x)^2 \cdot \sum\limits_{k=1}^{k=n}(y_k - m_y)^2}}$$

The correlation coefficient is a gauge of the reliability of repeated measurements from identical objects. The coefficient assumes values between zero and 1. If R is greater than 0.75, reliability is said to be excellent; values between 0.4 and 0.75 are accepted as satisfactory, and values below 0.4 are regarded as unsatisfactory (Fleiss, 1986). It can be shown that the correlation coefficient R of x and y is equal to the quotient of the biological variance σ_{bio}^2 and the total variance σ_{total}^2 (the proof of this formula is not detailed here)

$$(12) \qquad R = \sigma_{bio}^2 / (\sigma_{bio}^2 + \sigma_{measurement}^2)$$

If R and σ_{total}^2 are known, the magnitudes of the biological and the measurement variance can be obtained separately

$$(13) \qquad \sigma_{bio}^2 = R \cdot \sigma_{total}^2$$

$$(14) \qquad \sigma_{measurement}^2 = (1 - R) \cdot \sigma_{total}^2$$

By this means it can be checked whether the statistical measurement errors are, as required, much smaller in fact than the biological variance. R conveys no information on (potential) systematic errors.

Comparing precision among measuring methods or among investigators

Repetition of a measurement series is indicated if the precision of different measurement methods, precision of repeated measurements by one observer (intra-observer test), or the precision of two observers (inter-observer test) is to be compared. For comparison purposes, the repeated measurements are to be performed on a sample representing the typical range of the variable under investigation. The results of the first test are designated x_k, and those of the second test y_k. In order to judge the degree of agreement, it seems obvious to plot y_k in relation to x_k. If both measurement series are in good agreement, the points lie on a straight line. This diagram, however, is suitable only for a rough overview. Finer details become apparent when the differences in the measured values $v_k = y_k - x_k$ are plotted in relation to their mean values $u_k = (x_k + y_k)/2$. If systematic deviations can be neglected, and on the assumption that one method is much more precise than the other, the standard deviation s_v of the variable v represents an upper limit for the statistical measurement error of the less precise method (Bland and Altman, 1986).

The assessment of measurement precision in the case of two observers repeating a measurement (inter-observer test) or of one single observer repeating his or her own measurement (intra-observer test) is identical in principle with the comparison of two different measurement apparatuses. Potential technical differences between the apparatuses are merely replaced by individual differences between the observers (or in one observer at different points in time). Individual differences may result from differences in readings from scales, in estimates of length or time intervals, or in ratings of gray shades in radiographs. In addition, subjective influences such as learning (and, potentially, forgetting) come into play. In the case of an intra-observer test it is important to ensure that some time elapses between the first and the second measurement series and that measurements are performed in a different sequence in the second series, in order to avoid memory effects.

For two sets of measured data, no matter whether the sets have been obtained by two measurement apparatuses, by two observers, or by one single observer working on two separate occasions, it holds that, if the measurement series agree (the ideal case), the expectation value for the difference in the measurements is equal to zero, $< v_k > = < y_k - x_k > = 0$. From the sample of size n, the mean m_v and the variance s_v^2 are determined. The question now to be answered is whether or not the actual deviation m_v from the expectation value zero is due to chance. To this end the t test is applied. If the value of t calculated from

(15)
$$t = \frac{m_v}{s_v / \sqrt{n}}$$

proves to be too large, we conclude that one measurement series exhibits a systematic shift with respect to the other. In this case, the data of one series can be systematically corrected by m_v, in order to enforce agreement between the two series.

If the measurement variance of one investigator is known from an intra-observer test, and if an inter-observer test furthermore showed only a negligible systematic deviation, if any, between the two observers, the measurement variance of the second observer can be estimated from these data. The variance of the first observer from the intra-observer test is designated s^2_{intra}. The measurement errors of this observer in the first and second measurement series are assumed to be equal. It then holds that

(16)
$$s^2_{intra} \approx s^2_{observer\,1,\,measurement\,1} + s^2_{observer\,1,\,measurement\,1}$$
$$s^2_{observer\,1} \approx 1/2 \cdot s^2_{intra}$$

From this value and the variance of the inter-observer test s^2_{inter} we calculate the measurement variance of the second observer $s^2_{observer\,2}$

(17)
$$s^2_{inter} \approx s^2_{observer\,1} + s^2_{observer\,2}$$
$$s^2_{observer\,2} \approx s^2_{inter} - s^2_{observer\,1}$$

Up to this point it was tacitly agreed that the measurement resulted in continuous variables.

In contrast to variables on continuous scales, findings in medicine and psychology are often assigned to classes or categories. For the sake of completeness it is pointed out that in such cases the agreement (or disagreement) of observers is judged from contingency tables and quantified by the so-called kappa ratio (Fleiss, 1981).

Error propagation

The rules of error propagation quantify the error of a result combined from a number of parameters, each subject to measurement error. This can be illustrated by the error of a velocity measurement of

a subject measured in a gait test. To determine the velocity, distance and time are measured. Length measurement may be performed with an error of $\Delta L = \pm 5$ cm and time measurement with an error of $\Delta t = \pm 0.2$ s. Velocity is a function of distance L and time t

(18)
$$v = f(L, t) = L/t$$

As distance and length can only be measured within certain error limits, it follows that velocity can only be obtained within certain error limits. The inaccuracies of L and t are 'propagated'.

The error of a compound result is obtained by first inspecting the individual contributions. In the example discussed here, the velocity error Δv resulting from the distance error ΔL amounts to

(19)
$$\Delta v = (L + \Delta L)/t - L/t = \Delta L/t$$

The relation between the velocity error and the distance error can be written as

(20)
$$\Delta v \approx \Delta L \cdot (\partial f / \partial L)$$

$\partial f / \partial L$ designates the partial differentiation of v with respect to L. When performing a partial differentiation of the function $v = f(L,t)$ to L, the variable t is regarded as constant and an 'ordinary' differentiation with respect to L is performed. For the velocity error as a function of the time error Δt we obtain

(21)
$$\Delta v \approx \Delta t \cdot (\partial f / \partial t)$$

Once the individual error influences are known, we can estimate their combined effect. The maximum error is given by the sum of the magnitudes of the individual errors

(22)
$$\Delta v_{max} = \pm(|\Delta L \cdot (\partial f / \partial L)| + |\Delta t \cdot (\partial f / \partial t)|)$$

This estimate rests on the unfavorable assumption that both the distance error and the time error occur with maximum magnitude and that both errors shift the velocity result in the same direction. If time and distance measurements are independent of each other and occur with random errors, the mean error of the velocity is stated

(23)
$$\Delta v = \pm\sqrt{(\Delta L \cdot (\partial f / \partial L))^2 + (\Delta t \cdot (\partial f / \partial t))^2}$$

This equation is also termed Gauss' law of error propagation. The fact that the individual errors are not statistically correlated permits the squares of these errors to be added. The mean error is smaller than the maximum error. The formula for the mean error is generally valid for all functions f (x,y,z,...)

of the variables x, y, z, ..., measured with errors Δx, Δy, Δz, ...

$$(24) \quad \begin{aligned} (\Delta f(x, y, z, \dots))^2 &= (\Delta x \cdot \partial f / \partial x)^2 + \\ (\Delta y \cdot \partial f / \partial y)^2 &+ (\Delta z \cdot \partial f / \partial z)^2 + \dots \\ \Delta f(x, y, z, \dots) &= \pm \sqrt{(\Delta f(x, y, z, \dots))^2} \end{aligned}$$

Calculation of a propagated error using the example of an angle defined by the end points of two straight lines

Chapter 4 discussed the example of a rotation simulated by measurement errors (Fig. 4.9). The appertaining numerical calculation is detailed below. In the example, a body with reference points P and Q is moved in a plane. The final locations of the reference points are designated P′ and Q′. If the angle between the lines PP′ and QQ′ were zero, the motion would be a pure translation. The problem is to determine the accuracy of the angle measurement when the locations of the reference points are known only within certain error limits. To solve the problem, a rectangular xy-coordinate system is introduced. Using the above-quoted formulae, the error of the angles between the two lines and the x-axis, and in a second step employing Gauss' formula (24) the error of the angle difference (i.e. of the angle between PP′ and QQ′) is obtained.

Point P (Fig. **4.9**) may have the coordinates x_1, y_1 and point P′ the coordinates x_2, y_2. The measurement error for the coordinates is assumed to be equal for all coordinates and to amount to σ. The angle α between the line PP′ and the x-axis amounts to

$$(25) \quad \alpha = \text{atan} \frac{(y_2 - y_1)}{(x_2 - x_1)}$$

The partial derivative of the angle α with respect to x_1, calculated by means of the chain rule for derivation, amounts to

$$(26) \quad \frac{\partial \alpha}{\partial x_1} = \frac{1}{1 + \left(\frac{y_2 - y_1}{x_2 - x_1}\right)^2} \cdot \frac{(y_2 - y_1)}{(x_2 - x_1)^2}$$

Re-writing this equation with L_1 designating the distance PP′

$$(27) \quad \frac{1}{1 + \left(\frac{y_2 - y_1}{x_2 - x_1}\right)^2} = \frac{(x_2 - x_1)^2}{L_1^2}$$

$$(28) \quad L_1^2 = (x_2 - x_1)^2 + (y_2 - y_1)^2$$

gives us for the partial derivative

$$(29) \quad \frac{\partial \alpha}{\partial x_1} = \frac{1}{L_1^2} \cdot (y_2 - y_1)$$

In an analogous way we obtain for the partial derivatives of the angle α with respect to x_2, y_1, y_2

$$(30) \quad \frac{\partial \alpha}{\partial x_2} = -\frac{1}{L_1^2} \cdot (y_2 - y_1)$$

$$(31) \quad \frac{\partial \alpha}{\partial y_1} = -\frac{1}{L_1^2} \cdot (x_2 - x_1)$$

$$(32) \quad \frac{\partial \alpha}{\partial y_2} = \frac{1}{L_1^2} \cdot (x_2 - x_1)$$

According to the law of error propagation (24) we obtain for the error of the angle α in dependence on the 4 variables x_1, y_1, x_2, y_2

$$(33) \quad \begin{aligned} (\Delta \alpha)^2 &= \left(\frac{\sigma}{L_1^2} \cdot (y_2 - y_1)\right)^2 + \\ & \left(\frac{\sigma}{L_1^2} \cdot (y_2 - y_1)\right)^2 + \\ & \left(\frac{\sigma}{L_1^2} \cdot (x_2 - x_1)\right)^2 + \left(\frac{\sigma}{L_1^2} \cdot (x_2 - x_1)\right)^2 \end{aligned}$$

after adding the terms, and with (28) we obtain

$$(34) \quad \Delta \alpha = \pm \sqrt{2} \cdot \frac{\sigma}{L_1}$$

An analogue expression is obtained for the angle error Δβ of the line QQ′; instead of the length L_1, the length L_2 is to be inserted there. The error of the angle difference γ = α − β is calculated from Gauss' formula of error propagation as

$$(35) \quad \Delta \gamma = \pm \sqrt{(\Delta \alpha)^2 + (\Delta \beta)^2}$$

If the lengths of the lines PP′ and QQ′ are approximately equal and if the distances L_1 and L_2 are large compared with the error σ, L_1 and L_2 may be replaced by their mean L. We then obtain

$$(36) \quad \Delta \gamma = \pm 2 \cdot \frac{\sigma}{L}$$

This result can be intuitively understood: the error of the angle increases as the error of the coordinate measurement increases, and decreases as the length of the lines connecting the reference points increases.

In this example error propagation was explicitly calculated. In complex cases, such calculations can become be very long and confusing. In such instances, a computer simulation using random numbers is more appropriate. In a computer simulation the measured quantities (here the coordinates of the four points) are changed by adding or subtracting errors produced by means of the computer's random number generator. The effect of such changes on the final result is observed and documented. In principle, this is equivalent to an actual physical experiment. If we could repeat an experiment a large number of times (each time getting a slightly different result), we would finally arrive at a representative estimate of the error. The advantage of a computer simulation is that a result can be obtained quickly. The disadvantage of the simulation is that the individual factors influencing the error (in the example above the accuracy of the coordinate measurement and the length of the lines PP' and QQ') are not explicitly identified.

A procedure where one or more input parameters are varied with the aim of observing the effect of such a variation on the final result is termed a 'sensitivity study'. The factor tested is the sensitivity of the final result to changes in input parameters. Performing a sensitivity study is recommended especially in those cases where the input parameter errors are known only imprecisely, if at all. If the sensitivity study demonstrates that the final result depends only weakly on the unknown errors, our confidence in the correctness of the result is corroborated. If, in contrast, the final result depends strongly on the unknown errors, we are inclined to have reservations regarding the final result.

Method of least squares

It was shown earlier that the mean m_x of n repeated measurements x_k constitutes an improved approximation to the true, but unknown value, x. We can now ask whether m_x does in fact constitute the best approximation, i.e. the value closest to the true value. This question can be answered using the 'method of least squares'. It is postulated that the value w, for which the sum of the squared deviations assumes a minimum value, is this best approximation

$$(37) \quad Q = (w - x_1)^2 + (w - x_2)^2 + ... + (w - x_n)^2$$

All terms in this sum are positive (as squares are always positive); thus Q is a positive number. It can be shown (the proof not being detailed here) that Q assumes a minimum value when the mean m_x is inserted in place of w in this equation. It follows that the mean constitutes the best approximation to the true value. The method of least squares can be generalized by demanding an optimal fit of a given function to measured data, when the sum of the squared deviations from this function assumes a minimum value. This procedure is very useful when processing measured data.

Regression line

Stating a quantitative relation between two measured variables x and y is a frequently occurring task. We can, for example, observe the motion of a body moving at constant velocity, take n measure-

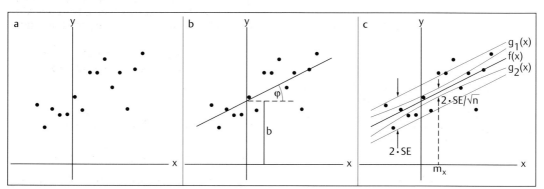

Fig. B3.1 Fit of a regression line to data points. **a:** data points (x_k, y_k) in an xy-coordinate system. **b:** regression line y = f(x) = a · x + b fitted to the data points (x_k, y_k) with slope a = tanφ and intercept b. **c:** The deviation of the data points with respect to the regression line is depicted by two lines parallel to the regression line f(x), i. e. f(x) + SE and f(x) – SE. The uncertainty (potential error of the fit) of the regression line f(x) is depicted by the functions $g_1(x)$ and $g_2(x)$. These two functions enclose a waisted region; the true, but unknown regression line passes somewhere inside this region. The diameter of the region at the waist (the point of minimum width) is equal to 2 · SE/$\sqrt{n}$; in this formula n designates the number of data points. The waist is located at x = m_x, i. e. at the geometric center of the x-coordinates of the data points.

ments of time (x_k) and distance covered (y_k), and plot these data in a rectangular coordinate system (Fig. B3.**1a**). In the case of constant velocity we expect a linear relation between x and y. As both time and distance are fraught with measurement errors, it is impossible to find a line on which all points are exactly located.

Based on the principle of least squares, the line $y = f(x) = a \cdot x + b$ is to be searched for where the sum Q of the squared deviations

(38) $$Q(a, b) = (a \cdot x_1 + b - y_1)^2 + (a \cdot x_2 + b - y_2)^2 + \dots + (a \cdot x_n + b - y_n)^2$$

assumes a minimum value. The designation Q(a,b) means that Q depends on ('is a function of') the slope a and the intercept b of the line. If a and b are chosen as

(39) $$a = S_{xy}/S_{xx}$$

(40) $$b = m_y - a \cdot m_x$$

Q assumes a minimum value (the proof of this is not detailed here). The terms in equations (39) and (40) are calculated as follows

(41) $$S_{xx} = (x_1 - m_x) \cdot (x_1 - m_x) + (x_2 - m_x) \cdot (x_2 - m_x) + \dots + (x_n - m_x) \cdot (x_n - m_x)$$

(42) $$S_{xy} = (x_1 - m_x) \cdot (y_1 - m_y) + (x_2 - m_x) \cdot (y_2 - m_y) + \dots + (x_n - m_x) \cdot (y_n - m_y)$$

(43) $$m_x = (x_1 + x_2 + \dots + x_n)/n$$

(44) $$m_y = (y_1 + y_2 + \dots + y_n)/n$$

The straight line $f(x) = a \cdot x + b$ is designated 're-gression line' (Fig. B3.**1b**). Representing the functional relation by this line compensates for the statistical measurement errors.

The standard error of estimate SE

(45) $$SE^2 = \sum_{k=1}^{n} (a \cdot x_k + b - y_k)^2/(n-2)$$

constitutes an estimate of the mean deviation of the original data points from the fitted regression line in y-direction, i.e. for the mean of the y-deviation of the data points y_k from the value of the regression line at the arguments x_k. (To facilitate writing, equation 45 states the square of SE). The denominator n – 2 (instead of n) in this equation

indicates that this formula makes sense only in the case of a line fitted to more than two data points. With only two data points, the line would pass exactly through these points and the y-deviation would be zero. Fitting a regression line and calculating a standard estimate error thus makes sense only in cases of at least three data points.

In addition to the error in the y-direction, we can estimate the error of the coefficients a and b. At first sight it seems out of place to consider such errors, because the coefficients are given exactly by equations (39) and (40). If, however, we imagine an experiment to be repeated, the n measured data points of the second experiment will differ slightly from those of the first experiment; we are then also left with different parameters a and b. As a and b are not independent, due to the relation $m_y = a \cdot m_x + b$, the deviations Δa and Δb are not independent either. Besides errors for a and b, a value exists for the correlated error between a and b

(46) $$< \Delta a \cdot \Delta a > = (1/S_{xx}) \cdot <SE^2>$$

(47) $$< \Delta b \cdot \Delta b > = (1/n + m_x^2/S_{xx}) \cdot <SE^2>$$

(48) $$< \Delta a \cdot \Delta b > = -(m_x/S_{xx}) \cdot <SE^2>$$

In the special case where the origin of the coordinate system is located at m_x, Δa and Δb are uncorrelated; in this case $<\Delta a \cdot \Delta b>$ is equal to zero. (Proof of this relation is provided in the context of the theory of normal equations.) Relations (46) to (48) permit the statistical reliability of a regression line to be depicted diagrammatically. For each x- and related y-value $f(x) = a \cdot x + b$ an error limit $\Delta f(x)$ can be stated in the form of an expectation value

(49) $$< (\Delta f(x))^2 > = < \Delta a \cdot \Delta a > \cdot x^2 + 2 \cdot < \Delta a \cdot \Delta b > \cdot x + < \Delta b \cdot \Delta b >$$

In practice, the curves

(50) $$g_1(x) = f(x) + \sqrt{<(\Delta f(x))^2>}$$

(51) $$g_2(x) = f(x) - \sqrt{<(\Delta f(x))^2>}$$

are plotted in addition to the regression line (Fig. B3.**1c**). Instead of the expectation value, $<SE^2>$ the estimate for SE^2 (equation 45) is inserted in equations (46) to (48).

When discussing the reliability of the regression line, the question can be raised of whether it might be better to fit the function $x = h(y) = c \cdot y + d$ instead of the function $y = f(x) = a \cdot x + b$. Notwithstanding special applications, the convention is to represent the variable with the larger measurement error as a function of the variable with the smaller error. A special case (dictated by the type of experiment to be interpreted) is encountered when the measured data points are to be fitted 'geometrically' to a straight line. In this case, the deviation of the points from the fitted line is not specified by the distances in y-direction but by the perpendicular distances of the points from the line. This case is subject to an adapted set of equations (differing from the set quoted above).

Fit of two sets of points by translation and rotation

In the following, we assume that reference points are fixed on a rigid body. If the rotation matrix and translation vector are specified, the change of location of the reference points in the final state with respect to the initial state can be calculated exactly. In orthopedic biomechanics one is often confronted with the inverse problem. From locations of reference points in the initial and final state, the rotation matrix and translation vector have to be determined. This already complex task is further complicated by the fact that locations of points cannot be measured exactly but only with experimental errors. Consequently there is no description of the motion (rotation matrix and translation vector) effecting an exact superposition of the points in the initial and final state. One can only search for a description resulting in a best fit. In the following, the fitting procedure is described for the two-dimensional as well as for the three-dimensional case; the illustrations depict the two-dimensional case. Vector and matrix notation permits a largely uniform formulation for the plane and the spatial problem.

A number of n reference points are fixed on the body. The minimum number of points in the plane case is two, and in the three-dimensional case three. In both cases it is advantageous if the number of reference points chosen is larger than the required minimum (Spoor and Veldpaus, 1980). In the initial state the radius vectors of the reference points are designated r_{ak}, and in the final state r_{ek}. The index k assumes values from 1 to n. The aim of the calculation is to superimpose the initial locations r_{ak} of the points as closely as possible on to the final locations r_{ek}. We imagine the fit to be performed in two steps. In the first step the radius vectors r_{ak} are translated by a translation vector t

$$(52) \qquad r'_{ak} = r_{ak} + t$$

The geometric center of the reference points in the initial state is designated R_a, and after the transla-tion, R'_a. In the second step the translated points r'_a are rotated about their geometric center R'_a by the rotation matrix D

$$(53) \qquad r''_{ak} = D \cdot (r'_{ak} - R'_a) + R'_a$$

The quantity Q

$$(54) \qquad Q = \sum_k (r''_{ak} - r_{ek})^2 = \\ \sum_k (D \cdot (r'_{ak} - R'_a) + R'_a - r_{ek})^2$$

as a function of the translation vector t and the matrix D is to be minimized. To start with, it can be shown that the translation vector is given by $t = R_e - R_a$. This means that the geometric center of the radius vectors in the initial state is to be shifted to the location of the geometric center of the radius vectors in the final state. If this value for t is inserted in equation (54) and a change is made to coordinates relative to the geometric center

$$(55) \qquad p'_{ak} = r'_{ak} - R'_a \quad \text{with} \\ R'_a = \sum_k r'_{ak}/n \ \text{ and } \ \sum_k p'_{ak} = 0$$

$$(56) \qquad p_{ek} = r_{ek} - R_e \quad \text{with} \\ R_e = \sum_k r_{ek}/n \ \text{ and } \ \sum_k p_{ek} = 0$$

then the minimum of Q as a function of the rotation matrix D is to be determined

$$(57) \qquad Q = \sum_k (D \cdot p'_{ak} - p_{ek})^2$$

In the two-dimensional case, there is only one single parameter, the angle of rotation φ, to be fitted. In this case, there is an explicit solution

$$(58) \qquad \varphi = \text{atan}(S/C) \pm 180°$$

with

$$(59) \qquad S = \sum_k \xi'_a \cdot \eta_e - \eta'_a \cdot \xi_e \\ C = \sum_k \xi'_a \cdot \xi_e + \eta'_a \cdot \eta_e$$

In these equations ξ'_a, η'_a designate the relative coordinates of the vectors p'_{ak}, and ξ_e, η_e the relative coordinates of vectors p_{ek}.

Fig. B3.**2** illustrates these steps for the two-dimensional case. Fig. B3.**2a** depicts the initial and final state. In the first step (Fig. B3.**2a, b**) the geometric centers are superimposed. In the second

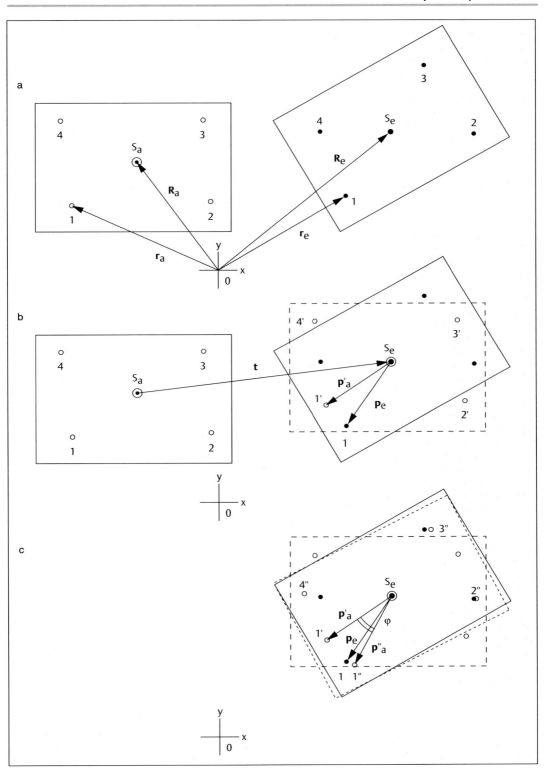

step (Fig. B3.**2c**) the relative vectors $\mathbf{p}'_a$ are rotated through the angle φ with the aim of superimposing them as closely as possible on the relative vectors $\mathbf{p}_e$. The reference points in the initial and final state were assumed to have been measured with random errors. Thus, it is hardly surprising that an exact superposition of the two sets of points (in the initial and final state) cannot be achieved.

In three dimensions the rotation matrix **D** depends on three parameters (angles of rotation). For example, the matrix **D** can be represented according to Bryant-Cardan as a product of three rotation matrices about the three coordinate axes

(60) $$\mathbf{D} = \mathbf{D}_x(\phi_1) \cdot \mathbf{D}_{y'}(\phi_2) \cdot \mathbf{D}_{z''}(\phi_3)$$

The minimum condition for Q requires solving three nonlinear, coupled equations for the angles of rotation ϕ_1, ϕ_2, ϕ_3.

An iterative procedure is best suited to this problem. Such a procedure starts with an approximation of the solution and delivers an improved solution in its first step, i.e. a set of angles resulting in a value of Q (equation 57) smaller than the first approximation. This improved approximation is again used as input for a further improvement and so on, until Q becomes acceptably small. (Due to measurement errors Q will never be exactly equal to zero.) As iterative procedures are usually well suited to computer processing, they are in common use. The relevant formulae and algorithms (sequences of mathematical operations) are not listed here; the reader is referred to textbooks on numerical methods.

Once the parameters of three-dimensional motion, **t** and **D**, are known, the motion can, according to Chasles' theorem, also be interpreted as helical motion. For this description the axis of rotation **n** and the angle of rotation φ (both determined from the rotation matrix **D**) have to be specified. A point $\mathbf{r}_A$ on the axis and the translation vector $\mathbf{t}_p$ in the direction of the axis can then be calculated (see Chapter B2).

Further reading

Textbooks and review papers

Fleiss JL. *Statistical methods for rates and proportions.* 2nd ed. New York: Wiley; 1981

Fleiss JL. *The design and analysis of clinical experiments.* New York: Wiley; 1986

Scientific papers, cited in the text or the figures

Bland JM, Altmann DG. Statistical methods for assessing agreement between two methods of clinical measurement. *Lancet.* 1986; **8**: 307–310

Spoor CW, Veldpaus FE. Rigid body motion calculated from spatial coordinates of markers. *J Biomechanics.* 1980; **13**: 391–393

Fig. B3.2:   Fit (superposition) of two sets of data points in a plane. **a**: a rectangular, plane object equipped with four reference points is moved from an initial position (open symbols) to a final position (solid symbols). The locations of the object are described in an xy-coordinate system with origin O. The radius vectors of the reference points in the initial and final state are designated $\mathbf{r}_a$ and $\mathbf{r}_e$; those of the geometric centers S_a and S_e are designated $\mathbf{R}_a$ and $\mathbf{R}_e$. **b**: In a first step the object is translated from its initial location by the vector $\mathbf{t} = \mathbf{R}_a - \mathbf{R}_e$ (dashed outline, points with single primes). Thus, the geometric centers are superimposed. The relative vectors $\mathbf{p}'_a$ and $\mathbf{p}_e$ are still rotated with respect to each other. **c**: In a second step the object is rotated about its geometric center through the angle φ (object now outlined with fine dashed lines, rotated points with double primes). The rotated relative vectors $\mathbf{p}''_a$ are now fitted to the relative vectors $\mathbf{p}_e$ in the final state. A perfect fit cannot be achieved because the reference points were measured with experimental errors.

Designations and units

	designation in the text or the figures	unit (dimension)
length	L, D, E, ...	m (meter)
mass	m	kg (kilogram)
time	t	s (second)
area	A	m^2
volume	V	m^3
velocity (vector, magnitude)	**v**, v	m/s
acceleration (vector, magnitude)	**a**, a	m/s^2
angle	$\alpha, \beta, \gamma, ...$	degree or radian
angular velocity	ω	degree/s or radian/s
angular acceleration	α	$degree/s^2$ or $radian/s^2$
force (vector, magnitude)	**F, H, R,** ... F, H, R, ...	$kg \cdot m/s^2 = N$ (newton)
moment (vector, magnitude)	**M**, M	$N \cdot m$
mechanical work, energy	E	$N \cdot m = J$ (joule)
power	P	$N \cdot m/s$ (watt)
gravitational acceleration	g	m/s^2
gravitational force (weight)	$m \cdot g$	$kg \cdot m/s^2 = N$
pressure	p	$N/m^2 = Pa$ (pascal)
compressive or tensile stress	σ	$N/m^2 = Pa$
shear stress	τ	$N/m^2 = Pa$
strain	ε	dimensionless
moment of inertia	I	$kg \cdot m^2$
section modulus	Z	m^3
polar moment of inertia	I_p	m^4
polar section modulus	Z_p	m^3
modulus of elasticity	E	N/m^2 or N/mm^2
shear modulus	G	N/m^2 or N/mm^2
Poisson's ratio	μ	dimensionless

Additional designation for units

prefix (symbol and name)	factor by which the unit is multiplied
n (nano-)	10^{-9}
μ (micro-)	10^{-6}
m (milli-)	10^{-3}
k (kilo-)	10^{3}
M (mega-)	10^{6}
G (giga-)	10^{9}

Notation of vectors and matrices, illustrated by the example of vectors **F** and **G** and a matrix **D**

	notation
vector	**F**
magnitude of the vector	$|\mathbf{F}|$ or F
components of the vector with respect to a xyz-coordinate system	F_x, F_y, F_z
coordinates of the vector with respect to an xyz-coordinate system	F_x, F_y, F_z
matrix	**D**
element of a matrix (i-th row, k-th column)	D_{ik}
scalar product of vectors **F** and **G**	$\mathbf{F} \cdot \mathbf{G}$
vector (cross) product of vectors **F** and **G**	$\mathbf{F} \times \mathbf{G}$

Index